Leading and Managing Health Services

An Australasian perspective

Leading and Managing Health Services: An Australasian perspective provides a comprehensive overview of leadership and management in health services, with a particular focus on the Australasian context. This text aims to help students from a broad range of health studies disciplines to develop leadership and management skills, and to critically analyse the issues they will face in practical health service settings.

The book features a contemporary approach to learning, in line with the Health LEADS Australia framework, which focuses on five key leadership attributes: Leads self, Engages systems, Achieves outcomes, Drives innovations and Shapes systems. Further, it offers a rich pedagogy both in the text and on its companion website. Each chapter includes case studies to provide practical examples of management and leadership issues in healthcare settings, as well as reflective and self-analysis questions to extend student learning.

Written by respected Australian academics and industry experts, this text will equip students of the health professions with practical skills to successfully manage change and innovation. *Leading and Managing Health Services* is an indispensable resource for students in the ever-changing healthcare industry.

Comprehensive instructor resources – including further reading, multiple-choice and short-answer questions, and additional case studies and reflective questions – are available online at http://www.cambridge.edu.au/academic/leadinghealth.

Gary E. Day is Professor of Health Services Management in the Centre for Health Innovation, School of Medicine at Griffith University.

Sandra G. Leggat is Professor of Health Services Management in the School of Psychology and Public Health at La Trobe University.

Leading and Managing Health Services

An Australasian perspective

Edited by

GARY E. DAY and SANDRA G. LEGGAT

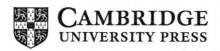

CAMBRIDGE
UNIVERSITY PRESS

University Printing House, Cambridge CB2 8BS, United Kingdom

One Liberty Plaza, 20th Floor, New York, NY 10006, USA

477 Williamstown Road, Port Melbourne, VIC 3207, Australia

314-321, 3rd Floor, Plot 3, Splendor Forum, Jasola District Centre, New Delhi - 110025, India

79 Anson Road, #06-04/06, Singapore 079906

Cambridge University Press is part of the University of Cambridge.

It furthers the University's mission by disseminating knowledge in the pursuit of education, learning and research at the highest international levels of excellence.

www.cambridge.org
Information on this title: www.cambridge.org/9781107486393

First published 2015 (version 4, February 2019)

Cover design by Marianna Berek-Lewis
Typeset by Aptara Corp.

A catalogue record for this publication is available from the British Library

A Cataloguing-in-Publication entry is available from the catalogue of the National Library of Australia at www.nla.gov.au

ISBN 978-1-107-48639-3 Paperback

Additional resources for this publication at www.cambridge.edu.au/academic/leadinghealth

....

Every effort has been made in preparing this book to provide accurate and up-to-date information which is in accord with accepted standards and practice at the time of publication. Although case histories are drawn from actual cases, every effort has been made to disguise the identities of the individuals involved. Nevertheless, the authors, editors and publishers can make no warranties that the information contained herein is totally free from error, not least because clinical standards are constantly changing through research and regulation. The authors, editors and publishers therefore disclaim all liability for direct or consequential damages resulting from the use of material contained in this book. Readers are strongly advised to pay careful attention to information provided by the manufacturer of any drugs or equipment that they plan to use.

All chapters in this text have been peer reviewed by academic and industry experts.

For Linda, Alex, Emily, Teri, Georgia and Tobin
For Will, Evan, Sarah and Geoffrey

Contents

Contributors

Editors

Gary E. Day RN, EM, DipAppSc (Nurs Mgt), BNurs, MHM, DHSM, FCHSM, FGLF
Professor, Health Services Management, and director, Centre for Health Innovation, School of Medicine, Griffith University.

Professor Gary E. Day is a senior executive with over 30 years' experience as a consultant, project manager, director and chief executive officer as well as a clinician, academic, researcher and author. Gary has worked in both the for-profit and the not-for-profit healthcare sectors across three Australian states and in the higher education sector, including project lead roles in major infrastructure and change management, and organisation-wide roles in workforce development and learning and medical education.

Sandra G. Leggat MHSc, MBA, PhD, FCHSM
Professor, Health Services Management, and director, Building Healthy Communities Research Program, La Trobe University.

Professor Sandra G. Leggat has worked as a senior health executive in management and consulting roles in both Australia and Canada. She has studied healthcare systems around the world, with a focus on human resource management and leadership. Sandra has written a large number of journal publications and book chapters, and she has editorial experience with the *Australian Health Review* and the *Asia Pacific Journal of Health Management*.

Authors

Ben Archdall RN
Manager, Workforce Mapping, Analysis, Planning, Projections Project, Department of Health, Queensland Government.

Mark Avery BHA, MBus (Res), AFACHSM, FAIM, FAICD, CHM
Senior lecturer and discipline head, Health Services Management, Centre for Health Innovation, School of Medicine, Griffith University.

Cathy Balding MBus, PhD, FCHSM, GAICD
Adjunct associate professor, Health Services Management, La Trobe University; founder and director, Qualityworks Pty Ltd.

Richard Baldwin RN, AssDipNursAdmin, BHlthAdmin, MBA, PhD, FCHSM
Chief examiner, fellowship program, Australasian College of Health Service Management; associate, Faculty of Health, University of Technology, Sydney.

Melanie Bish BN (Hons), MN, PhD
Senior lecturer, Department of Rural Nursing and Midwifery, La Trobe Rural Health School.

David S. Briggs BHA, MHM (Hons, 1st class), PhD, Dr PH (Hon. NU) FCHSM, FCHKCHSE
Adjunct associate professor, Schools of Rural Medicine and Health, University of New England; editor, *Asia Pacific Journal of Health Management*; president, Society of Health Administration Programs in Education.

Sharon Brownie RN, RM, BEd, MEd Admin, M Hth S Mgt, GAICD, FCNA, DBA
Professor, Workforce and Health Service, Griffith University; and head of nursing, Fatima College of Health Sciences.

Gian Luca Casali BBA, MBA, PhD
Senior lecturer, School of Management, Queensland University of Technology.

Martin Connor PGDipHServMgt, PhD
Executive director, Centre for Health Innovation, and professor, School of Medicine, Griffith University.

Ian Edwards Ass Dip Bus (Mgnt), BBus (HRM), MHSA
Senior lecturer, Health Services Management, Centre for Health Innovation, School of Medicine, Griffith University.

John Adamm Ferrier CertGenNurs, DipAppSci (P&O), GradCertNurs (Periop), GradDipNurs (Periop), RN, PGradDipHSM, MHA, MACN
Lecturer, China Health Program, and School of Psychology and Public Health, La Trobe University.

Janna Anneke Fitzgerald RN, GradDipAdultEd (VET), MClinPrac, PhD
Professor, Health Management, Griffith Business School, Griffith University.

Linda Fraser RN, BHSc, MAdvPrac (Critical Care), MBA
Assistant director of nursing, Anaesthetic and Critical Care Service Specialty and Procedural Services, Gold Coast Hospital and Health Service.

Audrey Holmes BA, MA
Adjunct research fellow, Population and Social Health Research Program, Griffith Health, Griffith University.

Godfrey Isouard BSc, MHA, PhD, MLE, FCHSM, FACBS
Associate professor, Health Services Management, School of Health, University of New England.

Denise M. Jepsen BPsych (Hons), PGCertHE, MOrgPsych, PhD, MAPS, FAHRI
Organisational psychologist; associate professor, Business and Economics, Macquarie
University.

Jennifer (Jenny) Jones BA (Hons, 1st class), PhD
Clinical ethicist, Metro South Health Service; academic titleholder, School of Medicine,
Griffith University.

Leila Karimi PhD (OrgPsych), MAPS, ACHSM
Senior lecturer, Health Services Management, School of Psychology and Public Health,
La Trobe University.

Mark Keough BA, CertIVTAA, DComm
Director, Meechi Road Consulting.

Zhanming Liang MSc, MBBS, PhD, FCHSM
Senior lecturer, Health Service Management, School of Psychology and Public Health,
La Trobe University.

Chaojie (George) Liu MB, MPH, PhD
Associate professor and director, China Health Program, School of Psychology and Public
Health, La Trobe University; lecturing professor, Sichuan University and Hubei University
of Chinese Medicine.

Kirsty Marles GradCert Health Services Management, GradDip Public Health
Interprofessional learning and service design innovator, ACH Group.

Nicola McNeil BCom (Hons), LLB, PhD
Senior lecturer, Human Resource Management, La Trobe Business School, La Trobe University.

Eleanor Milligan GradDipEd, BA (Hons, 1st class), BSc, PhD
Associate professor and discipline lead, Ethics and Professional Practice, School of
Medicine, Griffith University.

Jiri Rada BA, BPHE, MSc, PhD
Academic, Health Services Management and Organisational Behaviour, La Trobe
University.

Katrina Radford BPsych (Hons), MHRM, PhD
Lecturer, Griffith Business School, Griffith University.

John Rasa BA, GD (Industrial Law and Industrial Relations), MHP, MAICD, FCHSM
Adjunct associate professor, Health Services Management, La Trobe University; chief
executive officer, Networking Health Victoria.

Elizabeth Shannon PhD
Manager, Leadership and Management Development, Tasmanian Department of Health
and Human Services; senior lecturer, Health Services Innovation, School of Medicine,
University of Tasmania.

Mindaugas Stankunas MPH, PhD
Professor, Department of Health Management, Lithuanian University of Health Sciences; adjunct senior lecturer, School of Medicine, Griffith University; visiting professor, CAPHRI: School of Public Health and Primary Care, Maastricht University.

Lorraine Venturato RN, BBusHlthAdmin, BN (Hons), PhD
Chair, Gerontology, Faculty of Nursing, University of Calgary.

Ged Williams RN, RM, CritCareCert, GradCertPSM, BachAppSc (Adv Nurs), GradCertLaw, LLM, MHA (UNSW), MAICD, FACN, FACHSM, FAAN
Nursing and allied health consultant, SEHA: Abu Dhabi Health Service Company; professor, Nursing, Griffith University.

Preface

This book is a culmination of over 30 years of studying, practising, researching and observing leadership and management within the Australasian healthcare industry. Over this period, a range of industry and system factors has made working, managing and leading in health services more challenging and complex. These factors include greater scrutiny of the spending on health and the resulting outcomes, which has led to substantial reform initiatives; recognition of the importance of good governance and individual, organisational and system accountability; reliance on technology to support clinical and non-clinical healthcare decision-making; workforce shortages and role substitution; and better understanding of the ways to improve clinical safety and quality, and overall health outcomes. These factors have been driven by greater public interest and political scrutiny of the healthcare system, focused on quality and safety, access and equity, and the roles of the various levels of government and private operators. We have seen funders, regulators and other agencies requiring increasing levels of effectiveness, efficiency and better health outcomes.

To navigate the complexity of the industry and national and international factors, it is not enough to just be a good manager or a good leader. Being successful as a manager or a health professional requires a combination of both management and leadership skills and aptitudes. *Leading and managing health services: An Australasian perspective* provides a critical and concise overview of the important skills, aptitudes and content areas required to successfully lead and manage in a wide range of healthcare settings, no matter where you sit in the organisational structure. It provides insights into aspects of healthcare leadership and management applicable to Australasian health systems from highly experienced healthcare managers, leaders and academics.

To assist in the understanding and development of the skills and aptitudes required to successfully lead and manage health services, the content of this book has been organised around Health Workforce Australia's Health LEADS Framework (see Figure 0.1). This framework was developed by Health Workforce Australia after extensive research and industry consultation and was adopted by all Council of Australian Governments health ministers in 2012. Setting out the book in this way provides a contemporary approach to understanding the key leadership and management attributes across the five critical domains: leading self, engaging others, achieving outcomes, driving innovation and shaping systems.

According to Health Workforce Australia (2013, p. 5), 'Leadership requires reflection and improvement of self (Leads self), fostering growth in and influencing others (Engages others), and communicating a vision for the future and enabling decisions to align with the goal (Achieves outcomes). To achieve outcomes, leaders embrace the spirit of change and innovation (Drives innovation) and strategically understand and align complex systems with the goal (Shapes systems)'. This accepted leadership framework provides a clear

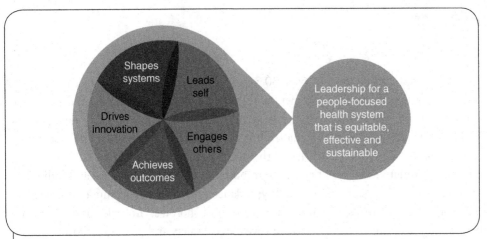

Figure 0.1 Health LEADS Framework. Health Workforce Australia. (2013). Health LEADS Australia: The Australian health leadership framework (p. 1). Retrieved from http://www.hwa.gov.au/sites/uploads/Health-LEADS-Australia-A4-FINAL.pdf.

approach to leadership and management that is applicable to both developed and developing countries. Additionally, the LEADS Framework helps cement the five key domains for healthcare leadership and management development. The LEADS Framework, by providing this book's chapter and section structure, ensures it is a definitive resource for leading and managing health services in Australasia.

The text commences with a broad understanding of a range of leadership and management theories and frameworks that underpin past and current practice in the chapters 'Concepts of leadership and management in health services' and 'Leadership and management frameworks and theories'. These two chapters provide a sound theoretical and contextual basis from which to explore the content areas around leading self, engaging others, achieving outcomes, driving innovation and shaping systems.

Leads self

Leaders need to be constantly learning about their own strengths and limitations through self-appraisal and reflection. These activities are critical elements in the development of successful leadership. These chapters provide a foundation in the self-awareness and personal attributes that are essential for successful health leadership and management:

- ethical leadership
- self-management
- emotional intelligence and self-awareness
- exploring values
- ambiguity and leadership
- leadership and critical reflective practice.

These chapters aim to highlight the importance of self-reflective and critical self-assessment in terms of an individual's own performance as a leader. The chapters also form the basis for reflecting on one's own performance around these important personal leadership qualities.

Engages others

Health leaders have a critical role in engaging others to seek solutions to complex health and systems challenges. Successfully engaging others is a critical component in having influence as a healthcare leader and manager. The seven chapters in this section provide a detailed foundation in aspects of engaging others to successfully influence staff, stakeholders and the broader community. The chapters are designed to assist the reader in engaging others through:

- communication leadership
- leading interprofessional teams
- clinical governance
- partnering with stakeholders
- power and political astuteness
- influencing strategically
- networking.

Achieves outcomes

Healthcare leaders and managers are increasingly being held to account for results and outcomes. Achieving outcomes is critical not only for system sustainability but also to balance effectiveness and efficiency in line with resource allocations. The six chapters in this section highlight important skills and aptitudes associated with achieving outcomes:

- holding to account
- critical thinking and decision-making
- managing and leading staff
- project management
- financial management
- negotiating.

Drives innovation

Strong leadership is required to build teams that are effective in the development of new approaches and solutions to entrenched health system challenges. Driving innovation includes 'fundamental changes to business and models of care to achieve people-centred quality services. A key factor for successful innovation is passionate leadership, without which the status quo cannot be challenged' (Health Workforce Australia, 2013, p. 9). The chapters in this section detail important aspects of leading innovation and change through:

- creativity and visioning
- evidence-based practice
- successfully managing conflict
- building positive workplace cultures
- leading and managing change
- quality and service improvement.

Shapes systems

Healthcare leaders play a vital role in shaping the systems in which they work. In many ways, shaping systems is a culmination of self-reflective and informed leaders engaging others, driving innovation and achieving outcomes. 'Health is a complex evolving system where all the parts, including services, legislation[, policy] and funding, are interconnected [and interdependent]. A change in one part has implications for the whole. Leaders who recognise patterns of interdependency are able to explain trends and facilitate strategies that achieve maximum benefits and minimise unintended harm or negative consequences' (Health Workforce Australia, 2013, p. 9). The three chapters in this section demonstrate the system interdependencies and the need for today's healthcare leader and manager to understand the interplay between planning and strategy to create an equitable, accessible, effective and efficient healthcare system, which includes:

- workforce-planning
- strategic planning
- health service planning.

This book is designed to be used as a whole, to develop and revise a range of skills and aptitudes for successful healthcare leadership and management, or to review individual leadership and management content areas. Additional reading and resources, case studies, reflective and self-analysis questions in each chapter assist in combining the theory, practice and real-life application of healthcare leadership and management.

Gary E. Day and Sandra G. Leggat

Reference

Health Workforce Australia. (2013). *Health LEADS Australia: The Australian health leadership framework*. Retrieved from http://www.hwa.gov.au/sites/uploads/Health-LEADS-Australia-A4-FINAL.pdf

Acknowledgements

The authors and Cambridge University Press would like to thank the following for permission to reproduce material in this book.

Table 2.1: Table reproduced with permission from University of Exeter Centre for Leadership Studies; **Chapter 11**: Some material in this chapter first published in the journal *Australian Health Review* 32(3), pp. 383–391, published by CSIRO Publishing: http://publish.csiro.au/nid/270/paper/AH080383.htm; **Figures 19.1, 19.2**: J. Dwyer, Z. Liang, V. Thiessen & A. Martini (2013). *Project management in health and community services: Getting good ideas to work with* (p. 2). Sydney: Allen & Unwin. Reproduced with permission; **23.1**: Z. Liang, P.F. Howard, S.G. Leggat & G. Murphy (2012). A framework to improve evidence-informed decision-making in health service management. *Australian Health Review* 36(3), 284–289. doi: 10.1071/ah11051. Reproduced with permission; **28.1**: Reproduced with the permission of the publisher, from World Health Organization (2010). Models and tools for health workforce planning and projections. *Human Resources for Health Observer*. Issue no. 3, p. 4, fig. 1. Retrieved from http://whqlibdoc.who.int/publications/2010/9789241599016_eng.pdf?ua=1

Part 1

Introduction

Concepts of leadership and management in health services

Mindaugas Stankunas

Learning objectives

How do I:
- define management and leadership in healthcare organisations?
- distinguish between the functions of top-level, middle-level and first-line managers?
- understand the concept of power and how it is used in management and leadership?
- determine the skills I would need for effective running of healthcare facilities?

Introduction

Intense debate surrounds the differences between the roles, functions and even superiority of leadership and management (Lease, 2006). Leadership is not something wholly different from management; indeed, it is a component of management and a responsibility of management, especially for senior managers. The present situation in health systems suggests that effective managers need to be effective leaders, and that the most effective leaders are also good managers.

Definitions

Most people think they know what management is. However, if they are asked to explain or describe the term management, they will give different answers. Some of them will say that it is a science; others will argue that it is an art; still others will vote for its being a practice. In addition to these answers, they will give examples of successful entrepreneurs like Jack Welch or world-class companies like Apple. It is also tough to explain differences between management and leadership. In many non-English-speaking countries, there is no term for leadership. This suggests that common words like management and leadership could have confused meaning for many of us. Therefore, it is important to discuss the definitions and functions of management and leadership.

Organisations

Why do we need management? Let's say that someone has been asked to prepare a health promotion project highlighting the dangers of skin cancer. If they decide to do everything by themselves, most likely they will not need to think about planning, organising and controlling. However, the situation changes if five or six fellow staff members join them. They will need to plan activities and organise their colleagues, to monitor the process. In this case, they become a manager. The second situation differs from the first because there is an **organisation**. The management function normally appears only within organisations.

> **Organisation**
> A group of individuals who inter
> each other to achieve a commor

Researchers have identified many different types of organisations (McKenna, 1998). The term organisation includes a hunting tribe in Papua New Guinea, a primary healthcare unit somewhere in the Northern Territory, a university in New Zealand, a sophisticated cancer research institute in France and the World Health Organization itself. What do these organisations have in common? First, they have one or more objectives. This means that their activity has a direction and purpose. The French institute tries to better understand cancer and its treatment. The tribe has a mission to hunt for food and to survive. The university exists to train new specialists and health professionals. Second, all of these organisations have two or more members within them. Third, all of these members are organised. The primary healthcare centre has a doctor (or several doctors), a nurse (or several nurses), a receptionist and a practice manager. All these people have different responsibilities, but all these activities are targeted at achieving a common goal. The World Health Organization has a more sophisticated organisational structure, with different specialists and functions. Therefore, an organisation could be described as a group of individuals who interact with each other in an interdependent relationship towards achieving a common goal or goals.

Organisations are platforms for management. For a better understanding of this, we need to discuss the structure of organisations. All organisations (from primeval tribes to international corporations) have certain similar structures, presented in Figure 1.1. All organisations are targeted to achieve a series of agreed goals. This means that all organisations produce results, or outcomes. For example, results for a tribe will be hunted game; for a hospital, healthy patients; for a pharmaceutical company, a new drug against hypertension. However, we cannot expect these desired results to occur without doing something. Therefore, we always have to develop some process before seeing results. Processes for a hospital may be the examination, treatment and rehabilitation of patients;

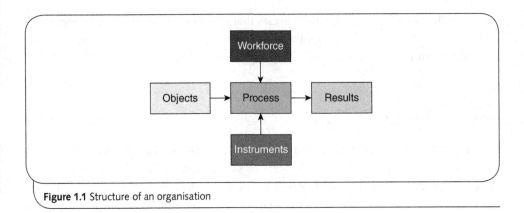

Figure 1.1 Structure of an organisation

for a university, the teaching of students; and for a non-governmental organisation, running a project against smoking.

These processes (a core of any organisation) are possible if we have objects, people and tools. A hospital will stop functioning if it does not have patients admitted with health issues. We can define these patients as objects. Little will happen to these patients if there are no health specialists, which we define as the workforce. The workforce ensures a process within the organisation. In this case, doctors, nurses and other allied health specialists take care of the patients. However, for most of the processes we need tools, or instruments. Doctors and nurses would not be able to do much without facilities, technologies and drugs. All these instruments help the workforce in the process towards achieving the common goals or outcomes.

A disorganised group of people will not be able to achieve their organisation's goals. If we want a group to work effectively and in one direction, we need to have adequate management.

Management

As we have already seen, there are many definitions of **management**. Literally every author provides their own definition; however, the main principle is the same in all definitions and lies in the classic works of French mining engineer Henri Fayol, known for his theory on the fundamental functions of management. According to Fayol (1917), every manager plans, organises, commands (or leads), coordinates and controls. This definition of management is generic: it should be suitable for all industry sectors. Can it be applied to the healthcare sector?

Management happens in organisations, so **health management** happens in health organisations. According to the World Health Organization (2000), all the organisations, institutions and resources that are

ement
, organising, leading and
ng resources in order to achieve
isation's goals

management
, organising, leading and
ng resources in order to
, restore or maintain health

devoted to producing health actions are components of a **health system**. Based on this, we can define health management as planning, organising, leading and controlling resources in order to promote, restore or maintain health. It is noteworthy that some authors use the terms healthcare management and health services management; these emphasise the focus on the organisation and delivery of services (Fulop, Allen, Clarke & Black, 2001). Health management covers management and organisation of the health system and its various subsystems and components (Hunter & Brown, 2007).

Health system
Combined activities whose prim purpose is to promote, restore o maintain health

However, health management has an unfortunate reputation. It is often regarded as an unnecessary activity that at best diverts resources from the real frontline activities of providing healthcare or preventing ill health (Green, Collins & Mirzoev, 2012). Nevertheless, scientific data oppose this. A recent systemic review has proven clear positive correlation between the performance of healthcare systems and their organisation and management practices, leadership and manager characteristics (Lega, Prenestini & Spurgeon, 2013).

Health management is a social process and reflects national social, political and cultural values. It cannot be transferred easily from one country to another. Most likely, successful health management practices in New Zealand will not work in Tajikistan. This is not because of any ineffectiveness in New Zealand's principles; simply, these two countries have different histories of development.

What kinds of managers do health systems need?

The World Health Organization's (1999) regional office for Europe has identified the most crucial functions for public health managers. Although these principles are targeted at the European region, they are relevant in the Australasian context.

> Essentially what is needed are public health managers, with the skills to manage partnerships and coordinated multisectoral action within alliances. They must … be trained in population-based analysis of health problems, be grounded in the approaches to deal with problems of lifestyles, the environment and health care, and be capable of the advocacy and networking needed to bring many partners together. They must also be skilled in creating excellent public health information for the general public, professionals and politicians.

> Within the health service itself they must be trained in policy and programme planning, including target-setting, outcome measurement and evaluation, and instrumental in shaping the pattern of services provided. They must be able to help plan, monitor and evaluate broad health development programmes, defined by disease category or client group, making scientifically informed judgements about the balance to be struck … between health promotion, disease prevention, therapy and rehabilitation.

Organisations, then, need management. Therefore, all organisations have formal managerial positions – for example, chief executive officer, director, president, vice-chancellor and director of nursing. A 2011 survey found that 22 400 managers were employed in all health services in Australia (Martins & Isouard, 2014), and this number had increased by 15.6 per cent since 2006.

For many years, there was a common understanding that all management functions should be delegated to formal managers with the power to manage organisations, and their departments and units. However, new approaches suggest that these responsibilities should not be concentrated in formal positions but shared within the organisation (for example, see Czabanowska, Smith, Stankunas, Avery & Otok, 2013). This means that more people in organisations should have a chance to participate in decision-making in and the running of organisations.

Leadership

This has inspired a discussion on the importance of leadership. According to the classic work of Abraham Zaleznik (1977), managers are reactive, and while they are willing to work with people to solve problems, they do so with minimal emotional involvement. On the other hand, leaders are emotionally involved and seek to shape ideas instead of reacting to others' ideas.

Moreover, leadership is not locked to formal positions in organisations. This means that everybody can be a leader, and there can be more than one leader in an organisation. Many academics and managers emphasise the growing importance of leadership in the healthcare sector (Beaglehole, Bonita, Horton, Adams & McKee, 2004; Simpson & Calman, 2000). According to the literature, every public health and healthcare organisation should be engaged in developing leaders at every level and creating collaborative organisational cultures (Czabanowska et al., 2013).

What it is **leadership**? Researchers mostly define it according to their individual perspectives and the aspects of the phenomenon of most interest to them (Yukl, 2013), leading to many and varied views. Ralph Stogdill (1974, p. 7) reviewed over 3000 studies directly related to leadership and suggests that there are almost as 'many different definitions of leadership as there are persons who have attempted to define the concept'. In this text, we use the definition of leadership devised by Peter Northouse (2007, p. 3): 'a process whereby an individual influences a group of individuals to achieve a common goal'. This definition emphasises the main elements of leadership: it is a process, it entails influence, it occurs within a group setting or context, and it involves achieving goals that reflect a common vision.

| **ship** |
| ss whereby an individual |
| es a group of individuals to |
| a common goal' (Northouse, |
| 5) |

According to Rowitz (2003, as cited in Stankunas et al., 2012, p. 582), health leadership 'includes commitment to the community and the values it stands for'. Grainger and

Griffiths (1998, as cited in Stankunas et al., 2012, p. 582) argue that 'health leaders differ from leaders in other sectors, as they are required to balance corporate legitimacy, while also existing outside the corporate environment'. Kimberly (2011, as cited in Stankunas et al., 2012, p. 582) suggests that a flatter, 'more distributed and collaborative world will require a new generation of leaders in public health with new mind sets, an appetite for innovation and interdisciplinary collaboration and a strong dose of political savvy'. Koh (2009, as cited in Stankunas et al., 2012, p. 582) believes that a health leader 'must be the transcendent, collaborative "servant leader" who knits and aligns disparate voices together behind a common mission, pinpoints passion and compassion, promotes servant leadership, acknowledges the unfamiliarity, ambiguity, and paradox, communicates succinctly to reframe, and help understand the "public" part of public health leadership'. Another study emphasises that health leaders must be 'exceptional "networker–connectors" capable of "putting the pieces of the jigsaw together"; they combine administrative excellence with a strong sense of professional welfare and actively develop the profession, articulate its shared values and build for the future' (Day et al., as cited in Stankunas et al., 2012, p. 582).

This short discussion of health leadership reveals that most authors agree on the presence of Northouse's (2007, p. 3) leadership elements in health leadership. However, they also emphasise health leadership's specific characteristics, such as a servant leader approach with community and specific orientation to public health values, which make it unique and important in the health sector (Stankunas et al., 2012, p. 582).

Challenges

The specificity of the health sector creates many challenges for leadership. According to McAlearney (2006), there are two main challenges to developing leadership in healthcare settings: environment and organisation. Environmental challenges arise because healthcare organisations are faced with a myriad of regulatory influences, some largely out of their control. Therefore, provider organisations rarely have much power or influence over some areas – for example, reimbursement for hospital and doctor services.

McAlearney (2006, p. 968) suggests that 'multiple hierarchies of professionals, on both the clinical and administrative sides of the organization, generate special challenges for directing the organization and coordination of work in healthcare. Often noted is the cultural chasm between administrators and clinicians'. McAlearney also says that the healthcare industry is behind other sectors in implementing new leadership and management methods. This suggests a need for competent managers and leaders in healthcare organisations.

Power and skills

Both leadership and management are about influencing people in order to achieve organisational goals. The outcome (effectiveness) of the influence process depends largely on the

power of the leader or manager over their followers or staff. Two major types of power have been identified: positional and personal (Rahim, 1988). Positional power is based on legitimate authority, control over resources, rewards, punishments, information and the physical work environment. Personal power comes from task expertise, friendship and loyalty. Gary Yukl (2010) claims that personal and position power have different subpowers, brief descriptions of which are presented in Table 1.1.

's ability to influence the target

Table 1.1 Types of powers

Power	Subpower	Description
Position	Legitimate	Formal authority and the right to set rules and directions for followers
	Reward	The right to control resources and give rewards to followers
	Coercive	The right to enforce punishments, penalties and sanctions
	Information	The right to control important information
	Ecological	The right to control the physical environment and organisation of work
Personal	Referent	Control through followers' positive feelings about the leader
	Expert	Control through competency in the particular field

Source: Adapted from G. Yukl (2010). *Leadership in organizations* (7th ed., pp. 201–211). Upper Saddle River, NJ: Pearson / Prentice Hall.

Power studies suggest that expert and referent power are more effective (for example, see Schriesheim, Hinkin & Podsakoff, 1991). However, other powers do not show any positive correlation with followers' satisfaction and performance. It could be concluded that leaders use more expert and referent power to influence followers, while managers use more position power (see Figure 1.2).

How much power do managers and leaders need? The most common answer would be 'as much as possible'. However, more power is not always better. More power is necessary in organisations where major change is required. On the other hand, managers with too much position power may be tempted to rely on it instead of developing personal power and using other approaches (for example, consultation or coalitions).

It is important to have the skills necessary to use available power. These can reduce the need to have a lot of power. Robert Katz (1955) suggests effective management is based on three types of skills. Technical skills come from specific knowledge in a particular area of work, human skills involve working and communicating with people, and conceptual skills help in developing ideas and vision, and in understanding economical principles.

Three levels of management can be identified in healthcare organisations, and this classification presents the most common hierarchical management structure found in organisations (see Figure 1.3). Top-level (executive or senior) managers are responsible for the performance of all departments and the organisation (for

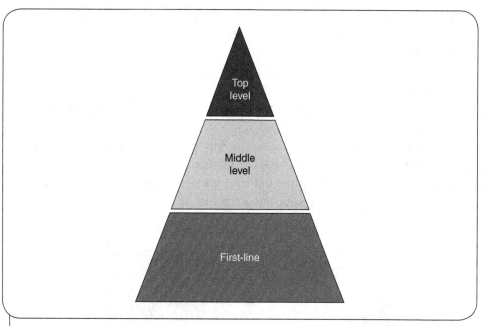

Figure 1.2 Power distribution between managers and leaders

example, chief executive officer). Middle-level managers supervise first-line managers and non-managerial employees (for example, director of obstetrics and gynaecology). Finally, first-line managers are responsible for the daily supervision of the non-managerial employees (for example, the nurse manager in the obstetrics department).

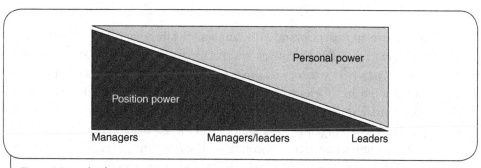

Figure 1.3 Levels of management within an organisation

Liang and Howard (2010) identify four tiers of top-level managers in the health sector in New South Wales: director-general, deputy directors-general, department of health division directors and chief executive officers of an area health service. The Australian Bureau of Statistics (2013) uses another classification, identifying a different four groups of managers in the health sector: chief executive officers and general managers, specialist managers (who work in specialist areas such as finance, human resources, information technology, medical and other clinical services, nursing and allied health services), service managers (who are concerned with catering, cleaning, maintenance and other support services), and managers not further defined. Australian census 2011 data show that 12.3 per cent of all health managers in Australia are chief executive officers and general managers, 68.3 per cent are specialist managers, 15.2 per cent are service managers, and 4.1 per cent are not defined.

The management skills identified earlier are required in different proportions depending on the manager's position within the organisation (see Figure 1.4). First-line managers need more technical skills, while top-level managers need more conceptual skills. However, human skills have the same importance for all levels.

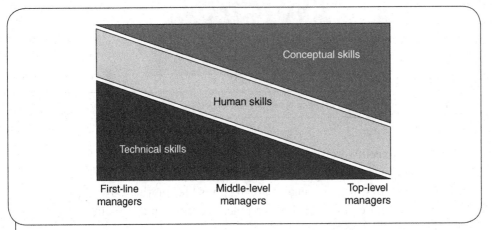

Figure 1.4 Katz's three-skills approach to management in relation to management level. Adapted from R. L. Katz (1955). Skills of an effective administrator. *Harvard Business Review, 33*(1), 33–42.

In an alternative approach, Mumford, Campion & Morgeson (2007) identify four types of management skills: cognitive, interpersonal, business and strategic. This work reinforces Katz's (1955) theory that management skills are important for all leaders and managers but in different proportions. According to Mumford et al. (2007), different management skill requirements emerge at different organisational levels, and jobs at higher levels of an organisation require higher levels of all of the skills. Certain cognitive skills are important across organisational levels, while certain strategic skill requirements fully emerge only at the highest levels in an organisation.

Functions

As mentioned earlier, one of the essential components of an organisation is the people, or workforce (see Figure 1.1). The group of staff that works directly with patients – such as doctors, nurses and other allied health specialists – is called the direct group. Other groups provide support for the direct group, ensuring that doctors and nurses have adequate equipment and supplies, clean facilities, care taken of financial issues and patient bookings attended to, freeing the direct group from all these duties and responsibilities. The support groups do not have direct contact with patients but undoubtedly are valuable to the functioning of the organisation. Because of the other groups' supportive role, the direct group can focus on the tasks it knows best. However, all direct and support staff need to be organised. They have to know what, when, where and how to do tasks. Therefore, there is another group of staff in an organisation, which we can call the executive group. This group undertakes the main responsibilities of management and leadership in the organisation.

What do managers actually do? As mentioned earlier, Fayol (1917) proposed a list of five primary functions of management: planning, organising, commanding (or leading), coordinating and controlling. Later authors have added further functions, like staffing and decision-making (Longest, Rakich & Darr, 2000), or have merged some of the functions (Waddell, Devine, Jones & George 2009). Following on from the definition of health management given above, we can say that managers have four functions:

Planning identifies the goals of the organisation and the courses of action that will best achieve these goals.

Organising establishes tasks and authority relationships that allow people to work together to achieve the organisational goals.

Leading articulates a clear vision, energising, motivating and enabling staff so they will contribute to achieving the organisational goals.

Controlling evaluates how well an organisation is achieving its goals and indentifies ways to improve performance.

It is obvious that different managers have different roles, meaning that for each manager the relative importance (or daily use) of these four managerial functions depends on their position in the organisation. Results from studies show that the amount of time managers spend planning and organising resources to maintain and improve organisational performance increases as they ascend the hierarchy. So first-line managers spend significantly less time on planning and organising, and more time on leading and controlling, than top-level managers (Gomez-Mejia, McCann & Page, 1985; Mahony, Jerdee & Carroll, 1965).

The difference between the functions of leaders and managers is, as stated earlier, the subject of intense debate. Some people use the terms management and leadership interchangeably, but this is not correct. While management has four main functions, leadership implements only one of these. It could be perceived that health leaders' roles and responsibilities are relatively glamorous (for example, setting the vision for the organisation, inspiring and motivating people), while managers are required to undertake boring tasks like staffing and budgeting. However, some leadership roles are not very exciting. Alvesson & Sveningsson (2003) have found that leaders often engage in passive, mundane activities, such as listening to employees, and that these activities are critical to the leaders' effectiveness.

According to John Kotter (1990), each system of action in an organisation has three main steps: deciding what needs to be done, creating networks of people and relationships that can accomplish the agenda, and trying to ensure that those people actually do the job. Leaders and managers are involved in every step, but in different ways. For the first step, managers do planning and budgeting, while leaders set directions. For the second, managers are concerned with organising and staffing, whereas leaders try to align people. For the last, managers do some controlling and problem-solving, while leaders try to motivate and inspire people.

Louis Rubino (2011) contributes to this discussion by arguing that running healthcare organisations has two 'foci', external and internal, and that leaders usually have an external focus, while the focus of managers is more internal. Leaders tend to spend the majority of their time communicating and aligning with outside groups that can benefit their organisation (partners, community, vendors) or influence them (media, government, public agencies). Meanwhile, managers are concerned more with internal stakeholders (administrators, professionals, operators).

In summarising, we could say that managers are concerned with today – with delivery, targets, efficiency, utilisation and authority – focusing on internal organisational issues, on control and on doing things right. Leaders are focused on tomorrow – on development, direction, purpose and vision, and driving innovation (Iles & Preece, 2006).

Summary

- The main functions of managers are planning, organising, leading and controlling, and health management is about planning, organising, leading and controlling resources in order to promote, restore or maintain health.
- There are three levels of management in healthcare organisations: first-line, middle and top.
- Effective management is based on three types of skills: technical, human and conceptual.
- Leaders and managers use positional and personal power to influence followers.
- Leaders influence individuals to achieve a common goal. Health leadership has specific characteristics, including a servant leader approach with the community and specific orientation to public health values.

Reflective questions

1 What first comes to your mind when you hear the words 'leadership' and 'management'? Why?

2 Are leadership and management different from one another? If so, how?

3 What are the differences between the functions of leaders and mangers?

4 Do you agree that everyone can be a leader? Explain your answer.

5 How can healthcare organisations select and develop effective leaders?

Self-analysis questions

Think about the most effective leader you have ever worked with, observed closely or know well from the media or other sources. List the five key traits, skills or practices of this leader. In addition, think about the person who in your understanding is the least effective leader you have come across. List the five traits, skills or practices of this person that you think are most important in determining that they are a poor leader. Now consider how they could develop, improve or change these characteristics to become more effective in their leadership.

References

Alvesson, M. & Sveningsson, S. (2003). Managers doing leadership: The extra-ordinarization of the mundane. *Human Relations, 56*, 1435–1459. doi: 10.1177/00187267035612001

Australian Bureau of Statistics. (2013). *2011 census of population and housing* [Customised report]. Canberra: Author.

Beaglehole, R., Bonita, R., Horton, R., Adams, O. & McKee, M. (2004). Public health in the new era: Improving health through collective action. *Lancet, 363*, 2084–2086. doi: 10.1016/S0140-6736(04)16461-1

Czabanowska, K., Smith, T., Stankunas, M., Avery, M. & Otok, R. (2013). Transforming public health specialists into public health leaders. *Lancet, 381*, 449–450. doi: 10.1016/S0140-6736(13)60246-9

Fayol, H. (1917). *Administration industrielle et générale: Prévoyance, organisation, commandement, coordination, contrôle* [French]. Paris, France: H. Dunod & E. Pinat.

Fulop, N., Allen, P., Clarke, A. & Black, N. (2001). Issues in studying the organisation and delivery of health services. In N. Fulop, P. Allen, A. Clarke & N. Black (Eds), *Studying the organisation and delivery of health services: Research methods* (pp. 1–23). London, United Kingdom: Routledge.

Gomez-Mejia, L., McCann, R. C. & Page, R. C. (1985). The structure of managerial behaviours and rewards. *Industrial Relations, 24*, 147–154. doi: 10.1111/j.1468-232X.1985.tb00986.x

Green, A., Collins, C. & Mirzoev, T. (2012). Management and planning for global health. In M. H. Merson, R. E. Black & A. J. Mills (Eds), *Global health: Diseases, programs, systems, and policies* (3rd ed., pp. 653–706). Burlington, MA: Jones & Bartlett Learning.

Hunter, D. J. & Brown, J. (2007). A review of health management research. *European Journal of Public Health, 17*(Suppl 1), 33–37. doi: 10.1093/eurpub/ckm061

Iles, P. & Preece, D. (2006). Developing leaders or developing leadership? The Academy of Chief Executives' programmes in the north east of England. *Leadership, 2*, 317–340. doi: 10.1177/1742715006066024

Katz, R. L. (1955). Skills of an effective administrator. *Harvard Business Review, 33*(1), 33–42.

Kotter, J. P. (1990). What leaders really do. *Harvard Business Review, 68*(3), 103–111.

Lease, D. R. (2006). *Management reviled: Is leadership just a good management repacked?* Paper presented at the Academy of Business Education Conference, San Antonio, TX.

Lega, F., Prenestini, A. & Spurgeon, P. (2013). Is management essential to improving the performance and sustainability of health care systems and organisations? A systematic review and a roadmap for future studies. *Value in Health, 16*, S46–S51. doi: 10.1016/j.jval.2012.10.004

Liang, Z. & Howard, P. F. (2010). Competencies required by senior health executives in New South Wales, 1990–1999. *Australian Health Review, 34*, 52–58. doi: 10.1071/AH09571

Longest, B. B., Rakich, J. S. & Darr, K. (2000). *Managing health services organizations and systems.* Baltimore, MD: Health Professions.

Mahony, T. A., Jerdee, T. H. & Carroll, S. J. (1965). The job(s) of management. *Industrial Relations, 4*, 97–110. doi: 10.1111/j.1468-232X.1965.tb00922.x

Martins, J. M. & Isouard, G. (2014). Health service managers in Australia: Progression and evolution. *Asia Pacific Journal of Health Management, 9*, 35–52. Retrieved from http://www.achsm.org.au

McAlearney, A. S. (2006). Leadership development in healthcare: A qualitative study. *Journal of Organizational Behavior, 27*, 967–982. doi: 10.1002/job.417

McKenna, E. (1998). *Business psychology and organisational behaviour: A student's handbook.* Hove, United Kingdom: Psychology.

Mumford, T. V., Campion, M. A. & Morgeson, F. P. (2007). The leadership skills strataplex: Leadership skill requirements across organizational levels. *Leadership Quarterly, 18*, 154–166. doi: 10.1016/j.leaqua.2007.01.005

Northouse, P. G. (2007). *Leadership: Theory and practice* (4th ed.). Thousand Oaks, CA: Sage.

———. (2013). *Leadership theory and practice* (6th ed.). Los Angeles, CA: Sage.

Rahim, M. A. (1988). The development of a leader power inventory. *Multivariate Behavioural Research, 23*, 491–502. doi: 10.1207/s15327906mbr2304_6

Rubino, L. (2011). Leadership. In S. B. Buchbinder & N. H. Shanks (Eds), *Introduction to health care management* (pp. 17–38). Burlington, MA: Jones & Bartlett Learning.

Schriesheim, C. A., Hinkin, T. R. & Podsakoff, P. M. (1991). Can ipsative and single-item measures produce erroneous results in field studies of French and Raven's (1959) five bases of power? An empirical examination. *Journal of Applied Psychology, 76*, 106–114. doi: 10.1037/0021-9010.76.1.106

Simpson, J. & Calman, K. (2000). Making and preparing leaders. *Medical Education, 34*, 211–215. doi: 10.1046/j.1365-2923.2000.0650a.x

Stankunas, M., Sauliune, S., Smith, T., Avery, M., Sumskas, L. & Czabanowska, K. (2012). Evaluation of leadership competencies of executives in Lithuanian public health institutions. *Medicina (Kaunas), 48*(11), 581–587.

Stogdill, R. M. (1974). *Handbook of leadership: A survey of theory and research.* New York, NY: Free.

Waddell, D., Devine, J., Jones, G. R. & George, J. M. (2009). *Contemporary management.* North Ryde: McGraw-Hill Australia.

World Health Organization. (1999). *Health21: The health for all policy framework for the WHO European region* (European Health for All Series no. 6). Retrieved from http://www.euro.who.int/__data/assets/pdf_file/0010/98398/wa540ga199heeng.pdf?ua=1

——. (2000). *The world health report 2000: Health systems; Improving performance.* Geneva, Switzerland: Author.

Yukl, G. (2010). *Leadership in organizations* (7th ed.). Upper Saddle River, NJ: Pearson / Prentice Hall.

——. (2013). *Leadership in organizations* (8th ed.). Harlow, United Kingdom: Pearson Education.

Zaleznik, A. (1977). Managers and leaders: Are they different? *Harvard Business Review, 55*(3), 67–78.

2

Leadership and management frameworks and theories

Melanie Bish

Learning objectives

How do I:
- determine the leadership approach I might take in my organisation?
- decide when I might need to change my leadership approach to a different style?
- learn about how management theory has changed over time?
- consider how best to develop my own leadership and management skills?
- integrate knowledge of leadership and management theory to inform future practice?

Introduction

Effective leadership and management are crucial for healthcare services to meet the expectation to provide high-quality, accessible, affordable care that will result in improved health outcomes (Fehr, 2011) in the context of health reform. Healthcare professionals must understand the main theories of leadership and management and how these approaches translate into improving work practices in order to develop their own work capacity. This chapter presents leadership and management theories that healthcare professionals currently use to inform their practice.

Definitions

Definitions that locate the concepts of leadership and management in a healthcare context are important. The concept of leadership in healthcare receives attention from government, policy-makers, organisational managers, clinicians and researchers (Kean & Haycock-Stuart, 2011). To be effective, leadership must be appropriate for healthcare in its broadest sense and see issues addressed in a political, social, policy and economic context (Swearingen, 2009). Gopee and Galloway (2014, p. 65) identify four possible meanings of the term **leadership**:

1   The activity of leading.
2   The body of people who lead a group.
3   The status of the leader.
4   The ability to lead.

> **Leadership**
> 'A process whereby an individual influences a group of individuals achieve a common goal' (North 2013, p. 5)
>
> **Management**
> Planning, organising, leading an controlling resources in order to an organisation's goals

The definition of leadership used in this book is 'a process whereby an individual influences a group of individuals to achieve a common goal' (Northouse, 2013, p. 5).

Management focuses on the organisation of people's endeavours as they work to achieve set goals that contribute to ensuring an organisation functions effectively and efficiently. A preference for approaches that emphasise employee empowerment is clear in current management practices, evidenced by a move away from hierarchical structures and the adaptation of contemporary leadership techniques.

Leadership theories

Evolvement

Leadership features in management, psychological and sociological sciences literature spanning over 100 years (Millward & Bryan, 2005). Early **theories** focus on the characteristics and behaviours of successful leaders. In later theories, consideration of the role of followers and the context for leadership is evident. Irrespective of their point in time, all theories have an individualistic viewpoint of leadership, discussing the concept in relation to one person's actions (Bolden, Gosling, Marturano & Dennison, 2003; Martin, 2007). The majority of the research generated may be categorised into one of four major approaches:

> **Theory**
> An idea or group of ideas based set of principles presented to exp a phenomenon, account for a sp situation or underpin an approac future actions

1   trait approaches;
2   situational approaches;
3   power-influence approaches; and
4   behavioural approaches. (Yukl, 1989, as cited in Rowden, 1999, p. 30)

Table 2.1 offers an overview of the evolvement of leadership theories.

Leadership theories in contemporary healthcare

Leadership involves the facilitation of change, the creation of a learning environment, the shaping of the cultural norms and values of an organisation and the sharing of a

Table 2.1 Overview of the evolvement of leadership theories

Great man theories	Based on the belief that leaders are exceptional people, born with innate qualities, destined to lead. The use of the term man was intentional since until the latter part of the twentieth century leadership was thought of as a concept which is primarily male, military and Western.
Trait theories	The lists of traits or qualities associated with leadership exist in abundance and continue to be produced. They draw on practically all the adjectives in the dictionary to describe a positive or virtuous attribute.
Behaviourist theories	These concentrate on what leaders actually do rather than on their qualities. Different patterns of behaviour are observed and categorised as 'styles of leadership'. This area has probably attracted the most attention from practising managers.
Situational leadership	This approach sees leadership as specific to the situation in which it is being exercised. It also proposes that there may be differences in required leadership styles at different levels in the same organisation.
Transactional theory	This approach emphasises the importance of the relationship between leader and followers, focusing on mutual benefits attained from a form of contract through which the leader delivers reward and recognition in return for the commitment or loyalty of the followers.
Transformational theory	The central concept being change and the role of leadership in envisioning and implementing the transformation of organisational performance.

Source: R. Bolden, J. Gosling, A. Marturano & P. Dennison (2003). *A review of leadership theory and competency frameworks* (Edited version of a report for Chase Consulting and the Management Standards Centre). Retrieved from University of Exeter, Business School website: http://business-school.exeter.ac.uk/documents/discussion_papers/cls/mgmt_standards.pdf. Reproduced with permission from University of Exeter Centre for Leadership Studies.

vision (Barr & Dowding, 2012). These components are essential in assisting all professionals to navigate their work in the complexities of the healthcare delivery context.

Today's healthcare leader needs 'to create space for other people to generate new and different ideas; to encourage meaningful conversation between people; and to assist people in becoming more effective, agile, and prepared to respond to complex challenges' (Martin, 2007, as cited in Singh & Sahay, 2009, p. 434). Healthcare leaders may utilise a mixture of theories, models and conceptual **frameworks** to guide their conduct.

Servant leadership

Servant leadership places emphasis on 'leadership as service' (Parris & Peachey, 2013; Sendjaya et al., 2008; van Dierendonck, 2011; all as cited in Orazi et al., 2014, p. 39) that relies heavily on 'relationship-orientated behaviours' (Northouse, 2009, as cited in Orazi et al., 2014, p. 39). Yoshida, Sendjaya, Hirst and Cooper (2013, as cited in Orazi et al., 2014, p. 39) describe it as 'a holistic approach to leadership that encompasses the rational, relational, emotional, moral, and spiritual dimension of the leader–follower relationship such that followers enhance and grow their capabilities', which results in the development of a greater sense of self-worth. This approach is suitable for leading multidisciplinary teams through change processes, as it relies on the establishment and maintenance of 'mutual trust and empowerment of followers' (Howatson-Jones, 2004, p. 22).

Howatson-Jones (2004, pp. 23–24) claims that 'trust is the cornerstone of the servant leader model of leadership, in that collegiate relationships are based on mutual respect and feedback, and direct in-the-field access to leaders … This model of leadership can help build trust and provide the support structures required to negotiate change successfully, while developing those involved to move forward and mature … The interdependence of this model contrasts with the traditional power models, and requires considerable maturity'. Servant leadership supports the role of a values-based approach to leadership, as it promotes positive organisational and individual outcomes.

Transactional leadership

In transactional leadership, the leader acts as an agent of change, making meaningful exchanges with employees that result in improvements in productivity (Al-Mailam, 2004). Characteristics of this approach are focused on the activities taking place at a daily operations level, with employee motivation being achieved through financial remuneration in exchange for services (Bass & Avolio, 1990).

A task-orientated style of leadership can have a positive influence on performance specifically, as an increased quality of internal communication through goal-setting, monitoring and feedback ensures that knowledge is generated to improve effectiveness and increase efficiencies (Bryant, 2003). The degree to which the leader and followers agree on the transactional aspects of the work equates to the level of the leader's positive influence on performance and organisational commitment, and on the level of trust in the leader (Whittington, Coker, Goodwin, Ickes & Murray, 2009).

Transactional leaders operate well in structured environments, where goal-setting and efficient routines can lead to positive outcomes. Transactional leadership is effective in crisis situations, when a clear direction is needed for the common good and deviance is not tolerated (Orazi et al., 2014).

Transformational leadership

The crux of transformational leadership is being able to inspire a commitment among colleagues to collectively achieve the vision of a preferred future (Leach, 2005).

Transformational leaders infuse pride and motivation in others, create a shared understanding and ownership of the future vision of an organisation and demonstrate open consideration of employees' ideas (Burns, 1978). They engage peers across periods of change and prioritise the provision of resources needed to achieve goals (Hocker & Trofino, 2003), which makes the approach suitable in organisations requiring change, development, initiative and creativity in turbulent and uncertain environments (Bass & Avolio, 1990).

Collaborative decision-making, mentoring, a patient focus and the use of ethical frameworks are all supported by transformational leadership (Hocker & Trofino, 2003). Specific constructs that see it feature predominantly in healthcare management include participatory management, individual consideration, charisma and intellectual stimulation (Upenieks, 2003). The creation of a shared values system and sense of purpose provides transformational leaders with opportunities to mould how staff at individual and group levels may view themselves and their organisation (Martin & Henderson, 2001).

The approach of the transformational leader encourages an evolvement of the basic values, beliefs and attitudes of followers that informs their approach to work, which results in a greater level of empowerment to achieve the vision and mission of the organisation. The benefits are visible in a greater level of productivity, heightened employee morale and positive personal and professional growth (Gopee & Galloway, 2014).

Charismatic leadership

In an early study of charismatic leaders, charisma was defined as a particular persona that an individual can have that sets them apart and, as a consequence, sees them treated as the host of some exceptional qualities (Weber, 1947). The qualities credited to charismatic leadership may also be attributed to transformational leadership and include refined interpersonal skills, self-confidence, courage, the ability to imagine different and better futures, the ability to communicate vision and a willingness to take risks (Taylor, 2007a). Charismatic leaders demonstrate a preference for relationship-oriented behaviours (Northouse, 2009). They are highly motivated leaders characterised by a confidence in their skills and have a disposition that projects determination and inspires followers to cope in times of uncertainty. In this sense, charismatic leaders are entrepreneurial, making sacrifices and taking risks to achieve what they believe is the most beneficial outcome for the organisation (Orazi et al., 2014).

A leadership style that often emerges in times of crisis, charismatic leadership has a capacity to generate excitement, enthusiasm and loyalty while exhibiting the skills required to carry out the identified tasks (Taylor, 2007b). Given the investment required of those who opt for this leadership style, concern exists over their ability to retain its enchantment over a sustained period, strengthening the argument that organisations are more effective if they invest in the development of leadership capacity across all levels of staff (Conger & Kanungo, 1988).

Authentic leadership

Regarded as being in the formative phase of development and a newcomer to leadership research, authentic leadership is highly desirable in a period in which people are seeking genuine and trustworthy leaders (Northouse, 2013). It suggests that to be able to lead, individuals must be true to themselves and to their guiding values system, or set of principles, and must act in accordance with them in a consistent manner (Marquis & Huston, 2015). Authentic leaders have distinguishing characteristics that include understanding of their own purpose through ongoing self-reflection, consistency between their beliefs and actions, genuine compassion for their followers, establishment of strong connections and practice of self-discipline through striving for professional and personal balance (Shirey, 2006). A high level of self-knowledge, commitment to enhancing their own leadership capacity and engagement in an interpersonal process with colleagues to nurture skills in others feature in this style of leadership (Northouse, 2013; Shirey, 2006).

Clear benefits of authentic leadership are the inspiration and excitement it can generate in others to achieve a level of performance that is regarded as success. Such success confers benefits at an individual and an organisational level. It results in favourable personal outcomes that may include feelings of self-efficacy and job satisfaction, which creates increased organisational commitment, with the positive organisational outcomes verified by growth, meeting of financial targets and fulfilment of a service need (Shirey, 2006). Individuals and organisations benefit from authentic leaders who demonstrate transparency in their intentions and exhibit a seamless link between espoused values, actions and behaviours (Luthans & Avolio, 2003).

E-leadership

E-leadership occurs in a context where work is mediated by information technology. The introduction of advanced information technology in healthcare organisations is changing the approach to healthcare leadership (Avolio & Kahai, 2003), and given the continued growth and application of information technology in the healthcare sector, theorists suggest that e-leadership will become routine rather than the exception in organisational leadership (Zaccaro & Bader, 2003).

In response to greater reliance on technology to interact with colleagues, leaders find themselves conducting many of the processes of leadership through electronic channels (Zaccaro & Bader, 2003). Leaders and followers have a greater level of access to information and to each other, which is changing the nature and content of their interactions. The purpose of e-leadership is to enhance the relationships among organisational members that are defined by an organisation's structure (Avolio & Kahai, 2003).

The challenges facing leaders who operate in circumstances where communication is no longer an interaction in person extend to building trust, maintaining open lines of communication and being open to subtle cues of concern (Barr & Dowding, 2012). Leaders adopting this approach are encouraged to facilitate communication and provide opportunities for shared learning (Avolio & Kahai, 2003).

Management theories

Skilled management has significant positive effects on productivity, profitability and the ability of organisations to adapt and change to meet emerging challenges. To achieve this in healthcare services, approaches to management need to be based on investment in skills, opportunities for employee engagement in the workplace and quality positions that provide incentives for employees to contribute (Orazi et al., 2014). In their practice, healthcare managers may use a combination of the theories discussed below.

Evolvement

During the Industrial Revolution, Frederick Winslow Taylor developed the four principles of scientific management that, if adhered to, would see productivity increase (see below). The works of Henri Fayol and Max Weber, produced in the late 19th and early 20th century, sought to combine theory with practice in addressing the fundamental issue of how organisations should be structured (Wren & Bedeian, 2009). The 'management functions of planning, organisation, command, coordination and control' were first identified by Henri Fayol (1925). These were expanded by Luther Gulick (1937) with the introduction of the seven activities of management: planning, organising, staffing, directing, coordinating, reporting and budgeting (Marquis & Huston, 2015).

A shift occurred during the 1920s when the focus turned to people rather than equipment. Several theories were generated in the human relations era, including participative management, the Hawthorne effect, theory X and theory Y, and employee participation (Marquis & Huston, 2015).

Approaches

Scientific management

A branch of the classical management perspective, scientific management theory proposes that efficiency and labour productivity are improved by scientifically determined jobs and management practices. Applying the four principles of management developed by Fredrick Winslow Taylor in the late 1800s, scientific management aims to improve the performance of individual workers through the use of analytical procedures to increase workplace efficiency (Daft & Marcic, 2013). Taylor's (1911, pp. 12–77) four principles of management are listed below:

- Develop a science for each element of the job to replace the old rule-of-thumb method.
- Scientifically select employees and then train, teach and develop them to do their job.
- Supervise employees to ensure that the work is completed in accordance with the prescribed methods for doing their job.
- Divide the work and responsibility almost equally between managers and employees.

Organisational behaviour

Contemporary views on motivation, leadership, trust, teamwork and conflict management are informed by research on organisational behaviour (Robbins, Bergman, Stagg & Coulter, 2011), which addresses individual, group and organisational processes in terms of the impact of the individual on the organisation and the impact of the organisation on the individual (Davidson & Griffin, 2006). Advocates of the approach believe that people are the most important asset of an organisation and should be managed accordingly. Theorists' work in this area has served as a foundation for management practices such as employee selection procedures and employee motivation programs (Robbins et al., 2011).

Hawthorne effect

A series of studies conducted in the 1920s and 1930s at the Hawthorne Works, at the Western Electric Company in Chicago, provide insight into individual and group behaviour (Mayo, 1953). Experiments established that psychological factors are an important variable in worker output and that the need for social acceptance affects output more than financial incentive (Davidson & Griffin, 2006). There is some debate concerning the rigour of several of the studies, but there is consensus that their importance in stimulating interest in seeing employees as more than extensions of production machinery far outweighs how academically sound the research was (Daft & Marcic, 2013). The studies are viewed as having had a significant impact on management beliefs about the role of human behaviour in organisations (Robbins et al., 2011). They identified the need for a new paradigm of management thought and have led to managers being equipped to handle the human element in the workplace (Davidson & Griffin, 2006).

Human relations movement

Instigated by the findings of the Hawthorne studies, the human relations movement is based on the notion that truly effective control comes from within the individual worker as opposed to an authoritarian approach (Daft & Marcic, 2013). The importance of employee satisfaction resulting in improved performance is advanced by the philosophies of Abraham Maslow and Douglas McGregor.

Maslow (1943) observed that individuals' problems often stem from an inability to satisfy their needs. This resulted in his creating a hierarchy of needs that starts with psychological needs and progresses to safety, belonging, esteem and self-actualisation needs. The theory remains influential in contemporary approaches to management (Daft & Marcic, 2013).

McGregor's (1960) work challenges the classical perspective and human relations assumptions about human behaviour through theory X and theory Y, which specify the extreme attitudinal position held by managers. Theory X represents the negative view of workers consistent with scientific management, and theory Y the positive approach, which aligns with the human relations perspective. McGregor advocates a theory Y approach to managing people (Davidson & Griffin, 2006).

Systems approach

In the 1960s, attention turned to analysing organisations from a **systems** perspective, generating a theory that focuses on systems and how they work and function within an organisation. The relationships between the parts are seen as equally important as the properties of the parts themselves (Davidson & Griffin, 2006).

interrelated and interdependent
anged in a manner that
a unified whole' (Robbins,
, Stagg & Coulter, 2011, p. 56)

Organisations are viewed as being composed of interdependent factors that include, but are not limited to, individuals, groups, attitudes, goals, motives, formal structure, status and authority. The approach argues that managers need to coordinate the work of various parts of their organisation and ensure that all of its interdependent parts are working together so that the organisation's goals are achieved (Robbins et al., 2011). Managers are also encouraged to understand the synergy of the whole organisation rather than just its separate elements, so that the organisation is managed as a whole (Daft & Marcic, 2013).

Managing a hospital with a systems approach

A large metropolitan public hospital exemplifies how the systems approach to management is used. Consider the role of an after-hours manager when a group of road trauma patients comes in via the emergency department. The assessments at triage reveal that the driver requires emergency surgery for a ruptured spleen, an adult passenger has suffered a myocardial infarction, and a child passenger has suffered concussion and a laceration to the forehead that requires suturing. To ensure the delivery of quality care, the management of these patients will require the coordination of several departments. The manager must have an understanding of the respective units throughout the organisation that will need to be engaged:

- There must be enough vacant beds in the respective units (intensive care, cardiac care, child and adolescent care) to admit the patients.
- The operating suite will need to have a theatre vacant to deal with the emergency case.
- The necessary qualified staff must be on shift to care for the patients.

This scenario also provides an example of how units need to work together to achieve a common goal.

Situational management

Situational management takes the position that there is no singular management theory that has universal application, as there are always numerous factors that are specific to each situation that will directly influence organisational performance. As there is no optimum state in any organisation, the management approach used and its success are dependent upon the nature of the task that needs to be undertaken or the situation that needs to be dealt with at a particular point in time and under prevailing environmental circumstances (Gopee & Galloway, 2014). Known also as the contingency approach, this theory is widely adopted in the healthcare sector. Contingency means that one thing depends on other things; the manager's response to a situation depends on identifying key contingencies in an organisational situation (Daft & Marcic, 2013).

Summary

- Leadership and management theories are broad constructs with variation in definitions to suit the context and purpose.
- The study of leadership has progressed from broad conceptualisations of traits and behaviours of leaders to an approach that focuses on the sphere of influence and development of interdependent relationships to impact on the culture of a workplace.
- The effectiveness and efficiency of services are influenced by the application of leadership and management theories.
- Healthcare professionals may use a combination of different leadership and management theories in their practice.

Reflective questions

1 Why is it so important to underpin practice with theory?

2 What do you think needs to feature in future leadership and management theory for them to be relevant to health professionals?

3 Based on the content in this chapter and your experience, what do you perceive to be the strengths and weaknesses of transactional leadership?

4 Which of the leadership theories presented do you align with?

5 Can you identify the leadership theory that underpins the conduct of one of your colleagues?

Self-analysis question

How does your leadership style impact on your colleagues? Provide examples.

References

Al-Mailam, F. F. (2004). Transactional versus transformational style of leadership: Employee perception of leadership efficacy in public and private hospitals in Kuwait. *Quality Management in Health Care, 13*, 278–284. doi: 10.1097/00019514-200410000-00009

Avolio, B. J. & Kahai, S. S. (2003). Adding the 'E' to E-leadership: How it may impact your leadership. *Organizational Dynamics, 31*(4), 325–338. doi: 10.1016/S0090-2616(02)00133-X

Barr, J. & Dowding, L. (2012). *Leadership in health care* (2nd ed.). London, United Kingdom: Sage.

Bass, B. & Avolio, B. (1990). The implications of transactional and transformational leadership for individual, team and organizational development. In R. W. Woodman & W. A. Passmore (Eds), *Research in organizational change and development* (Vol. 4, pp. 231–272). Greenwich, CT: JAI.

Bolden, R., Gosling, J., Marturano, A. & Dennison, P. (2003). *A review of leadership theory and competency frameworks* (Edited version of a report for Chase Consulting and the Management Standards Centre). Retrieved from University of Exeter, Business School website: http://business-school.exeter.ac.uk/documents/discussion_papers/cls/mgmt_standards.pdf

Bryant, S. E. (2003). The role of transformational and transactional leadership in creating, sharing and exploiting organizational knowledge. *Journal of Leadership & Organizational Studies*, 9(4), 32–44. doi: 10.1177/107179190300900403

Burns, J. M. (1978). *Leadership*. New York, NY: Harper & Row.

Conger, J. A. & Kanungo, R. N. (1988). *Charismatic leadership: The elusive factor in organizational effectiveness*. San Francisco, CA: Jossey-Bass.

Daft, R. L. & Marcic, D. (2013). *Understanding management* (8th ed.). Independence, KY: Cengage Learning.

Davidson, P. & Griffin, R. W. (2006). *Management* (3rd Australasian ed.). Milton: Wiley.

Fayol, H. (1925). *General and industrial management*. London, United Kingdom: Pittman.

Fehr, L. (2011). The future of nursing: Leading change, advancing health. *Colorado Nurse, 111*, 6–7.

Gopee, N. & Galloway, J. (2014). *Leadership & management in health care* (2nd ed.). Los Angeles, CA: Sage.

Gulick, L. (1937). Notes on the theory of the organisation. In L. Gulick & L. Urwick (Eds), *Papers on the science of administration* (pp. 3–13). New York, NY: Institute of Public Administration.

Hocker, S. M. & Trofino, J. (2003). Transformation leadership: The development of a model of nursing case management by the army nurse corps. *Lippincott's Case Management, 8*(5), 208–213. doi: 10.1097/00129234-200309000-00006

Howatson-Jones, I. L. (2004). The servant leader. *Nursing Management, 11*(3), 20–24. doi: 10.7748/nm2004.06.11.3.20.c1978

Kean, S. & Haycock-Stuart, E. (2011). Understanding the relationship between followers and leaders. *Journal of Nursing Management, 18*(8), 31–35. doi: 10.7748/nm2011.12.18.8.31.c8843

Leach, L. S. (2005). Nurse executive transformational leadership and organizational commitment. *Journal of Nursing Administration, 35*(5), 228–237. doi: 10.1097/00005110-200505000-00006

Luthans, F. & Avolio, B. J. (2003). Authentic leadership: A positive developmental approach. In K. S. Cameron, J. E. Dutton & R. E. Quinn (Eds), *Positive organizational scholarship* (pp. 241–261). San Francisco, CA: Berrett-Koehler.

Marquis, B. L. & Huston, C. J. (2015). *Leadership roles and management functions in nursing theory and application* (8th ed.). Philadelphia, PA: Wolters Kluwer.

Martin, A. (2007). The future of leadership: Where do we go from here? *Industrial and Commercial Training, 39*(1), 3–8. doi: 10.1108/00197850710721345

Martin, V. & Henderson, E. (2001). *Managing in health and social care*. London, United Kingdom: Routledge / Open University.

Maslow, A. (1943). A theory of human motivation. *Psychological Review*, (July), 370–396.

Mayo, E. (1953). *The human problems of an industrial civilization*. New York, NY: Macmillian.

McGregor, D. (1960). *The human side of enterprise*. New York, NY: McGraw-Hill.

Millward, L. J. & Bryan, K. (2005). Clinical leadership in health care: A position statement. *Leadership in Health Services, 18*(2–3), xiii–xxv. doi: 10.1108/13660750510594855

Northouse, P. G. (2009). *Leadership: Theory and practice* (5th ed.). Thousand Oaks, CA: Sage.

——. (2013). *Leadership: Theory and practice* (6th ed.). Los Angeles, CA: Sage.

Orazi, D., Good, L., Robin, M., van Wanrooy, B., Butar, I., Olsen, J. & Gahan, P. (2014). *Workplace leadership: A review of prior research*. Retrieved from Centre for Workplace

Leadership website: http://www.workplaceleadership.com.au/app/uploads/2014/07/ Workplace-Leadership-A-Review-of-Prior-Research-20142.pdf

Robbins, S., Bergman, R., Stagg, I. & Coulter, M. (2011). *Foundations of management* (Vol. 6). Frenchs Forest: Pearson Education.

Rowden, R. W. (1999). The relationship between charismatic leadership behaviors and organizational commitment. *Leadership & Organizational Development Journal, 21*(1), 30–35. doi: 10.1108/01437730010310712

Shirey, M. R. (2006). Building authentic leadership and enhancing entrepreneurial performance. *Clinical Nurse Specialist, 20*(6), 280–282. doi: 10.1097/00002800-200611000-00007

Singh, S. K. & Sahay, S. S. (2009). Business excellence in global corporations through emotionally intelligent leadership. *International Journal of Value Chain Management, 3*(4), 431–445. doi: 10.1504/IJVCM.2009.031771

Swearingen, S. (2009). A journey to leadership: Designing a nursing leadership development program. *Journal of Continuing Education in Nursing, 40,* 107–114. doi: 10.3928/00220124 -20090301-02

Taylor, F. W. (1911). *The principles of scientific management.* New York, NY: Harper & Row.

Taylor, V. (2007a). Leadership for service improvement (part 1). *Nursing Management, 13*(9), 30–34. doi: 10.7748/nm2007.02.13.9.30.c4337

——. (2007b). Leadership for service improvement: Part 3. *Nursing Management, 14*(1), 28–32. doi: 10.7748/nm2007.04.14.1.28.c4342

Upenieks, V. (2003). Nurse leaders' perceptions of what compromises successful leadership in today's acute inpatient environment. *Nursing Administration Quarterly, 27*(2), 140–152. doi: 10.1097/00006216-200304000-00008

Weber, M. (1947). *The theory of social and economic organization.* New York, NY: Free.

Whittington, J. L., Coker, R. H., Goodwin, V. L., Ickes, W. & Murray, B. (2009). Transactional leadership revisited: Self–other agreement and its consequences. *Journal of Applied Social Psychology, 39*(8), 1860–1886. doi: 10.1111/j.1559-1816.2009.00507.x

Wren, D. A. & Bedeian, A. G. (2009). *The evolution of management thought* (6th ed.). Hoboken, NJ: Wiley.

Zaccaro, S. J. & Bader, P. (2003). E-leadership and the challenges of leading E-teams: Minimizing the bad and maximizing the good. *Organizational Dynamics, 31*(4), 377–387. doi: 10.1016/ S0090-2616(02)00129-8

Part 2

Leads Self

3

Ethical leadership

Gian Luca Casali and Gary E. Day

Learning objectives

How do I:
- understand the importance of ethics in the health manager's decision-making process?
- understand the different perspectives of the four schools of moral philosophy and how they can influence a health manager's decision-making?
- understand the concepts of moral courage and whistleblowing?
- identify the main factors that influence ethical decision-making?
- identify the eight steps in the decision-making framework?

Introduction

This chapter explores the notion of ethics and ethical decision-making frameworks in leading and managing health services. Chapter 1 outlined the four sets of skills, or functions, that every manager should possess, which are usually summarised under the acronym POLC: planning, organising, leading and controlling. With leadership being one of the four functions of management, it is important to understand both the management and the leadership aspects of ethical decision-making.

Ethical decision-making

For managers, ethical decision-making incorporates the development and dissemination of frameworks to assist staff to make decisions in line with the organisation's direction and values, ensuring current staff understand these frameworks and recruiting staff who will work within the frameworks. For leaders,

ethical decision-making is about taking action when it is needed, guiding others in working through difficult and complex decision-making processes and being a role model for other staff.

New managers in the healthcare system will be faced with multiple and sometimes competing frameworks that guide practice. These may include managerial ethical frameworks, clinical decision-making frameworks and in some cases reli-

> **Ethical decision-making**
> Decisions that take into account morals and norms

gious frameworks. All of these may come into play around single or multiple issues, increasing the complexity in finding an acceptable ethical solution satisfying all of the competing values, including those of the patient.

Health managers face many challenges in today's work environment, which is characterised by rapid changes, globalisation, tough competition and higher demands for socially responsible healthcare provision. In such a complex and uncertain milieu, managers must make decisions affecting not only their organisation, their personal career, their patients and their families, but also the wider community. Achieving an understanding of how those decisions are made is vital.

Research has shown that the likelihood of making unethical decisions in the workplace is relatively high. In Australia and New Zealand, results from KPMG's (2004, 2013) forensic fraud surveys in 2004 and 2012 indicate that unethical practice at both individual and organisation levels is real and alarming (see Table 3.1).

Table 3.1 Selected results from KPMG's Australian and New Zealand fraud surveys, 2004 and 2012

2004	2012
33% of employees had witnessed unethical or improper conduct at work during the previous two years.	43% of the respondent firms experienced fraud.
22% attributed unethical or improper conduct at work to senior management's lack of commitment to the organisational ethical code.	30% of the respondent firms detected less than 40% of frauds in their organisation.
18% believed a poor ethical culture contributed to unethical behaviours.	47% of the major frauds occurred due to deficient internal controls.

Source: KPMG. (2004). *KPMG fraud survey report*. Singapore: Author; KPMG. (2013). *A survey of fraud, bribery and corruption in Australia & New Zealand 2012*. Retrieved from https://www.kpmg.com/AU/en/IssuesAndInsights/ArticlesPublications/Fraud-Survey/Documents/fraud-bribery-corruption-survey-2012v2.pdf.

Even if these results reflect the actions of only a few bad managers, those unethical behaviours were widely visible to others and are likely to have influenced decision-making within the organisational culture that allowed them to exist. These statistics present a challenge to those wanting to promote virtuous or ethical management behaviour in organisations.

Despite best efforts to address the problem by introducing so-called ethics regimes into organisational culture (Preston, 1994), unethical practice can be as resistant to bureaucratisation as it is to legislation. While good regulations and sound organisational practices are important, ethics goes beyond good rules and good practices; it involves the ability to make value-based judgements appropriate to personal and professional identities and situational contexts, both regular and irregular.

Creating and sustaining procedural uniformity when dealing with ethical issues in organisations is a near impossible task. Ethical decision-making at the managerial level remains highly individualised work even when it necessitates collaboration, as the manager is often the one responsible for getting people together and facilitating groups to discuss problems, as well as monitoring and evaluating outcomes. In completing their tasks, managers are subjected to a wide range of influences; they can react differently to diverse situations, and, even if they are not guided by commitments to contrasting ethical principles, they may still prioritise them in varying ways.

A preference for a particular ethical approach is only one of the factors that can influence a decision-maker, and all of the individual differences that arise from the variable influences of these factors can increase complexity and uncertainty in an organisation, especially when it comes to predicting behaviour. Recently, organisations have introduced codes of ethics and codes of conduct as tools to minimise the likelihood of staff engaging in unethical behaviours. Nevertheless, as Guy (1990, pp. 25–26) argues, 'these cannot replace ethical decision making; they can only supplement what is within the individual, which is his or her own set of principles applied to each decision made'. The mere introduction of a code of ethics without taking into consideration these individual differences, then, could be detrimental for the organisation. Instead of achieving a higher degree of consistency across the organisation when facing particular ethical situations, codes could create more conflict between staff, as they will inevitably differ in their interpretations of the codes and the situations to which they are to be applied. The factors influencing these differing responses are embedded in each individual manager and are open to investigation.

Influential factors

Individual responses in the decision-making process are the results of numerous factors that have contributed to the creation of the personality of the person making the decision, and more specifically to their particular predispositions (or **heuristics**). It is not possible, for example, to separate nationality from the individual. But then, an individual from a particular ethnic background could act differently from another individual from the same ethnic background because of other factors, in addition to cultural norms and values that have contributed to the development of the two individuals' characters.

ics
al procedures, guidelines or rules
ɔ developed to assist people in
omplex problems (Bazerman,

Bazerman (2005) defines heuristics as individual procedures, guidelines or rules of thumb developed to assist people in solving complex problems. Skitmore, Stradling and Touhy (1989) additionally inform us that decision-makers use heuristics as shortcuts instead of carrying out detailed analyses of problems. As a result, when solving a problem, they tend to rely upon those principles and constructs that are embedded in them, rather than engaging in a totally new decision-making process. The various factors that contribute to people's predispositions and influence their decision-making are discussed in the sections below.

Ethical factors

The first group of factors that affect individuals' ability to make decisions can be described as ethical or moral – that is, beliefs about right and wrong. **Morality** can be taken to mean 'moral judgments, standards and rules of conduct' (Ferrell, Fraedrich & Ferrell, 2005, p. 5) or 'the principles, norms, and standards of conduct governing an individual or group' (Trevino & Nelson, 2007, p. 13).

> **Morality**
> The standards, principles and ru
> that govern an individual's or a
> conduct

Generally, people hold different sets of values, morals and norms; however, they all involve a claim that one ought to act in a certain way. Due to this normative propensity, ethics and morality tend to be constructed of shared understandings which are responsive to the demands of particular contexts. Being socially and historically embedded, the quest for shared understandings has led to the creation of various schools of moral philosophies. In everyday decision-making, we knowingly and unknowingly tend to draw on these philosophies.

Four major schools of moral philosophy have been used to profile the expression of morality in ethical decision-making: **egoism**, **utilitarianism**, **virtue ethics** and **deontology**. These cover a spectrum of ethical styles, from a focus on consequences (utilitarianism and egoism), through a focus on the moral traits within people developed from habit and education over time (virtue ethics), to a focus on universal principles and duties which ought to be applied in all like circumstances (deontology) (Ferrell, Fraedrich & Ferrell, 2008; Trevino & Nelson, 2007).

> **Egoism**
> A doctrine that maximises the g
> good or benefit for the individua
>
> **Utilitarianism**
> A doctrine that maximises the g
> good for the greatest number of
>
> **Virtue ethics**
> A system that focuses on the
> embodiment of virtues in the ind
>
> **Deontology**
> An ethical theory that applies ur
> principles and duties in all simila
> circumstances

The main difference between utilitarian and egoistic philosophies is one of scope. Utilitarians are concerned with creating the greatest good for the greatest number, while egoists commit to maximising the good for themselves alone. A similar difference of scope could be said to apply to deontology and virtue ethics. Deontologists focus on universal rights and duties, while virtue ethicists focus on the embodiment of virtues in the individual. These traits are acquired through learning and habits.

In the past, the virtue ethics approach has been most closely aligned with professional life when practitioners are trained in groups under apprentice-like conditions (such as nurses and doctors) but go on to practise mainly as individuals. In such a setting, codes of ethics expressing universal principles are also important, but until recently greater emphasis has been placed on the character and integrity of the practitioner and their ability to interpret the application of those rules independently.

The ethical dilemma

I once worked with a health manager who was making decisions predominantly based on the consideration of what would make him look good in front of his superiors, rather than the staff he had to manage and lead. His decision-making was driven by what would get him the next promotion (egoism) instead of what was best for the organisation as a whole (utilitarianism). It took the manager some time to realise his decision-making processes were selfish and not in the interests of the organisation as a whole. He eventually recognised that his decision-making approach hindered rather than enhanced his ability to take on more senior roles within the organisation.

There is animated debate in ethics over whether the focus should be on applying universal principles to all situations or on finding principles appropriate for each particular situation – in short, whether one should subscribe to an absolutistic or a pluralistic viewpoint. Both sides have strong supporting arguments.

A large portion of the current literature on ethical decision-making is based on Lawrence Kohlberg's (1979) cognitive moral development (or CMD) model (for example, Lind, 1995; Rest, 1979). Cognitive moral development is a theory that divides respondents into different categories based on their individual level of moral development. Typically, however, each respondent can belong to only one particular stage at any given time, reflecting the absolutistic view. Thus, if a person strongly identifies with only one school of morality, or has reached a certain level of moral development, they will mostly adopt principles and criteria from that particular approach or level in reaching an ethical decision. The problem with this approach is the underlying assumption that individuals perfectly fit into only one level or school. In reality, it seems more plausible that individuals could belong to different levels or schools in different situations or that even in the same situation they could act as a result of a combination of different levels or schools. With this approach, a person will reach an ethical decision by using a mix of principles from more than one school of moral philosophy or level of moral development. In order to reduce the likelihood of preconceived bias towards an absolutistic approach, the framework for managerial ethical decision-making proposed later in this chapter has been developed in such a way that it is flexible enough to capture a continuum of responses, from absolutism to pluralism.

For health managers, insisting on what is right requires perseverance. An important concept that has been supported frequently (Clancy, 2003; Kidder, 2005; Lachman,

2009) is that of **moral courage**. In ancient Greek epics the term courage was explained as the bravery that a person possesses and was illustrated in heroes' fearlessness about death so long as their values were put first. In a less heroic but more professional context, moral courage can be displayed by managers who stand by their values despite there being a cost in doing so. Kidder (2005) defines moral courage as being at the intersection of three acts: applying values, recognising risks and enduring the hardship. The last of these is the essential component of moral courage.

> **Moral courage**
> A quality of mind that allows in
> to stand by their values despite
> or professional cost
>
> **Whistleblowing**
> Openly disclosing organisational
> malpractice

A commonly understood example of moral courage is the concept of **whistleblowing**, the term used to describe the actions of employees who go outside their workplace to openly disclose to the public organisational malpractice such as fraud, theft, corruption, resource wastage, negligence (including medical negligence), misrepresentation and major safety violations. Whistleblowing demonstrates a high level of morale courage. Although whistleblowers are afforded protection under federal and state legislation, and while a whistleblower in a healthcare organisation may do the right thing by a patient or the organisation by revealing serious problems or breaches of policy or protocol, as a result of formally raising such issues they can encounter personal and professional costs, including a high level of stress, ostracisation, strained working relationships, blacklisting, vilification and the destruction of their professional reputation and career (Sawyer, Johnson & Holub, 2010).

Personal factors

Personal factors that affect people's ability to make decisions are all those that are directly related to the individual decision-maker, including their nationality, age, gender, education, professional experience, ethical training, cognitive moral development and personal values. Ford and Richardson (1994) argue that these factors can be subdivided into two groups: individual factors related to birth (such as gender, nationality and age) and individual factors related to human development and interactions with others (such as religion, employment, cognitive moral development, education and professional experience). An individual may be influenced by numerous personal factors; however, not every factor will necessarily impact on them to the same degree. In practice, when a person is put in a situation of making a decision, initially, the individual factors related to birth will start to shape the decision-making process, and the process will then be further shaped by the individual factors related to human development and interactions with others.

Organisational factors

Organisational factors comprise those inherent to a particular enterprise that are in some degree able to influence individual decision-making. The most common organisational factors are codes of ethics and codes of conduct, rewards and sanctions, ethical climate and culture, industry type, organisational size, referent groups and training. Organisational factors can influence decision-making in different ways. Organisational culture, for example, can affect an individual decision-maker's judgement by emphasising particular values that have been shared within the organisation.

But organisational values may come into conflict with values that individuals within the organisation usually hold and act upon outside the organisation. For example, Casali and Day (2010), researching problems that emerged from an investigation into hospital fatalities, have found that both the values of the staff and the espoused values of the organisation in question were similar and positive, whereas the values promoted by the organisational culture included bullying, fear, tokenistic consultation and power control.

External factors

External factors that affect people's ability to make decisions are those that belong neither to the individual nor to their organisation but impact on the decision-making process from the outside. They are also referred to by researchers as the general environment; they are seen as the background conditions in which an organisation operates. External factors can be grouped into six main categories: political and legal, economic, social and demographic, technological, environmental, and competitive (Jirasek, 2003; Peer & Rakich, 1999; Schermerhorn, 2005; Zentner & Gelb, 1991).

External factors, even though they may not influence decision-making directly, can indirectly play an important role in shaping it. Some external factors may be within the control of the decision-maker, while others may not. For example, government health policy and funding are not within the direct control or influence of the health manager, but the health manager will still be required to make decisions within the confines of both the budget and the health policy. Additionally, government health policy may be at odds with the manager's personal ethics and values, but there is an expectation that the health manager will nevertheless make decisions in the best interests of the organisation.

Frameworks for ethical decision-making

Decision-making is usually defined as a cognitive process that aims to choose a course of action between different alternative options (Bazerman, 2005). The word cognitive is derived from a Latin word, *cognoscere*, which means to know; therefore, a cognitive process is a process that through knowledge and analysis of available information arrives at a final choice.

n-making
ive process that aims to choose
of action from a number of
or alternatives

Only when processed raw data have offered some useful insights can they be called information (Davenport & Prusak, 2000), and only at a further stage of analysis, when the use of information has created value for the organisation, does that information become knowledge (Kanter, 1999). Knowledge has been defined as 'a fluid mix of framed experience, values, contextual information, and expert insight that provides a framework for evaluating and incorporating new experiences and information' (Davenport & Prusak, 2000, p. 5). Therefore, it is essential to understand how information is processed and knowledge created.

This has been attempted by Kolasa (1982) and further modified by Maqsood (2006). Both researchers highlight the importance of knowing that human information-processing occurs as a series of essential stages (conceptualisation, judgement, perception and reasoning), which need to be undertaken before a person can make a decision. At any one of the stages, if it is based on raw data and sensory inputs, a different decision may be made. For the experienced manager, past experiences and knowledge assist in framing the final decision. For the new manager, who may not have experienced similar inputs or situations before, the reasoning process has to rely more heavily for guidance on available frameworks, procedures, protocols and guidelines.

In information-processing, the information is firstly recognised (perceived) and is secondly compared with existing similar or inherent information (existing knowledge). Therefore, it is assumed that knowledge is not only created, used and reused throughout the process, but also heavily influenced by individual perceptions that, acting as catalysts, can affect every step of the process. More specifically, as discussed earlier, individual perceptions are affected by a large number of factors – such as values, nationality, education, work experience and gender – that ultimately underpin the overall process.

A well-accepted framework for decision-making is provided below. Its creators, Robbins and Coulter (2005), describe the decision-making process in a sequential series of eight steps. There are many frameworks similar to this one, but not all include the last two steps (Bazerman, 2005).

Identify the problem   Conduct a full analysis of the problem.

Identify the decision criteria   Create a list of criteria in order to assess the alternative options.

Allocate weights   Rate the criteria from the most important to the least important.

Develop alternatives   Generate alternative options in order to resolve the problem.

Analyse alternatives   Assess the alternative options against the weighted criteria.

Select an alternative   Choose the alternative with the highest score.

Implement the alternative   Plan how to act out the decision, and inform the people responsible for implementing it.

Evaluate the decision's effectiveness   Conduct research to find out if the decision and its implementation have fixed the problem.

If health managers use heuristics as shortcuts in their decision-making process, it can be assumed that they may use them on every one of the eights steps in the decision-making framework. Managers should be able to recognise as many of the factors that influence them as possible, in order to predict which heuristics they may use in reaching a decision. Understanding the cognitive process involved in decision-making is the theoretical foundation for the personal–structural element of the managerial ethical decision-making framework proposed above. The framework is flexible and allows attention to be given to a large number of different factors that have been found to be influential in ethical decision-making, as well as a step-by-step process that would allow the manager to consider ethical dimensions at each decision point.

For managers, the important steps to keep in mind to ensure decisions have a strong ethical underpinning include looking at issues from the perspective of all four schools of moral philosophy, in order to evaluate all possible ethical angles and minimise biases. It is important to remember that there are different types of factors that can influence decision-making and that managers have control over some (ethical and individual), less control over others (organisational) and no control over the rest (external). Using the decision-making framework helps managers to maintain consistency and to build self-confidence as decision-makers.

Summary

- Unethical behaviours such as theft and fraud can be the results of unethical decision-making.
- There are four schools of moral philosophy (ethical egoism, utilitarianism, virtue ethics and deontology), each of which presents a different perspective on how a person may arrive at a decision.
- Decision-making is influenced by ethical, personal, organisational and external factors.
- Moral courage is a combination of applying values, recognising risks and being persistent.
- There are eight distinct steps that should be taken in the managerial ethical decision-making framework.

Reflective questions

1 Why is an understanding of ethics important to the health manager in the decision-making process?
2 How might age and social culture influence decision-making? Provide some examples.
3 How might organisational culture influence decision-making?
4 What is a code of conduct, and what is its role in ethical decision-making?
5 Why is analysing alternatives an important step in the decision-making process?

Self-analysis question

From the perspective of a health service manager, consider the strengths and weaknesses of the four schools of moral philosophy (ethical egoism, utilitarianism, virtue ethics and deontology) in relation to your workplace. What are the risks to your organisation of making decisions from the perspective of each of the schools?

References

Bazerman, M. H. (2005). *Judgment in managerial decision making* (6th ed.). New York, NY: Wiley.

Casali, G. L. & Day, G. E. (2010). Treating an unhealthy organisational culture: The implications of the Bundaberg Hospital Inquiry for managerial ethical decision making. *Australian Health Review, 34*(1), 73–79. doi: 10.1071/AH09543

Clancy, T. R. (2003). Courage and today's nurse leader. *Nursing Administration Quarterly, 27*(2), 128–132. doi: 10.1097/00006216-200304000-00006

Davenport, T. H. & Prusak, L. (2000). *Working knowledge: How organizations manage what they know.* Boston, MA: Harvard Business.

Ferrell, O. C., Fraedrich, J. & Ferrell, L. (2005). *Business ethics: Ethical decision making and cases* (6th ed.). Boston, MA: Houghton Mifflin.

——. (2008). *Business ethics: Ethical decision making and cases* (7th ed.). Boston, MA: Houghton Mifflin.

Ford, R. C. & Richardson, W. D. (1994). Ethical decision making: A review of the empirical literature. *Journal of Business Ethics, 13*(3), 205–221.

Guy, M. (1990). *Ethical decision making in everyday work situations*. New York, NY: Quorum.

Jirasek, J. A. (2003). Two approaches to business ethics. *Journal of Business Ethics*, *47*(4), 343–347. doi: 10.1023/A:1027318120232

Kanter, J. (1999). Knowledge management, practically speaking. *Information Systems Management*, (Fall), 7–15. doi: 10.1201/1078/43189.16.4.19990901/31198.2

Kidder, R. M. (2005). Moral courage, digital distrust: Ethics in a troubled world. *Business and Society Review*, *110*(4), 485–505. doi: 10.1111/j.0045-3609.2005.00026.x

Kohlberg, L. (1979). *The meaning and measurement of moral development*. Worchester, MA: Clark University.

Kolasa, B. J. (1982). *Introduction to behavioural sciences for business* (3rd ed.). New Delhi, India: Wiley Eastern.

KPMG. (2004). *KPMG fraud survey report*. Singapore: Author.

——. (2013). *A survey of fraud, bribery and corruption in Australia & New Zealand 2012*. Retrieved from https://www.kpmg.com/AU/en/IssuesAndInsights/ArticlesPublications/Fraud-Survey/Documents/fraud-bribery-corruption-survey-2012v2.pdf

Lachman, V. D. (2009). *Ethical challenges in healthcare: Developing your moral compass*. New York, NY: Springer.

Lind, G. (1995). *The meaning and measurement of moral judgment revisited*. Paper presented at the American Educational Research Association, San Francisco, CA.

Maqsood, T. (2006). *The role of knowledge management in supporting innovation and learning in construction*. Melbourne: RMIT.

Peer, K. & Rakich, J. (1999). Ethical decision making in healthcare management. *Hospital Topics: Research and Perspectives on Healthcare*, *77*(4), 7–13. doi: 10.1080/00185869909596532

Preston, N. (1994). *Ethics for the public sector: Education and training*. Sydney: Federation.

Rest, J. (1979). *Development in judging moral issues*. Minneapolis, MN: University of Minnesota.

Robbins, S. P. & Coulter, M. K. (2005). *Management* (8th ed.). Upper Saddle River, NJ: Pearson / Prentice Hall.

Sawyer, K. R., Johnson, J. & Holub, M. (2010). The necessary illegitimacy of the whistleblower. *Journal of Business and Professional Ethics*, *29*(1–4), 84–107. doi: 10.5840/bpej2010291/46

Schermerhorn, J. R. Jr. (2005). *Management* (8th ed.). New York, NY: Wiley.

Skitmore, R. M., Stradling, S. G. & Touhy, A. P. (1989). Project management under uncertainty. *Construct Management and Economics*, *7*(2), 103–113. doi: 10.1080/01446198900000015

Trevino, L. K. & Nelson, K. A. (2007). *Managing business ethics: Straight talk about how to do it right* (4th ed.). New York, NY: Wiley.

Zentner, R. & Gelb, B. D. (1991). Scenarios: A planning tool for health care organizations. *Hospital & Health Services Administration*, *36*(2), 211–222.

4

Self-management

John Adamm Ferrier

Learning objectives

How do I:

- ensure a plan for self-management that helps my integration into the workforce and facilitates lifelong learning?
- motivate myself to strive for continual improvement through self-management?
- set personal and professional goals for self-management?
- plan to improve areas of intelligence that I have identified as not being as strong as needed?
- find and work with a mentor?

Introduction

Nurses and allied health personnel are held in high esteem by the general public, a fact confirmed consistently by rankings of trust and reliability in both the United States (Swift, 2013) and Australia (Roy Morgan Research, 2014). People may approach student health workers for advice because of this inherent trust and recognition of their status. Throughout their careers health professionals help people manage their own health, and they can be more effective if they understand how to manage themselves. People have varying abilities, talents, life experiences, upbringings and opportunities that shape their lives. While self-management is a foundational philosophy of lifelong learning, it comes more naturally to some than to others.

Some of the literature discusses self-management from a management perspective (Markham & Markham, 1995); and theorists come from a variety of backgrounds, including organisational development, psychology and sociology. An added complexity is the interchangeability of some of the terms found in the literature (self-management, self-leadership, self-control, self-efficacy, self-regulation and so on), so for the sake of clarity for this chapter, the terminology is restricted to facilitate understanding, acknowledging that others may have contradictory perspectives.

Patricia Benner (1982) describes the learning and acquisition of skills by nurses as they enter the workforce in five stages, and these can be applied to many professions. Novices are those entering the workplace with little or no experience, whereas advanced beginners 'demonstrate marginally acceptable performance' (p. 403) and need assistance in identifying priorities. The next stage, competency, requires two or three years of experience, in which 'the nurse begins to see his or her actions in terms of long range goals' (p. 404). With continued application and practice, proficiency is gained, where the nurse 'perceives situations as a whole' instead of as a series of sequential or consequential steps (p. 405). With further development, the nurse attains the expert level and, with the body of practical knowledge and skills amassed over time, can rely on intuitive understanding of issues as they arise. The transition from novice to expert does not occur without the active participation of the individual in a process of self-management.

The cycle of observation, planning, action and review are familiar to most students of health. We consciously and unconsciously monitor the external environment through our senses, process this information, make choices about how we will respond, and act (or not, as the case may be) in accordance with what might be the likely outcomes. We sense, think, act and react. If one practices a certain action sufficiently often, it may become habitual, thereby reducing cognitive demand; for example, experienced motor vehicle drivers may not recall actions that required intense concentration when they started learning to drive. The transition from student to the workforce is similar: tasks expected of new graduates that initially require significant concentration and guidance often need less conscious thought and planning over time as proficiency grows.

Definitions

Manz and Sims (1980) and Markham and Markham (1995) agree that **self-management** is a behavioural process involving the exercise of choice in which the individual is aware of possible alternative actions and appreciative of the consequences. Luthans and Davis (1979) suggest that self-control is dependent upon what we observe associated with consequential rewards or punishments, which hearkens back to operant conditioning theory, that learning is based on positive and negative experiences, which will shape the choices people make. Manz and Snyder (1983) note that individuals develop behaviours in three ways: through their own previous personal experience, their observation of other people around them and what might be considered 'socially endorsed performance criteria' (p. 69).

> **[self-ma]nagement**
> [a beha]vioural process involving the
> [exercise] of choice in which the individual
> [is aware] of possible alternative actions
> [and app]reciative of the consequences
> [(Manz &] Sims, 1980; Markham &
> [Markha]m, 1995)

Manz (1992, p. 1119) subsequently differentiated self-management from self-leadership, which aligns individuals into teams as contributing to 'organisational strategic processes'. This is an important link, because the collective contribution of team members adds to departmental achievements, which in turn contribute to organisational outcomes. Self-management, therefore, is not only of concern to the individual but has an impact on organisational performance. Houghton and Neck (2002) conceptualise self-leadership as encompassing self-regulation, self-control and self-management (Figure 4.1) through a process of cognition (or awareness) and motivation.

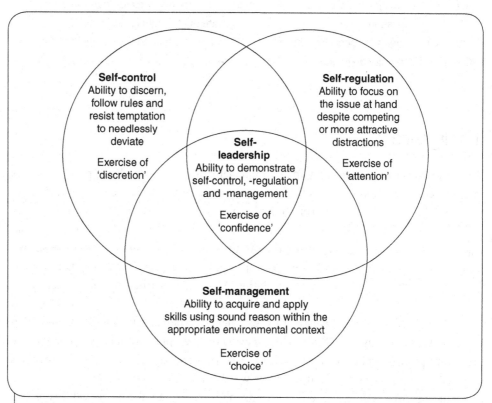

Figure 4.1 Relationships between self-control, self-regulation, self-management and self-leadership. Adapted from J. D. Houghton & C. P. Neck (2002). The revised self-leadership questionnaire. *Journal of Managerial Psychology, 17*(8), 672–691. doi: 10.1108/02683940210450484.

If self-management is characterised by making optimal choices, then it would be reasonable to expect that a person adept at self-management will become more effective in and valuable to their workplace (Baum, 1998). This is of paramount interest to organisations. A high-quality organisation is one where every employee knows what is expected of them, has the requisite skills and resources in which to achieve these expectations and is empowered so to do. Breevaart, Bakker and Demerouti (2014) conclude that individuals who are adept at self-management are most likely to be engaged with and in control of their immediate work environment, are secure in their resources, identify challenges and reduce workplace obstacles.

A different perspective?

I remember prizing logic above all else and getting frustrated with my fellow nurses who seemed – to me at least – more concerned with the collective sentiment or judgement regarding workplace issues rather than working through the issues systematically. Sometimes the outcome consensus opinion was completely divorced from reality, and it really irked me. On reflection, this was an awesome display and expression of power by my colleagues, often in defiance of 'logical' demands made by management that always seemed to require greater productivity for nothing in return. I now realise that the greatest part of my frustration was my inability to communicate my thoughts using language that resonated with my peers or to be able to sense the right time to say the right thing. Clearly, I lacked emotional intelligence.

Intelligence

What role does **intelligence** play in self-management? Sternberg (2012, p. 503) defines intelligence as the 'ability to learn from experience, and to adapt to, shape and select environments' expressed as either the individual changing to suit the circumstances (adaptation), the individual changing the circumstances (shaping) or, when these two strategies fail, opting for a new environment. The ancient Greek philosopher Aristotle described three distinct applications of intelligence: understanding, action (praxis) and production. Aristotle was investigating excellence, whereas Sternberg's focus is on success (Tigner & Tigner, 2000). This may seem like splitting hairs, except for one important point: excellence can be a subjective perspective, whereas success involves external or objective verification; in other words, it is relational. Sternberg's theory is by no means universally accepted: Gottfredson (2003) argues against its validity, citing a lack of data and the 'solid, century long evidentiary base' associated with psychometric approaches (p. 392).

Gardner states there is no single general intelligence (Sternberg, 2012) and describes a theory of multiple human intelligences, in that 'each human being is capable of seven relatively independent forms of information processing' (Gardner & Hatch, 1989, p. 4). Gardner's domains include interpersonal, intrapersonal, logical-mathematical, spatial, body kinaesthetic, linguistic and musical intelligences.

Let us consider a simplified model where intelligence could be described using three main themes: intellect (retention, recollection and application of facts), physicality (mastery of the physical body) and emotion (identification, recognition and mastery of emotional responses) (see Figure 4.2). Most of us have varying levels or abilities in relation to these areas, and some aspects of the multiple intelligences theory fit

> **ence**
> ty to learn from experience,
> dapt to, shape and select
> ents' (Sternberg, 2012, p. 503)

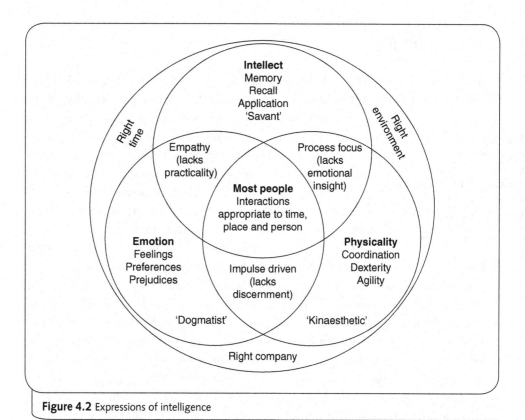

Figure 4.2 Expressions of intelligence

easily: spatial and body kinaesthesia are closely aligned with physical skills, as logical-mathematical and linguistic skills might be with intellect, and inter- and intrapersonal skills with the emotions. Musical skills cross all sectors.

It is not enough to be able to recall facts without being able to apply them. People with dogmatic views at variance with established facts may have a high emotional quotient: fundamentalism of any kind thrives on appeals to emotion, whereas emotion tempered with intellect produces a person who can sympathise and empathise appropriately, and if this is combined with physical skills it will result in non-verbal communication matching the words expressed. A person with intellect and good physical skills but without high emotion might have the capacity to design a highly efficient system, but without due concern or awareness of end user acceptability it is likely to be a failure.

Emotional intelligence is as important as physical or intellectual intelligence (Sternberg, 2012). Just as we need to tailor the words we use to best suit the person with whom we are hoping to communicate, our tone and mode of delivery should also try to anticipate the recipient's feelings if we are to communicate effectively and efficiently. An added complexity is the issue of context; for example, a particular conversation or action might be thoroughly appropriate in the company of friends at a social gathering and yet completely inappropriate or offensive in a professional or formal setting such as a staff meeting, even when the same people are involved.

Critical thinking

So how might one exercise the choice suggested by self-management? For people in the health professions, **critical thinking** is an essential skill. The most practical example in the healthcare system is the accurate gathering of a patient's changing signs and symptoms. A non–critical thinking approach would be to simply record observations and fail to understand their significance, or to treat each of the signs and symptoms independently, with the inherent danger of overlooking underlying conditions or the interplay between them.

> **thinking**
> ematic evaluation or
> on of beliefs or statements, by
> tandards' that forms the basis
> m-solving, decision-making
> tional intelligence (Vaughn &
> ald, 2010, p. 119)

Critical thinking is a common term but unfortunately there is no unified definition. A content analysis conducted by Geng (2014) identifies over 64 different definitions; however, the most common definitions included the exercise of judgement using reason. A particularly succinct definition is provided by Toplak, West and Stanovich (2014, p. 1039), who state that critical thinkers are people who 'decouple their prior opinions from the evaluation of evidence and arguments and … consider evidence in opposition to their own view'. A critical thinker never accepts things at face value and always seeks further information and validation. A critical thinking approach involves considering all the factors, identifying and exploring possibilities, weighing up probabilities, arriving at a considered conclusion and being prepared to alter one's viewpoint on further investigation. More information on critical thinking can be found in chapter 17.

Motivation

So far, we have explored the concepts related to intelligence, the gathering and processing of information, and what we may do as a result. It is timely to think about *why* we might choose to do certain things. Perhaps the most commonly known model of human motivation is Abraham Maslow's (1943) hierarchy (see Figure 4.3), which states motivation is driven by needs. Maslow stressed that the hierarchy is not linear, that there is fluidity between the levels.

The most basic needs are those related to biology, such as air, food and water; without these, a person could not survive. The next level of need relates to safety, so that potential harms associated with the natural environment (shelter from extremes of cold and heat, animal predation, avoidable disease) and with societal factors (violence arising from lawlessness, social inequity) are either avoided or minimised. Maslow (1943) suggests that after this, the next emergent need is for love – stressing that 'love is not synonymous with sex', as it is also a physiological need – and that love must be reciprocated. Esteem, the next level, relates to the capacity of people to enjoy not only a good opinion of themselves but also the regard of their peers. At the apex is the

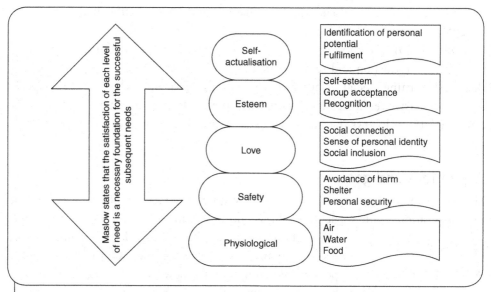

Figure 4.3 Maslow's hierarchy of human needs. Adapted from A. H. Maslow (1943). A theory of human motivation. *Psychological Review, 50*(4), 394–395. doi: 10.1037/H0054346.

need termed self-actualisation, relating to the identification of personal potential and (hopefully) personal achievement. Maslow states that self-actualisation is dependent upon satisfying prior needs, and that there will be variance in the perception of different individuals: some needs may be conscious, while others are unconscious.

Maslow (1943) acknowledges that needs influence behaviours, and that goals therefore become 'the [centring] principle in motivation theory' (p. 391), suggesting that needs generate aspirations, which are measured by and have meaning for the individual. The conclusion one may draw from this is that there are environmental factors required to achieve self-actualisation. It is unreasonable to expect a person to achieve optimal self-management in a workplace where there are, for example, physical hazards, discord, disunity or poor or ill-defined work practices. Individual self-management is not a solution for poor organisation design or a failure of general supervision or management.

Social learning

It is clear that learning from academic or evidentiary sources is valuable and necessary, but one often hears about the 'theory–practice gap' – that someone may have good conceptual understanding but fail to implement their knowledge in any practical manner. Social learning theory suggests that learning occurs not solely by memorisation of facts and figures but also by an individual modelling their behaviours on those of people admired for their skills and expertise – that is, learning by observing and doing (Bandura, 1971; Baum, 1998; Boyce, 2011; Brauer & Tittle, 2012; Markham & Markham, 1995).

Bandura (1971) acknowledges the four key components of learning – attention, retention, reproduction and reinforcement – but says that the defining difference is that *most* learning, social or otherwise, occurs by observing others, and that positive or persuasive reinforcement occurs when the model exhibits 'status, prestige and power' (p. 18). It follows that those with status, prestige and power are more likely to influence others.

Aspirations and goals

Most people have a general idea of what they want to achieve in life. Some approach their **aspirations** with single-mindedness and determination at the expense of other factors in their life. They have clearly defined plans and can describe to anyone exactly what they want to achieve and, perhaps more importantly, how they are going to do it and how they will know they have achieved it.

ion

ng we would like to achieve

oint or reward

Then there are those who have a clear idea of what they would like to achieve but may not have access to the resources or information needed to develop a clear pathway towards their **goals**. They may become discouraged and despondent because their ultimate goal or aspiration is complex and the preparatory steps may not be apparent. Alternatively, it may be that unexpected obstacles or barriers appear, or the person fails on their first attempt. At the other extreme, there are those who have little desire other than to meet their immediate needs. This might be described as opting out, and while it is a choice, those who do opt out may find they have less power and autonomy to shape their future lives. Most of us fall somewhere in between these extremes: we may find ourselves with a particular goal in mind but have no idea how to achieve it, or significant obstacles may appear.

Goal-setting influences performance: it focuses attention, energises the individual to achieve and encourages persistence. A person who sets personal goals is likely to develop an understanding of the strategies and tasks needed to achieve them, and it follows that increasingly difficult goals will lead to higher performance (Locke & Latham, 2002).

Successful people acknowledge they identify clear pathways to achieve their goals. They establish progressive or incremental goals on the pathway, sometimes called objectives, which help them identify if they are on the right track. For example, sportspeople refer to achieving 'personal bests' as they strive to match or emulate the achievements of others. These result in a number of achievements on the pathway to their ultimate goal. Each incremental goal achieved is something to celebrate. With each celebration comes further resolve to carry on. Often, the necessary pathway may not be clear or unexpected obstacles and setbacks may arise. Sometimes this can be catastrophic – or can have the *appearance* of being catastrophic – but experience teaches us that if we step back, often an alternate pathway becomes apparent.

Goals and objectives are most useful when they are measureable. Doran (1981), possibly basing his work upon the earlier ideas of Raia (1965), uses the acronym SMART to identify goals that are specific, measurable, achievable, realistic and time-related. SMART goals can be used by individuals and organisations (see Table 4.1) to effect change and are discussed again in chapter 29.

Table 4.1 Comparison of SMART goals in organisational and individual contexts

Organisational context	Individual context
Specific (capable of being exactly described)	Specific (capable of being exactly described)
Manageable (not too small but sufficient to build upon and develop existing skills)	Measurable (able to be measured against an external scale)
Assignable (within range of developing skills or competence of the team and able to be delegated)	Achievable (within range of developing skills or competence of the individual)
Realistic (likely to occur with the available resources open to the team)	Reasonable (within or slightly beyond the range of existing skills)
Time-related (predictable in terms of date of outcome)	Time-related (predictable in terms of date of outcome)

Source: Based on A. P. Raia (1965). Goal setting and self-control: An empirical study. *Journal of Management Studies, 2*(1), 34–53. doi: 10.1111/j.1467-6486.1965.tb00564.x; G. T. Doran (1981). There's a S.M.A.R.T. way to write management's goals and objectives. *Management Review, 70*(11), 35.

SMART goals are simple – for example, one might be 'In seven days I will have completed the first draft of my 2000-word assignment'. This goal is specific, measurable (the deliverable being the draft), achievable and reasonable (people setting their own goals are unlikely to have unrealistic expectations), and it is time-related (it will be achieved within seven days).

The benefit of measurable goals is that they provide an opportunity for both reflection and a sense of achievement. The more we achieve, the more likely we are to continue our progress. The more we do, the better we not only perform, but feel. Positive feedback loops can explain how and why some people thrive in certain jobs and others languish and harbour resentment or give up. Those who receive positive feedback are often motivated to continue to do better and feel more comfortable in taking calculated risks to expand their knowledge and capacities.

Aids for self-management

Prioritisation

We often have competing demands for our attention, but successful people learn to prioritise tasks to achieve their goals. A decision-making model has been attributed to Dwight D. Eisenhower, who planned Operation Overlord, the D-Day landings, during the Second World War and later became the president of the United States. He is attributed with a simple decision-making framework to determine importance and urgency that thereby permitted him to prioritise his time (see Figure 4.4). A model such as this helps identify what is needful. Using the examples in the figure, we would hope that one would attend to whatever crisis was happening before pursuing a leisure activity (Ciarnienė & Vienazindienė, 2014).

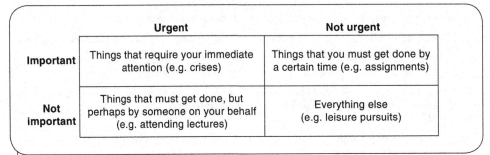

	Urgent	Not urgent
Important	Things that require your immediate attention (e.g. crises)	Things that you must get done by a certain time (e.g. assignments)
Not important	Things that must get done, but perhaps by someone on your behalf (e.g. attending lectures)	Everything else (e.g. leisure pursuits)

Figure 4.4 The 'Eisenhower' matrix. Based on R. Ciarnienė & M. Vienazindienė (2014). The conceptual model of time management. *Mediterranean Journal of Social Sciences*, 5(13), 45.

Mentors

Self-management need not be a solitary exercise. Social learning theory predicts that we will identify colleagues with more experience upon whom we may model behaviours, and some of whom may take an interest in us and our development (Kram, 1983). Mentors may provide advice or sometimes unwelcome or confronting truths, which on reflection are usually very valuable. They will not (and should not) complete work for mentees but rather help them understand how they are faring, be a source of external reflection and perhaps offer advice. The relationship is professional and nurturing. The reward to the mentor is their mentee's success, and generally little else other than satisfaction from helping another person. Mentoring is altruistic.

Preparation

The transition from university to the workplace is always challenging. It is not enough to expect to be nurtured; instead, new health professionals have to make an effort. As a result, they will find mentors appearing in the least likely places. It is important to be prepared and understand that new graduates are expected to have useful skills (they should be sure to be aware of what these might be) and to contribute immediately; this is the reason for hands-on clinical experience during training courses. In terms of Benner's (1982) model, new graduates should regard themselves as having advanced beginner status.

The decision to self-manage is an active process that we can only make for ourselves. Self-management is an ongoing process, not an event or something to get new graduates to the proficient stage. Developments in health and health technology are increasing at an almost exponential rate, and self-management is an important tool, if not the most important tool, to achieving lifelong learning.

Summary

- Integration into the workforce is a gradual process, and the acquisition of skills and learning is facilitated by self-management.
- Intelligence is not simply a matter of good memory; it also includes understanding of emotions and reflection on personal characteristics and actions.
- The development of shorter intermediate or incremental objectives is helpful in achieving detailed and challenging goals.
- We are more likely to be influenced by those we consider to have prestige and power, despite what we have formally learned.
- Identifying people we encounter through our career whose skills and knowledge are worthy of admiration and emulation may lead to our wanting to work with them in a mentoring relationship.

Reflective questions

1 To what extent do you agree that Maslow's (1943) hierarchy of needs is true when he suggests that one must be loved (or have the feeling of being loved) in order to develop self-esteem?

2 Do you think it takes two to three years to achieve proficiency, as Benner (1982) suggests? If not, why not? What could be done to expedite development?

3 Have you given up on a particular goal because it was just too hard? If you had been given assistance in developing smaller steps and incremental goals would it have made a difference? If so, how?

4 'Economic affluence is directly proportional to future options: those who are miserable and affluent have more options open to them than those who are miserable and poor.' Is this a statement with which you disagree, or is it simply a disagreeable statement? Is there a difference?

5 Has there ever been a time when something happened that from your perspective seemed like the world was about to end, but when you look back on it now you can see it was a blessing in disguise? What changed your perspective? Did this experience help you cope with later adversity?

Self-analysis questions

Where are you currently on Benner's (1982) spectrum of novice to expert? Are you where you expected to be at this stage? What things could accelerate your development? Do you actively look for ways to improve your skills, or do you expect them to develop over time?

References

Bandura, A. (1971). *Social learning theory*. New York, NY: General Learning.

Baum, F. (1998). *The new public health: An Australian perspective*. Melbourne: Oxford University.

Benner, P. (1982). From novice to expert. *American Journal of Nursing*, 82(3), 402–407.

Boyce, T. E. (2011). Applying social learning theory. *Training Journal*, (July), 31–34.

Brauer, J. R. & Tittle, C. R. (2012). Social learning theory and human reinforcement. *Sociological Spectrum, 32*(2), 157–177. doi: 10.1080/02732173.2012.646160

Breevaart, K., Bakker, A. B. & Demerouti, E. (2014). Daily self-management and employee work engagement. *Journal of Vocational Behavior, 84*, 31–38. doi: 10.1016/j.jvb.2013.11.002

Ciarnienė, R. & Vienazindiené, M. (2014). The conceptual model of time management. *Mediterranean Journal of Social Sciences, 5*(13), 42–48.

Doran, G. T. (1981). There's a S.M.A.R.T. way to write management's goals and objectives. *Management Review, 70*(11), 35.

Gardner, H. & Hatch, T. (1989). Multiple intelligences go to school: Educational implications of the theory of multiple intelligences. *Educational Researcher, 18*(8), 4–10. doi: 10.2307/1176460

Geng, F. (2014). An content analysis of the definition of critical thinking. *Asian Social Science, 10*(19), 124–128. doi: 10.5539/ass.v10n19p124

Gottfredson, L. S. (2003). Dissecting practical intelligence theory: Its claims and evidence. *Intelligence, 31*, 343–397.

Houghton, J. D. & Neck, C. P. (2002). The revised self-leadership questionnaire. *Journal of Managerial Psychology, 17*(8), 672–691. doi: 10.1108/02683940210450484

Kram, K. E. (1983). Phases of the mentor relationship. *Academy of Management Journal* [pre-1986], *26*(4), 608.

Locke, E. A. & Latham, G. P. (2002). Building a practically useful theory of goal setting and task motivation: A 35-year odyssey. *American Psychologist, 57*(9), 705–717.

Luthans, F. & Davis, T. R. V. (1979). Behavioral self-management: The missing link in managerial effectiveness. *Organizational Dynamics, 8*(1), 42–60. doi: 10.1016/0090-2616(79)90003-2

Manz, C. C. (1992). Self-leading work teams: Moving beyond self-management myths. *Human Relations, 45*(11), 1119–1140. doi: 10.1177/001872679204501101

Manz, C. C. & Sims, H. P. (1980). Self-management as a substitute for leadership: A social learning theory perspective. *Academy of Management Review, 5*(3), 361–367.

Manz, C. C. & Snyder, C. A. (1983). How resourceful entrepreneurs meet business challenges … and survive. *Management Review, 72*(10), 68.

Markham, S. E. & Markham, I. S. (1995). Self-management and self-leadership reexamined: A levels-of-analysis perspective. *Leadership Quarterly, 6*(3), 343–359. doi: 10.1016/1048-9843(95)90013-6

Maslow, A. H. (1943). A theory of human motivation. *Psychological Review, 50*(4), 370–396. doi: 10.1037/H0054346

Raia, A. P. (1965). Goal setting and self-control: An empirical study. *Journal of Management Studies, 2*(1), 34–53. doi: 10.1111/j.1467-6486.1965.tb00564.x

Roy Morgan Research. (2014). *Roy Morgan Image of Professions Survey 2014 – Nurses still most highly regarded – followed by doctors, pharmacists & High Court judges* (Article no. 5531) [Press release]. Retrieved from http://www.roymorgan.com/~/media/Files/Findings%20PDF/2014/April/5531-Image-of-Professions-2014-April-2014.pdf

Sternberg, R. J. (2012). *Intelligence. Wiley Interdisciplinary Reviews: Cognitive Science, 3*(5), 501–511. doi: 10.1002/wcs.1193

Swift, A. (2013). *Honesty and ethics rating of clergy slides to new low*. Retrieved from http://www.gallup.com/poll/166298/honesty-ethics-rating-clergy-slides-new-low.aspx

Tigner, R. B. & Tigner, S. S. (2000). Triarchic theories of intelligence: Aristotle and Sternberg. *History of Psychology*, *3*(2), 168–176.

Toplak, M. E., West, R. F. & Stanovich, K. E. (2014). Rational thinking and cognitive sophistication: Development, cognitive abilities, and thinking dispositions. *Developmental Psychology*, *50*(4), 1037–1048. doi: 10.1037/a0034910

Vaughn, L. & MacDonald, C. (2010). *The power of critical thinking* (2nd Canadian ed.). Ontario, Canada: Oxford University.

5

Emotional intelligence and self-awareness

Leila Karimi and Jiri Rada

Learning objectives

How do I:

- understand the meaning behind the models of emotional intelligence?
- enhance my emotional intelligence?
- improve my skills in self-awareness as a major component of emotional intelligence?
- compare intelligence quotient and emotional intelligence?
- use the concepts of emotional intelligence in the workplace to improve my own performance and that of staff working with me?

Introduction

Emotional intelligence (sometimes called EI or EQ) is a psychological construct that has attracted a lot of attention in the past 20 years. There have been many astonishing claims regarding emotional intelligence, many without scientific support. One popular claim is the notion that emotional intelligence is the most important factor for achieving success in life: in the workplace, at home or at school (Schulze & Roberts, 2005). Emotional intelligence – the ability to manage, understand, express and appraise emotions – is the theme of scientific controversy and investigation in spite of its huge appeal in business, education and popular literature.

Definitions

Intelligence has been defined in many different ways; however, most people associate it with the concept of testing for intelligence quotient (or IQ) and cognitive function. Throughout history, there have been attempts to recognise the importance of other forms of intelligence beyond the traditional intelligence quotient. In the 1920s, psychologist E. L. Thorndike (1920) coined the term social intelligence, referring to the skills of understanding and managing other people as well as engaging in adaptive social interactions and negotiating complex social relationships and environments. Sixty years later, developmental psychologist Howard Gardner (1983) described the idea of multiple intelligences, suggesting that all people have the capacity to possess different kinds of intelligences and that intelligence testing may be biased to certain types of individuals. He identified eight different types of intelligences, which may allow educators to identify differing strengths and weaknesses in students and provide suitable teaching and learning methods for them. Many experts believe that social intelligence, rather than quantitative intelligence, is important for quality of life and makes us what we are. It also appears that emotional intelligence can be developed rather than being biologically based (Goleman, 2000).

While the concepts of intelligence and intelligence quotient have been around for over 100 years, the field of **emotional intelligence** is relatively new. The term appeared in the literature for a few decades until it was formally defined by the United States psychologists Peter Salovey and John D. Mayer in 1990 (Salovey & Mayer, 1990). They define emotional intelligence as an 'ability to recognize the meanings of emotion and their relationships, and to reason and problem-solve on the basis of them' (Mayer, Caruso & Salovey, 1999, p. 267). Salovey and Mayer also developed the original test instruments to measure emotional intelligence. However, it was only after the publication of Daniel Goleman's (1995) popular book *Emotional intelligence: Why it can matter more than IQ* that the term emotional intelligence became widely used.

nal intelligence
ity to recognize the meanings of and their relationships, and to nd problem-solve on the basis (Mayer, Caruso & Salovey, 267)

Goleman (1995) argues that in the workplace, non-cognitive skills are just as important as intelligence quotient. He believes that employees with emotional intelligence skills are good communicators and have abilities to manage relationships, navigate social networks, influence and inspire others, and form strong emotional bonds with their organisations. Goleman also suggests that we would be better off if we understood our own emotions as well as those of others. By doing so, we might be able not only to more effectively control our emotional impulses but also to help others who are struggling, coping with grief or are angry, fearful or irritated. And, because emotional intelligence is easier to learn than cognitive abilities, Goleman says that companies might do well to invest in training people in the necessary emotional skills.

Characteristics of emotional intelligence

According to Goleman (1995), emotionally intelligent people tolerate high levels of stress, have a smoother life and experience more success. They are also curious about and enjoy meeting new people, know their strengths and weaknesses, and are aware of their emotions and impulses.

Emotional intelligence may even control so-called amygdala hijacks – any situation in which we respond grossly irrationally, even destructively, based on emotion rather than intellect. The amygdala is the emotional centre of the brain and can create havoc when under threat. In 1997, boxer Mike Tyson bit off part of Evander Holyfield's ear in the World Boxing Association's heavyweight championship in Las Vegas, and it cost him his boxing licence and $3 million. French superstar soccer player Zinedine Zidane headbutted Italy's defender Marco Materazzi during the 2006 World Cup final, sending him crashing to the ground. Rugby player John Hopoate had a troubled career but will always be remembered for forcibly inserting his fingers into the anuses of players. These are examples of extreme amygdala hijacks.

Researchers believe that emotional intelligence is a strong predictor of job performance. Emotionally intelligent people make better workers (O'Boyle, Humphrey, Pollack, Hawver & Story, 2010). Individuals who are emotionally intelligent are paid more and hold higher company positions than those with less emotional intelligence, and they receive higher peer and supervisor ratings of interpersonal facilitation and stress tolerance (Lopes, Grewal, Kadis, Gall & Salovey, 2006). In addition, people who accurately perceive others' emotions seem to be able to deal more easily with changes and build stronger social networks.

Gender differences

The results of some studies show that females seem to have higher emotional intelligence than males; high emotional intelligence in males is a predictor for achievement (Naghavi & Redzuan, 2011). This is probably due to the fact that females have traditionally been brought up to express their feelings, have better language skills and use more emotion regulation strategies. Most males have been encouraged to suppress their feelings and use physical reactions rather than words. Regardless of the cause, we know that appropriate emotional upbringing of children is an important factor in their future achievements and workplace success.

Some researchers believe that men and women have different types of emotional intelligence. While women tend to have stronger interpersonal skills, men seem to have a better sense of self and independence (Petrides & Furnham, 2000). This indicates that women may be better than men at being aware of their own emotions and those of others and are able to express their emotions more effectively. Men, on the other hand, tend to handle stressful events more successfully.

While there are no tests that produce a numerical emotional intelligence score, Block (1995) makes a comparison between people with theoretically high emotional intelligence and high intelligence quotient. Based on his research, the women with high emotional intelligence tend to be assertive, feel positive about themselves, express their feelings directly and handle stress well. Women with high intelligence quotient have intellectual confidence, value all things intelligent and are fluent in expressing their thoughts. They also tend to be more anxious, introspective, prone to guilt and not free to express anger.

Men who are high in emotional intelligence tend to be outgoing and cheerful, not fearful, and socially poised. They are also responsible, committed to good causes, caring in relationships and ethical. On the other hand, men with high intelligence quotient tend to have wide intellectual abilities and interests, are ambitious and productive and are not really concerned about themselves. They also tend to be critical, detached, cold and uneasy about sexual and emotional issues (Goleman, 1995).

Recent trends suggest that organisations are taking emotional intelligence seriously. In the past, top positions were dominated by those with independence and high stress tolerance, but more recently, people skills have become important as major changes take effect in organisations, such as competition, social responsibility, the culture of team working and partnerships. This may encourage more women to enter higher levels in organisations, especially if in addition to good interpersonal skills they have high stress tolerance.

Improving emotional intelligence

Plato said that all learning has an emotional base. Preliminary research shows that high emotional intelligence can boost happiness, career success, entrepreneurial potential, leadership talent, even health. It also shows that our level of emotional intelligence is firm but not rigid, which indicates that with practice and deliberate learning we can increase it (Chamorro-Premuzic, 2013). Some people may be naturally negative, shy or insecure, while others may be happy, with good personal skills; however, we all have the capacity to change and increase our emotional intelligence. There is evidence that emotional intelligence increases with age even without any special training, though the effect is not huge (Fariselli, Ghini & Freedman, 2008).

While improvement in emotional intelligence is possible, certain conditions apply. Firstly, the trainer or coaching program must be good. The most coachable ability is interpersonal skills, and evidence shows that the benefits of emotional intelligence coaching carry over to personal life, with improved happiness, health and relationships, and decreased stress levels (Chamorro-Premuzic, 2013).

Secondly, in order to improve, people need specific feedback – to see how they affect others, be aware of their own strengths and weaknesses and analyse their own behaviours. Thirdly, some techniques to enhance emotional intelligence produce better results than others. While the research is not conclusive, it seems that cognitive-behavioural therapy techniques are more effective than interventions designed to improve self-esteem or confidence (Chamorro-Premuzic, 2013). Finally, some people will benefit from emotional intelligence training, while others will not, depending on enthusiasm, personality, insecurity, willingness to change and other factors. Salovey (2007, p. 294), one of the original authors of the ability model, argues that

> schools, families and employers should encourage the development of the following competencies:

- Perceiving emotions in ourselves and others.
- Understanding and expressing our emotions.
- Managing our emotions.
- Using our emotions as sources of creativity, problem-solving, decision-making, and motivation. (Salovey & Grewal, 2005; Salovey & Sluyter, 1997; both as cited in Salovey, 2007, p. 294)

Models of emotional intelligence

Researchers disagree on a common definition of emotional intelligence. They also disagree on the terminology and how much of our behaviour is affected by emotional intelligence. Currently, there are three major schools of thought on emotional intelligence: the ability model, the trait model and the mixed model.

Ability model

Mayer, Roberts and Barsade (2008, p. 507) represent emotional intelligence as 'the ability to carry out accurate reasoning about emotions and the ability to use emotions and emotional knowledge to enhance thought'. The ability model of emotional intelligence (also called the four-branch model) describes four abilities that collectively illustrate the scope of emotional intelligence (Mayer & Salovey, 1997; Mayer, Salovey, Caruso & Sitarenios, 2003). These abilities are accurately perceiving emotions in oneself and others, using emotions to facilitate thinking, understanding emotional meanings and managing emotions.

According to the model, emotions are constructive sources of information. Every person has their own unique way of perceiving, understanding and dealing with emotions. The four abilities are arranged sequentially from areas specific to the emotions (perceiving emotions) to the areas more suited to personality (managing emotions). The capacity to accurately perceive nonverbal emotions in others is essential for more advanced understanding of emotions.

Trait model

This model, developed by Petrides (2009), is based on the individual's self-perceptions of their emotional abilities or their own emotional intelligence. According to the model, emotional intelligence is not a cognitive ability but 'people's perceptions of their own emotional abilities' (Petrides, 2011, p. 660). Petrides (2009) identifies 15 emotional intelligence traits measured by self-report, assuming that the respondents are able to accurately depict their own traits. The model suggests that people perceive their emotional abilities differently. Some people believe that they are in charge of their emotions, while others are astounded by them. Petrides believes that our perceptions are relatively stable and impact directly on our mood, achievements and behaviour.

Mixed models

In contrast to the ability model, mixed models represent emotional intelligence as a group of personality characteristics that predict personal or professional success (Schulze & Roberts, 2005). The mixed model that has received the most attention in the scientific literature was developed by Bar-On (1997). According to this model, emotional intelligence is defined as 'an array of noncognitive capabilities, competencies, and skills that influence one's ability to succeed in coping with environmental demands and pressures' (p. 14). To Bar-On, emotional intelligence explains why some people have better success in life than others. His self-report test is designed to measure factors such as awareness, stress, problem-solving and happiness.

Bar-On (1997) reviews personality characteristics in the mental health literature that are related to success beyond cognitive intelligence and identifies 5 dimensions and 15 subscales as key emotional intelligence factors. These are listed below:

Intrapersonal skills   include self-regard, emotional self-awareness, assertiveness, self-actualisation and independence. It is important to understand and accept oneself, as well as being able to recognise and express emotions.

Interpersonal skills   comprise empathy, social responsibility and interpersonal relationships. A person needs to be aware of and understand the emotions of others, be a constructive member of society and be able to form and maintain successful relationships.

Adaptability   refers to problem-solving, reality-testing and flexibility. Being able to solve problems constructively, being realistic and being able to manage change and ambiguity are the key factors here.

Stress management   includes stress tolerance and impulse control. The important abilities are managing stress effectively, resisting impulses and controlling one's emotions.

General mood   incorporates happiness and optimism. This dimension is about satisfaction with one's life and maintaining positive attitudes.

In 2000, Bar-On (2000) proposed an updated model that has become known as a model of emotional and social intelligence. Studies have shown that emotional social intelligence has an impact on overall subjective wellbeing (Bar-On, Maree & Elias, 2007). Also in 2000, Boyatzis, Goleman & Rhee (2000) introduced a conceptual approach to emotional intelligence within an organisational context. Their four competence clusters are self-awareness, self-management, social awareness and social skills (Schulze & Roberts, 2005). Similarly to Bar-On's (2000) work, Boyatzis et al.'s (2000) clusters are based primarily on broader social skills and wider personality constructs.

The most popular mixed model today was introduced by Daniel Goleman (1995). It is a mix of the ability and the trait models of emotional intelligence, emphasising emotional intelligence as a collection of skills and characteristics. It consists of five competencies: self-awareness, self-regulation, self-motivation, empathy and social skills. What is most important about Goleman's model is that the competencies are not seen as innate talents. There is a strong belief that general emotional intelligence is fixed by the time we become adults; on the other hand, Goleman believes that the competencies can be learned and developed over time in order to achieve outstanding performance.

Learning styles for immigrant nurses

I have been a nurse educator in oncology for over 10 years. I pride myself on my ability to integrate the student perspective and 'voice' into my classes. One day recently, I was walking past the lunchroom. I overhead some of the Asian student nurses saying that they didn't like going to classes because the teacher 'doesn't teach'. What really upset me was when I heard them saying that they 'didn't pay to hear their friends' opinions and to waste time playing games'.

As I walked on down the corridor I could feel my stomach tighten. How dare these students talk about my classes in these ways, when I'm such an experienced nurse educator? Part of me wanted to protest and to walk up to them and say, 'Don't you realise how carefully I plan your classes so that you can all participate?' Instead, I kept walking and let myself focus on my breath. As I did this I noticed just how upset I was. I also realised I was making several assumptions.

Firstly, these student nurses could have been talking about any of the nurse educators at the hospital and not necessarily about me. Secondly, I was judging the students as 'nurses who just didn't get it'. It occurred to me that I had complained to a friend about an evening class where I was a student learner. I had told my friend that the class was dull because it had no learning activities and very little interaction with student peers.

I also considered the fact that I did not know enough about the educational backgrounds of these immigrant student nurses. I had noticed, for example, that some of them had been less engaged in my classes, and I had not acknowledged this to myself. Perhaps they didn't view my classes as 'educational' compared with what they had experienced in their country of origin. I decided to have a conversation with one of my Asian colleagues. He could help me understand different ways to engage with these particular student nurses.

Leadership and emotional intelligence

Managers spend over 20 per cent of their time dealing with conflict. Conflict management skills are essential for managers, and there is evidence that people with high emotional intelligence are more effective in resolving conflict than those with low emotional intelligence. Managers who lack emotional intelligence and cannot see the problem through the eyes of others may contribute to conflict. Managers with high emotional intelligence contribute to better team and individual performances regardless of the levels of stress being experienced (Lopes et al., 2006).

Also, studies show that in conflicting situations, employees with high emotional intelligence are more likely to pursue collaborative solutions (for example, see Jordan & Troth, 2002). Joseph and Newman (2010) found that emotional intelligence is not consistently linked with job performance. People in jobs that are emotion intensive, such as selling things or ideas, benefit from higher emotional intelligence; handling stress well and providing service with a smile is of great benefit to them. These include teachers, healthcare professionals, managers, counsellors and real-estate agents. On the other hand, for those in jobs with fewer emotional demands, high emotional intelligence can be distracting or detrimental to work performance. The suggestion is that people with high emotional intelligence in low emotional intelligence jobs might concentrate more on emotions than on what they are supposed to be doing.

Does emotional intelligence make better leaders? Almost 150 years ago, Francis Galton described two basic concepts that affected popular thinking about leadership. Firstly, leadership was a characteristic ability of extraordinary individuals; and secondly, the special abilities of great leaders were genetically determined (McCleskey, 2014). Since then an enormous amount of research dealing with leadership has been produced, from the traits of individuals, through organisational constraints, to the notion of charisma and transformational leadership. We also know that leaders who have trouble perceiving and managing emotions may miss emotional clues from their co-workers and peers. Some evidence suggests that the leaders who gain the best outcomes achieve high scores on emotional intelligence ability tests, are open and are able to manage emotions well. The ability measure of emotional intelligence seems to predict effective leadership better than traditional measures such as personality and reasoning (Rosete & Ciarrochi, 2005).

George (2000, p. 1027) claims emotional intelligence is relevant because 'leadership is an emotion-laden process, both from a leader and a follower perspective'. She argues that emotional intelligence contributes to effective leadership through five essential elements of leader effectiveness: 'development of collective goals and objectives; instilling in others an appreciation of the importance of work activities; generating and maintaining enthusiasm, confidence, optimism, cooperation, and trust; encouraging flexibility in decision making and change; and establishing and maintaining a meaningful identity for an organization'.

Healthcare and emotional intelligence

Recent research shows that emotional intelligence may assist practitioners and organisations in delivering patient-centred care. Emotional intelligence positively contributes to the 'physician-patient relationship, increased empathy, teamwork, communication, stress management, organisational commitment, physician and nurse career satisfaction, and effective leadership' (Warren, 2013, p. 1). Many nursing studies have shown a high correlation between nurses' emotional intelligence and levels of performance. Karimi, Leggat, Donohue, Farrell and Couper (2014) found that both emotional labour and emotional intelligence had significant effects on wellbeing and perceived job stress among a group of Australian community nurses. Given the shortage of nurses in Australia, New Zealand and much of the world, effective emotional intelligence training may provide a key to keeping nurses in their jobs while helping them reduce job stress and burnout. Emotional intelligence also seems to correlate with both physical and emotional wellness in nurses, and their emotional intelligence skills correlate with professionalism and expert practice (Codier, 2012).

There is belief that healthcare leaders who possess high emotional intelligence will have the confidence to strengthen their organisations and lead them more effectively through difficult times such as budget and staff cuts. There is also a need to train all health and medical personnel in dealing with emotional issues, because every disease and health condition has an emotional component. Goleman (1995) believes that by treating people's emotional state together with their illness, medical effectiveness will increase.

Emotional intelligence is here to stay. We know that there are different types of emotional intelligence, and different tests and tools are being developed and validated in order to measure them. With more research, including in cultural impacts on emotional intelligence, recent developments in neuroscience, and leadership ethics, we will probably confirm that emotional intelligence is an important addition to intelligence quotient as well as to science in its own right.

Intelligence testing that is popular in many forms of educational practices may be extended to include emotional intelligence. Emotional intelligence, together with intelligence quotient, may also be used to identify how students or workers learn and to help in developing specialised learning tools and packages for them to improve and to achieve a higher level of success in both personal and professional life.

Emotional intelligence counters the negativism associated with the popular view that we are born with cognitive intelligence. It offers a 'hope for a more utopian, classless society, less constrained by biological heritage and conditions where assessment of it does not presuppose "destiny"' (Schulze & Roberts, 2005, p. 334).

Summary

- Emotional intelligence is seen to be as important as intellectual intelligence.
- There are three models of emotional intelligence: the ability model, the trait model and the mixed model.
- Self-awareness is a major component of emotional intelligence.
- Recent studies suggest that emotional intelligence can have a positive impact on the workplace.
- Individuals can improve their emotional intelligence through training.

Reflective questions

1 Why is it important to learn about emotional intelligence?

2 Daniel Goleman (1995) has identified five emotional intelligence competencies: self-awareness, self-regulation, self-motivation, empathy and social skills. Which competency or competencies do you think are the most important in becoming an emotionally intelligent individual, and why?

3 What is more important to you, intellect or emotional intelligence? Why?

4 Do you think that people who have high intelligence quotient tend to have lower emotional intelligence?

5 Is emotional intelligence dependent on basic living conditions such as food, shelter and education?

Self-analysis question

Many organisations believe that emotional intelligence is important for effective leaders, can be learned, increases work performance and improves profits. Based on the information covered in this chapter and your personal research, how would you improve your emotional intelligence, put it to practical use on a daily basis and be sure that it is working? In your answer, consider specific exercises and skills, such as becoming a better listener, observing how you react to people and handle stressful situations, how your actions affect others and what your strengths and weaknesses are.

References

Bar-On, R. (1997). *Bar-On Emotional Quotient Inventory (EQ-i): Technical manual*. Toronto, Canada: Multi-Health Systems.

——. (2000). Emotional and social intelligence: Insights from the Emotional Quotient Inventory. In R. Bar-On & J. D. A. Parker (Eds), *The handbook of emotional intelligence: Theory, development, assessment, and application at home, school, and in the workplace* (pp. 363–388). San Francisco, CA: Jossey-Bass.

Bar-On, R., Maree, J. G. & Elias, M. J. (2007). *Educating people to be emotionally intelligent*. Westport, CT: Praeger.

Block, J. (1995). A contrarian view of the five-factor approach to personality description. *Psychological Bulletin, 117*, 187–215. doi: 10.1037/0033-2909.117.2.187

Boyatzis, R. E., Goleman, D. & Rhee, K. (2000). Clustering competence in emotional intelligence: Insights from the Emotional Competence Inventory (ECI). In R. Bar-On and J. D. A. Parker (Eds), *The handbook of emotional intelligence: Theory, development, assessment, and application at home, school, and in the workplace* (pp. 343–362). San Francisco, CA: Jossey-Bass.

Chamorro-Premuzic, T. (2013). Can you really improve your emotional intelligence? *Harvard Business Review*, (May 29). Retrieved from https://hbr.org

Codier, E. (2012). Emotional intelligence: Why walking the talk transforms nursing care. *American Nurse Today*, 7(4). Retrieved from http://www.americannursetoday.com

Fariselli, L. Ghini, M. & Freedman, J. (2008). *Age and emotional intelligence* [White paper]. Retrieved from Six Seconds website: http://www.6seconds.org/sei/media/WP_EQ_and_Age.pdf

Gardner, H. (1983). *Frames of mind: The theory of multiple intelligences.* New York, NY: Basic Books.

George, J. M. (2000). Emotions and leadership: The role of emotional intelligence. *Human Relations*, 53(8), 1027–1055. doi: 10.1177/0018726700538001

Goleman, D. (1995). *Emotional intelligence.* New York, NY: Bantam.

——. (2000). Leadership that gets results. *Harvard Business Review*, 78(2), 78–90.

Jordan, P. J. & Troth, A. C. (2002). Emotional intelligence and conflict resolution: Implications for human resource development. *Advances in Developing Human Resources*, 4(1), 62–79. doi: 10.1177/1523422302004001005

Joseph, D. L. & Newman, D. A. (2010). Emotional intelligence: An integrative meta-analysis and cascading model. *Journal of Applied Psychology*, 95(1), 54–78. doi: 10.1037/a0017286

Karimi, L., Leggat, S. G., Donohue, L., Farrell, G. & Couper, G. E. (2014). Emotional rescue: The role of emotional intelligence and emotional labour on well-being and job-stress among community nurses. *Journal of Advanced Nursing*, 70(1), 176–186. doi: 10.1111/jan.12185

Lopes, P. N., Grewal, D., Kadis, J., Gall, M. & Salovey, P. (2006). Evidence that emotional intelligence is related to job performance and affect and attitudes at work. *Psicothema*, 18(Suppl 1), 132–138. Retrieved from http://www.psicothema.com

Mayer, J. D., Caruso, D. R. & Salovey, P. (1999). Emotional intelligence meets traditional standards for an intelligence. *Intelligence*, 27(4), 267–298. doi: 10.1016/S0160-2896(99)00016-1

Mayer, J. D., Roberts, R. D. & Barsade, S. G. (2008). Human abilities: Emotional intelligence. *Annual Review of Psychology*, 59, 507–536. doi: 10.1146/annurev.psych.59.103006.093646

Mayer, J. D. & Salovey, P. (1997). What is emotional intelligence? In P. Salovey & D. Sluyter (Eds), *Emotional development and emotional intelligence: Educational implications* (pp. 3–31). New York, NY: Basic Books.

Mayer, J. D., Salovey, P., Caruso, D. R. & Sitarenios, G. (2003). Measuring emotional intelligence with the MSCEIT V2.0. *Emotion*, 3(1), 97–105. doi: 10.1037/1528-3542.3.1.97

McCleskey, J. (2014). Emotional intelligence and leadership: A review of the progress, controversy, and criticism. *International Journal of Organizational Analysis*, 22(1), 76–93. doi: 10.1108/IJOA-03-2012-0568

Naghavi, F. & Redzuan, M. (2011). The relationship between gender and emotional intelligence. *World Applied Sciences Journal*, 15(4), 555–561.

O'Boyle, E. H., Humphrey, R. H., Pollack, J. M., Hawver, T. H. & Story, P. A. (2010). The relation between emotional intelligence and job performance: A meta-analysis. *Journal of Organizational Behavior, 32*(5), 788–818. doi: 10.1002/job.714

Petrides, K. V. (2009). *Technical manual for the Trait Emotional Intelligence Questionnaires (TEIQue)*. London, United Kingdom: London Psychometric Laboratory.

——. (2011). Ability and trait emotional intelligence. In T. Chamorro-Premuzic, A. Furnham & S. von Stumm (Eds), *The Blackwell-Wiley handbook of individual differences* (pp. 656–678). New York, NY: Wiley.

Petrides, K. V. & Furnham, A. (2000). Gender differences in measured and self-estimated trait emotional intelligence. *Sex Roles, 42*, 449–462. doi: 10.1023/A:1007006523133

Rosete, D. & Ciarrochi, J. (2005). EI and its relationship to workplace performance outcomes of leadership effectiveness. *Leadership Organizational Development, 26*, 388–399.

Salovey, P. (2007). Integrative summary. In R. Bar-On, J. G. Maree & M. J. Elias (Eds), *Educating people to be emotionally intelligent* (pp. 291–298). Westport, CT: Praeger.

Salovey, P. & Mayer, J. D. (1990). Emotional intelligence. *Imagination, Cognition, and Personality, 9*, 185–211. doi: 0.2190/DUGG-P24E-52WK-6CDG

Schulze, R. & Roberts, R. D. (Eds). (2005). *Emotional intelligence: An international handbook*. Göttingen, Germany: Hogrefe & Huber.

Thorndike, E. L. (1920). Intelligence and its use. *Harper's Magazine, 140*, 227–235.

Warren, B. (2013). Healthcare emotional intelligence: Its role in patient outcomes and organizational success. *Becker's Hospital Review*. Retrieved from http://www.beckershospitalreview.com

6

Exploring values

Eleanor Milligan and Jennifer Jones

Learning objectives

How do I:
* identify my personal values?
* learn how my personal values developed over time?
* consider the importance and role of values in healthcare leadership?
* ensure an organisational culture that is based on appropriate values?
* develop my skills in values-based leadership strategies in my organisation?

Introduction

As Mahatma Gandhi once said, 'Your beliefs become your thoughts, your thoughts become your words, your words become your actions, your actions become your habits, your habits become your values, your values become your destiny'. Values permeate every aspect of our lives, shaping individual actions and giving meaning, direction and scope to our work environments and organisational cultures. Defining positive behaviours and identifying unprofessional, disrespectful or negative behaviours, values permeate and define every aspect of our work and personal lives. Values also have an emotional component: when we act in accordance with our values, we experience positive emotions; conversely, when we act against our values or are placed in situations that compromise our values, we experience negative emotions. It is this emotional component that drives us to seek values alignment in our personal and professional lives.

In healthcare, values-based leadership is particularly important. Patients seek our care often at the most vulnerable time in their lives. In their vulnerability, they must trust us to provide competent and compassionate care. In reality, they have little choice but to trust that the healthcare system and those who work within it will act in their best interests. This power imbalance compels those who work within, manage and lead healthcare organisations to be trustworthy. The significant financial resources, paid for by the community at large through taxation, further reinforce the social obligation on healthcare organisations to be trustworthy and act in alignment with community values. The values of care, trust and reciprocity therefore define effective healthcare, as caring for vulnerable others makes the provision of health services a moral, value-laden practice.

In this chapter, we consider where values come from, why they are important, how they can be used to form the basis of ethically sound leadership to promote an organisation's ethical climate and culture, and how values-based leadership can build and maintain public trust in the healthcare sector.

Definitions

Due to the inextricable link between **values** and behaviour, the values we hold in our hearts inevitably become visible in our outward actions. The same is true for organisations: the values that shape the culture of an organisation are on display in the practices, norms, policies and codes that are endorsed within it. In his seminal work on organisational culture, *Culture's consequences: Comparing values, behaviors, institutions and organizations across nations*, Geert Hofstede (2001) proposes that our practices (heroes, symbols, rituals) are the outwardly visible representation of our hidden, or invisible, values.

> ng attitudes and beliefs
> rmine individual behaviour'
> ki, 2012, p. 29)
>
> **system**
> ring of values on the basis of
> tive importance to individuals
> sations

As a leader, it is important to reflect upon questions like the following: Who does your organisation hold as its heroes? Does your organisation reward competitiveness, while espousing collaboration? What symbols represent your organisation, and what do they say about your organisation's actual values? What rituals does your organisation adhere to?

Organisational values and **values systems** provide employees with norms that guide decision-making and behaviour in the workplace (Edwards & Cable, 2009). It is therefore important to give them careful attention.

In large and complex organisations, shared, common values, or values congruence, is recognised as an important factor in forming a coherent and successful organisation in ways that benefit individual staff and the organisation itself (Howell, Kirk-Brown & Cooper, 2012). Buchko (2007, p. 37) further explains, 'Values are the glue that binds people together in organisations. When a group of people share a set of beliefs about the goals that need to be achieved and the means to be used to attain those goals, there is a basis for organisation. In fact without some common beliefs or values, organisations could not exist; people need a common set of beliefs to come together and create social organisations'.

In the complex context of healthcare, it is almost inevitable that those in senior leadership roles will face challenges to their personal and professional values. Indeed, Graber and Kilpatrick (2008, p. 186) argue that 'challenges and crises are in a sense necessary to not only test, but to evoke, the leader's values'. In this environment, 'ethics and values may offer a more predictable, stable and sustainable base for leadership ... and provide a certain "warranty" on integrity and future prospects in organisations' (Viinamäki, 2012, p. 28). Becoming aware of, and clearly defining, their own personal and professional values empower and equip leaders to make principle-based decisions in a way that models ethical leadership to their staff, builds trust in them as a leader and promotes confidence in their organisation.

Personal values

Judging from the work of phenomenological philosophers such as Maurice Merleau-Ponty, Charles Taylor and Paul Ricoeur, the formation of a person's moral framework and values system is complex, multifaceted and highly individualised. Each of us, from the day we are born, experience the world on multiple different levels, each bringing knowledge, social expectations and norms which mould our moral development and values framework (Isaacs, 2003, 2010).

The experiences that shape our values arise from embeddedness in the areas discussed below. From the examples given, we can gain an appreciation of the complex factors that make up each person's individual moral framework and values system. Through appreciation and knowledge of our personal values, we can gain insight into the motivations of ourselves and others and begin to challenge unreflective or habitual responses to various situations (Clark, 2008).

The natural world

This affects us physically, spatially and biologically. With respect to health, for example, our expectations and values concerning disability or physical incapacity are influenced by our own lived reality. How we view disability in others is prejudiced by our assumptions, which are based on personal experience.

The social world

This is the area of multiple relationships, cultures, politics, economies, nations and communities of all shapes, moral understandings and identities. With respect to health, for example, if we have been embedded in a cultural and economic norm of 'free' healthcare, this may shape our values and expectations when it comes to decision-making about access to high-cost care for our patients. In a culture of presumed plenty, we may feel justified in dismissing the financial considerations of health resourcing, as our expectation is that no-one will, or should, miss out.

Temporal space

The area of temporal space asks us to consider the manner in which our cultural norms relate to the historical context we are in and invites us to consider how our historical place influences our perception of the present and imagining of the future. With respect to healthcare, for example, we may value the growth in scientific knowledge and expect that this body of knowledge will continue to be pursued. We may also expect that any technological advances made will be fully implemented for the benefit of our patients.

Language

Language mediates our relationships with others. It supports understanding, shapes our identities and allows us to express our future growth and desires. With respect to health, the choice of language can alter and define clinical relationships. We may, for example, choose to call those who seek our care patients, or we may call them consumers. The language adopted defines the terms of the relationship. We may interact with a consumer, who is purchasing a product or service. The use of different language, such as the word patient, may frame the interaction as one in which a moral duty of care exists beyond the transactional nature of supplying goods or services. Hence, language shapes the moral tenor, assumptions and expectations of healthcare interactions positively and negatively.

Spiritual horizons

These give direction and meaning to life for some. Many aspects of care evoke spiritual values which impact upon patients, staff and organisations. Issues concerning withdrawal of life-sustaining measures at the end of life or a patient's request for a termination of pregnancy may trigger challenges to the spiritual values of those involved (Isaacs, 2010).

....

Professional values

Once we enter a profession, another layer of socialisation is added to our existing values framework, potentially reducing some values differences among members of that profession (Hofstede, 2001). Similarly, when individuals become socialised in a particular organisation, another layer of shared experience and values is added. Like personal values, professional and organisational values are culminations of multiple layers of compounding and competing experience.

An essential first step in understanding and thoughtfully applying values-based leadership is to define one's own core values. (A helpful tool for this can be found on the Values in Action website: http://www.viacharacter.org. While it does not provide a definitive list, it is a starting point for recognising how values shape behaviour. It also enables users to reflect upon the origins of their values and can help foster appreciation of one's own motivations and the motivations of others' behaviours.) As an example, imagine that one of your strong personal values is gratitude. Your leadership style will be one in which you consciously show appreciation to your colleagues, and you are likely to flourish in an environment where you feel appreciated for your contribution. However, if you find yourself in a work environment where you feel undervalued, you are likely to interpret this as a negative workplace culture and experience significant distress. In interactions with patients, those you perceive as 'ungrateful' may trigger emotional reactions of resentment, or counter-transference. Understanding the source of these emotions as based on one of your values – that is, gratitude – and recognising the triggers can help you to manage their consequences. For example, to minimise the impact of counter-transference on patient care, strategies such as implementing team-based care or having regular supervision or debriefing with colleagues are helpful.

As a further example, imagine that one of your strong values is truthfulness. You will flourish in organisations which have a culture of transparency and openness, and your leadership style will model honesty and promote this in others. Moral distress may arise if you perceive that information is being withheld or an adverse event not disclosed on the grounds that others believe that disclosure would be harmful to a patient. In recognising your distress as based on one of your values – that is, honesty – you can frame discussions directly in language that identifies the ethical source of your concern.

Knowledge of your own values and those of your colleagues is therefore helpful not only in enabling you to manage your own emotional reactions but also in understanding team dynamics and building values congruence within your organisation and with your colleagues.

Leadership and values

Leaders are tasked with ensuring the efficient and financially responsible management of their organisations. However, they are equally responsible for ensuring that appropriate ethical standards are promoted, modelled and upheld. Edgar Schein (1992, as cited in Graber & Kilpatrick, 2008, p. 194) notes, 'The only thing of real importance that leaders do is to create and manage culture'. And Blanchard & O'Connor (1997, p. 3) claim that 'no longer is values-based organizational behavior an interesting philosophical choice – it is a requisite for survival'.

As staff take their cues from the actions of those in leadership positions, the ways in which values are modelled by managers and leaders are crucial. Leaders communicate organisational values to all employees; they have the opportunity to model values in action, empower others to make principled decisions, and promote trust. Individual leaders therefore have a significant influence over the ethical culture (Buchko, 2007). Positive role-modelling promotes confidence in leaders and improves values congruence for staff, which in turn promotes loyalty and optimism (De Hoog & den Hartog, 2008). The improved 'affective commitment' (Howell et al., 2012, p. 732) to an organisation as a result of improved trust and values congruence has also been correlated to the improved retention of staff (Buckley et al., 2001; Olson, 1995; Schluter, Winch, Holzhauser & Henderson, 2008). This has significant implications for organisational stability, which is especially important in healthcare organisations, where workforce instability can have negative impacts on patient care (Schluter et al., 2008).

At an organisational level, the ability to articulate shared values is an important strategy in managing complex organisations, as values are the foundation of shared principles of decision-making. Promoting shared values creates a vehicle through which the diverse views and expectations of individuals within an organisation can be focused towards a commonly agreed overarching goal. Authentic alignment to a set of organisational values or core values is consistently recognised as a characteristic of successful organisations (Viinamäki, 2012).

Climate and culture

It is clear that when ethical climate, organisational culture and the values of employees align in healthcare organisation there are significant benefits, including improved organisational stability, stronger emotional commitment and trust from staff and improved quality of care, confidence and trust for the public (Olson, 1995; Schluter et al., 2008).

Ethical climate

One of the most important enablers of individual ethical behaviour is being situated in a climate that supports ethical decision-making. The **ethical climate** is shaped by the prevailing organisational practices, procedures and codes that have ethical content or determine ethical action. In their seminal work, Victor and Cullen (1988) claim that ethical climates centre around three dimensions: egoism, benevolence and principles. Further research has confirmed that benevolent and principled climates are more likely to reduce unethical conduct. Ego-based climates, on the other hand, are more likely to create unethical behaviour (Kish-Gephart, Harrison & Triveno, 2010; Wimbush & Shepard, 1994). Hence, a leader's ability to promote a climate of acting on principle through values-based leadership with attention to the good of the whole can reduce unethical workplace behaviour (Kish-Gephart et al., 2010).

For further exploration of the ethical climate of an organisation, the Ethical Climate Questionnaire (Victor & Cullen, 1987, 1988; Cullen, Victor & Bronson, 1993) is a validated tool and useful resource.

climate
of prescriptive climates
the organisational procedures,
nd practices with moral
ences' (Martin & Cullen, 2006,

Organisational culture

Organisational culture is described as the shared values, meanings, beliefs, assumptions, rituals, myths, language and metaphors that describe an organisation. It predicts how people behave; it determines what behaviours are

ational culture
ed values, meanings, beliefs,
ions, rituals, myths, language
aphors that describe an
ion

rewarded or punished. It also demonstrates what values are actually at play within the organisation.

It follows that through ethical climate and organisational culture, organisations and their leaders can proactively create good or bad ethical environments that can promote or undermine ethical choices (Kish-Gephart et al., 2010). Employees look to leaders to display authenticity, to match their espoused values with their enacted values.

Values-based leadership

Values-based leadership provides a framework for making the inherent moral aspects of healthcare explicit, inviting and challenging healthcare leaders to model ethical behaviour, to make decisions based on ethical principles, to provide clear leadership, to strengthen the ethical climate and culture, and to improve alignment of organisational and personal values, reducing moral distress for staff and promoting alignment.

> **Values-based leadership**
> Leadership based on foundation
> principles (Viinamäki, 2012)

The defining feature of values-based leadership is communicating the values of the organisation and consistently acting in accordance with them. Leaders who lead from a values foundation are more effective than those who do not, as they provide credible and legitimate role models and effectively set standards of behaviour by rewarding ethical conduct. They also have the standing to identify and penalise unethical conduct. The four elements discussed below are crucial in ensuring the success of values-based leadership.

Values recognition

In order to act from a values base, a person must first recognise the situation as having an ethical, or values, dimension. Failure to do so results in the adoption of another decision-making schema, such as economic rationality or egocentric self-interest. Practical steps for healthcare leaders to promote recognition of values include knowing their own personal and professional values and increasing employee knowledge of values and ethics through education – for example, using public forums such as grand rounds, in which the values aspects of the organisation's work are openly discussed and modelled. Such forums can be used to explore ethically challenging clinical situations – for example, unlikeable patients, the withdrawal of life-sustaining measures and resource allocation. Willingness to openly discuss ethically laden issues demonstrates authenticity and transparency, promoting a culture of openness and honesty.

A further practical step is working with internal stakeholders to create a shared sense of values and link these to organisational values and principled decision-making. For example, if an organisational value is honesty, an open disclosure policy might outline an organisational pathway for principled decision-making with respect to sharing information concerning adverse events.

Values awareness

Leaders model values awareness when they demonstrate concern for the collective good of the whole group and for the impact of the means and ends of the decision-making process, consideration of the long- and short-term consequences of the decision and commitment to seek the views and input of multiple stakeholders who will be impacted by any decision.

Practical steps for healthcare leaders in promoting values awareness include clarifying the extent to which the organisation actually promotes the values its leaders aspire to implement. For example, if an organisation's values include justice, its leaders might consider pathways to promote access for socially and financially disadvantaged patients. Healthcare leaders can also facilitate discussions that communicate the enduring values of the organisation. For example, during staff meetings, decision-making should be linked to organisational values. If one of the organisation's values is community, a proactive invitation of external stakeholders to decision-making bodies within the organisation will demonstrate promotion of that value. Other practical steps involve committing to ensure that organisational values are embedded into the ethical codes, procedures and practices adopted by the organisation; ensuring that organisational values are visible to employees – for example, through a footer on all email correspondence or the design of a logo that has meaning related to the values; making organisational values visible to the community through a public website and communications; and monitoring feedback and evaluation systems, and acting upon what they say about the enactment of organisational values.

Resource allocation

A 59-year-old male, Joe, presents to the emergency department of a hospital breathless and blue and appears confused and weak on examination. His history reveals a diagnosis of an aggressive form of renal cancer two years previously, which has been treated aggressively at his request. It further reveals that Joe has refused palliative care despite being deemed terminal six months earlier, and that since that time his condition has continually deteriorated.

Despite his obviously terminal situation, Joe's wife and carer is advocating for 'all possible treatments', citing Joe's wishes and the family's financial security: the amount of Joe's superannuation payment decreases significantly if he is not alive on his 60th birthday, now six days away. Following the accidental death of their son and daughter-in-law, Joe and his wife are the legal guardians of their 12-year-old grandson.

As Joe's condition deteriorates further, a decision needs to be made in relation to the allocation of resources to care for him. He requires more care than can be provided on a regular ward, but can the hospital afford to care for him in the intensive care unit?

In considering Joe's case, it is evident that there are competing demands. For instance, if equitable healthcare for all is a major value, the use of a finite resource

continued ›

continued ›

to delay death will be a primary concern. If, however, patient autonomy, the right to self-determination, is also a main value, consideration of what is in Joe's best interests will be calling for attention. Add to these two competing and compelling demands the value of caring understood as the amelioration of suffering – be that physical, mental, emotional or spiritual – and the multilayered nature of the ethical challenge becomes evident.

In making sense of the situation and in seeking a best practice outcome, practitioners should be guided and supported by the personal, professional and organisational values which have arisen from multiple layers of compounding and competing experience. In respect to values-based leadership, they are also supported and guided by leaders who understand and appreciate 'the moral convictions of care providers, as well as the moral obligations care providers have to patients' (Rathert & Phillips, 2010, p. 502). Such leaders are committed to the development, implementation and maintenance of an organisational culture with an ethical climate that is underpinned by a strong sense of the personal, professional and institutional values embedded within it.

Values practice

As ethical problems are often characterised by uncertainty and ambiguity, leaders must have the skills to make principled decisions and demonstrate the practical application of values. Steps that demonstrate competence include the following:

- communicating and re-enforcing values through strategic avenues within the organisation
- rewarding behaviour that aligns with organisational values
- seeking consensus when values clash
- providing feedback to strengthen capacity and understanding
- providing organisational structures at all levels where values can be shared, debated and agreed.

Values commitment

Commitment to values-based leadership requires the ongoing communication of values, establishment of reward systems that re-enforce organisational values and authentic modelling of organisational values by those in leadership positions. If any of these steps is weak or missing, the success of values-based leadership implementation will be compromised and may ultimately fail (Graber & Kilpatrick, 2008; Olson, 1995; Viinamäki, 2012).

Summary

- Values are underlying attitudes and beliefs that shape our behaviour.
- Values arise from multiple sources and are related to our individual experiences with respect to the natural world, our social norms, the time and historical context of our experiences, the language we are exposed to and choose, and the spiritual dimensions that give meaning to these experiences.
- Organisational values evolve in response to internal and external factors that shape the purpose, role and expectations held by the organisation and the expectations held by external stakeholders.
- Important values inherent in effective leadership are authenticity, integrity, trustworthiness and social responsibility.
- The organisational and individual benefits of values in healthcare leadership include improved confidence, commitment, trust, loyalty and retention, and less likelihood of unethical behaviour.
- The promotion of values through strong ethical climates and organisational cultures can create healthy ethical environments that can promote sound ethical choices.

Reflective questions

1 What are your core values? What did you learn when you took the Values in Action survey?

2 Think of a time when your individual values were at odds with the values of a colleague or with the organisational values of your workplace. How did this make you feel? What steps, if any, did you take to resolve the tension?

3 If you were faced with a situation today in which your individual values were at odds with the values of a colleague or with the organisational values of your workplace, what new understanding could you bring to your decisions?

4 Think about a time when you felt most effective in your professional or personal life. What made this time memorable? What values were foremost at this time?

5 Do you believe values-based leadership would benefit your organisation? What are the barriers and enablers to values-based leadership in your organisation?

Self-analysis questions

Consider how your values, identified by the Values in Action survey, are evident in your personal and professional behaviours. Are there any inconsistencies in your list? Do you feel this list has evolved and changed as you have grown in your personal and professional life? How can you use your awareness of your values to understand the motivations and behaviours of others?

References

Blanchard, K. & O'Connor, M. (1997). (With J. Ballard.) *Managing by values*. San Francisco, CA: Berrett-Koehler.

Buchko, A. (2007). The effect of leadership on values-based management. *Leadership & Organization Development Journal, 28*(1), 36–50. doi: 10.1108/01437730710718236

Buckley, R. M., Beu, D. S., Frink, D. D., Howard, J. L., Berkson, H., Mobbs, T. A. & Ferris, G. R. (2001). Ethical issues in human resources systems. *Human Resource Management Review, 11*, 11–29. doi: 10.1016/S1053-4822(00)00038-3

Clark, L. (2008). Clinical leadership: Values, beliefs and vision. *Nursing Management, 15*(7), 30–35. doi: 10.7748/nm2008.11.15.7.30.c6807

Cullen, J. B., Victor, B. & Bronson, J. W. (1993). The ethical climate questionnaire: An assessment of its development and validity. *Psychological Reports, 73*, 667–674. doi: 10.2466/pr0.1993.73.2.667

De Hoog, A. H. B. & den Hartog, D. N. (2008). Ethical and despotic leadership, relationships with leader's social responsibility, top management team effectiveness and subordinates' optimism: A multi-method study. *Leadership Quarterly, 19*, 297–311. doi: 10.1016/j.leaqua.2008.03.002

Edwards, J. R. & Cable, D. M. (2009). The value of value congruence. *Journal of Applied Psychology, 94*(3), 654–677. doi: 10.1037/a0014891

Graber, D. & Kilpatrick, A. (2008). Establishing values-based leadership and value systems in healthcare organizations. *Journal of Health and Human Services Administration, 31*(2), 179–197.

Hofstede, G. (2001). *Culture's consequences: Comparing values, behaviors, institutions and organizations across nations*. Thousand Oaks, CA: Sage.

Howell, A., Kirk-Brown, A. & Cooper, B. K. (2012). Does congruence between espoused and enacted organizational values predict affective commitment in Australian organizations? *International Journal of Human Resource Management, 23*(4), 731–747. doi: 10.1080/09585192.2011.561251

Isaacs, P. (2003). *Doing ethics: An action based approach*. Paper presented at the Peninsula Behavioural Health Conference, Gatlinburg, TN.

——. (2010). Ontology, narrative and ethical engagement. In E. Milligan & E. Woodley (Eds), *Confessions: Confounding narrative and ethics* (pp. 121–142). Newcastle-upon-Tyne, United Kingdom: Cambridge Scholars.

Kish-Gephart, J., Harrison, D. & Triveno, L. K. (2010). Bad apples, bad cases and bad barrels: Meta-analytic evidence about sources of unethical decisions at work. *Journal of Applied Psychology, 95*(1), 1–31. doi: 10.1037/a0017103

Martin, K. D. & Cullen, J. B. (2006). Continuities and extensions of ethical climate theory: A meta-analytic review. *Journal of Business Ethics, 69*, 175–194. doi: 10.1007/s10551-006-9084-7

Olson, L. (1995). Ethical climate in health care organizations. *International Nursing Review, 42*(3), 85–90.

Rathert, C. & Phillips, W. (2010). Medical error disclosure training: Evidence for values-based ethical environments. *Journal of Business Ethics, 97*(3), 491–503. doi: 10.1007/s10551-010-0520-3

Schluter, J., Winch, S., Holzhauser, K. & Henderson, A. (2008). Nurses' moral sensitivity and hospital ethical climate: A literature review. *Nursing Ethics*, *15*(3), 304–321. doi: 10.1177/0969733007088357

Victor, B. & Cullen, J. B. (1987). A theory and measure of ethical climate in organizations. In W. C. Frederick (Ed.), *Research in corporate social performance and policy* (pp. 51–71). Greenwich, CT: JAI.

——. (1988). The organisational basis of ethical work climates. *Administrative Science Quarterly*, *33*(1), 101–125. doi: 10.2307/2392857

Viinamäki, O. (2012). Why leaders fail in introducing values-based leadership? An elaboration of feasible steps, challenges, and suggestions for practitioners. *International Journal of Business and Management*, *7*(9), 28–39. doi: 10.5539/ijbm.v7n9p28

Wimbush, J. C. & Shepard, J. M. (1994). Toward an understanding of ethical climate: Its relationship to ethical behaviour and supervisory influence. *Journal of Business Ethics*, *13*(8), 637–647. doi: 10.1007/BF00871811

7

Ambiguity and leadership

Mark Avery

Learning objectives

How do I:

- develop a clear understanding of how ambiguity in organisational settings impacts management and leadership?
- reduce ambiguity?
- develop confidence in the identification and articulation of ambiguity in healthcare organisations?
- acquire skills and knowledge in useful approaches to managing positions, directions and outcomes related to ambiguous circumstances and problems?

Introduction

Complexity is a feature of healthcare organisations. Irrespective of the role, size, processes and governance of these organisations, the internal and external environments in which they operate and the number of associated stakeholders represent significant challenges in managing clinical and social processes and outcomes, resources, workforces, decision-making and ethics. Within this complex framework, healthcare leaders need not only skills and strategies to manage their organisation, but also resources and personal competencies to lead individuals, groups and workforces.

Definitions

Ambiguity is defined as lack of certainty or dependability of meaning of communication, action or knowledge. It describes a situation in which information could be interpreted, construed or understood in more than one way. It is a natural aspect of the operations of healthcare facilities and the environments in which they engage with many stakeholders. Leading and managing health organisations requires awareness, understanding and focused action to ensure that ambiguous situations are managed for impact and usefulness to the health facility.

Three important elements align with **ambiguity**: uncertainty, clarity and vagueness. The purpose of a strong understanding of the roles of these elements in dealing with ambiguous situations in organisations relates to the leader's strength of understanding and comprehension of information and knowledge.

Firstly, **uncertainty** has been associated with human conceptions and understandings that may not be objective. For example, health managers may be uncertain whether the services provided to consumers are valued or seen as high quality. These are situations which can be addressed through obtaining facts from consumers (directly or indirectly), but given the large and varied number of consumers, there can be ambiguity in understanding their views on service needs and quality of care. Secondly, **clarity** is important in leadership, as it is the mechanism by which to ensure that staff or followers in an organisation understand requirements, directions, interpretations and purposes. The opposite of clarity is ambiguity. Health managers aim for clarity in direction and communication. Finally, **vagueness** – where communication and language about facts in a matter or situation are not certain or firm in imparting understanding – is also relevant. A healthcare leader might aim to use feedback from consumers as part of the organisation's quality review process. A vague approach here might result in consumer feedback that is not useful.

....

Healthcare

In health organisations and in leading them, two aspects of ambiguity are important.

Organisation ambiguity

Organisation, or bureaucratic, ambiguity concerns the development and values of the organisation. Best (2012) highlights the central role that ambiguity plays in the complex organisation. Organisations are formed for many reasons, and it is in the architecture and operation of their structures that ambiguity can be both identified and valued.

Health organisations operate in uncertain, risky and changing service and environmental contexts (Leatt & Porter, 2003). They need to work towards dealing with uncertainty (addressing and mitigating an environment of uncertainty through key activities including planning, developing systems and processes, and setting strategic and operational directions), standardisation to support efficiency and effectiveness (developing policies and procedures for the whole organisation and for localised and specific applications) and measuring and quantifying processes, goals and outcomes (expressing and valuing activities to support planning, operations and achievements).

Standardisation and development of policies and procedures support effective management in these contexts and enable clear communication and agreement with staff members. Quantification supports both operational clinical and non-clinical activities and establishes the basis for process and outcome evaluation. Leaders in health organisations are able to capitalise on the management of ambiguity through a bureaucratic organisational framework of systems and planning, policies and procedures, and qualification of performance. Casting of situations and paradigms onto these frameworks enables the leader to reduce complexity and ambiguity and therefore focus on interpretation and action.

Role ambiguity

Problems associated with ill-defined or ill-formed roles and lack of understanding about roles have a negative impact on organisation performance, as well as causing stress and lowered job satisfaction for individuals (Rizzo, House & Lirtzman, 1970). Key requirements associated with **role ambiguity** in an organisation or among workers include the existence of comprehensive role delineation, management of new or changing roles, and general or wide communications regarding roles. In relation to healthcare, a study of nurse executives found that role conflict and ambiguity can be associated with stress in professional roles (Tarrant & Sabo, 2010).

Role ambiguity
Lack of clarity about expected ac and behaviours associated with positions in an organisation

When discussing ambiguity in health organisations, it is useful to consider ambiguity in the role of leadership. Leadership is a complex role with complex actions. At times and in some contexts, leadership is difficult to define and evaluate. Leadership behaviours, characteristics and styles can make assessing the effectiveness of leadership and its impact on the performance of an organisation difficult. Pfeffer (1977) examines the concepts of leadership, the effectiveness of leaders and the attribution of leadership. This brings into focus the need for leaders to connect impact and effectiveness to the key organisational issues, including dealing with ambiguity.

The healthcare organisation and the key resource of the health system – its workforce – are important elements in the management of ambiguity. Complex healthcare organisations (as opposed to complexity in the organisation) provide both an operational and an environmental setting for ambiguity, but they also provide structures, processes and problem-solving constructs that can be used to address the issues of ambiguity.

Ambiguity in workforce-planning

Stromlo, in the Australian Capital Territory, is a relatively large health service and has a broad spectrum of care, across primary, secondary and tertiary sectors. The development of long-term regional health workforce plans presents several ambiguous elements. There are two key long-term goals. Firstly, the workforce will do things differently, in working within different models of patient and client care and organising operations and the business of healthcare differently. Secondly, to be effective, with new and dynamic models of care and operations, the workforce will need to have different skills, training, abilities and roles. Stromlo's health professionals will have a significant influence in the health workforce development agenda and will be affected by the workforce environment in over the next 10 to 15 years.

Stromlo managers understand that there are key areas where ambiguity exists as it relates to their long-term planning. These include the following:

- different models and arrangements of delivering care
- responses of professional bodies and groups in relation both to their own profession and to interprofessional aspects
- which practices regulators and licensing bodies will support and authorise
- what the national and international markets will do in response to the recruitment of current and new professionals in healthcare
- how training and education bodies will respond in respect to the long lead times associated with health professional education.

Stromlo managers need to seek clarification in all of these areas, as a key aspect of implementing new ways of working in professional groups is ensuring clarity, in order to avoid role ambiguity.

Management and ambiguity

Ambiguity affects key areas of planning, development and decision-making and requires a comprehensive approach. In most complex organisations, the management of ambiguity is not handled alone or in a simple, straightforward way. Two key areas where ambiguity interrelates are in an organisation's change management program and processes and in strategies and processes of evaluation. Both are discussed below.

Change management approaches

Healthcare managers use change management approaches with varying degrees of sophistication. The nature and complexity of the reform and development agenda that organisations face and develop influence the different types of changes and transformation approaches. Related here is the issue of ambiguity, which can be affected by timeframes (planning over medium and longer terms), the clarity of the growth and development agenda and the capacity of the organisation in the development of the change process and in all forms of its resourcing.

Changes in an organisation evolve at different rates, and variations in the organisation's activity levels, tolerance and resourcing affects these rates. The ability to describe and instil key aspects of organisational development is an important factor in the change management process. Whether processes enable review and understanding of internal and external environments will affect the content, quality and rates of change. Nadler and Tushman (1995) identify four key types of changes in organisations:

Tuning   is the seeking of better ways of performing or defending, and these are generally initiated internally.

Adaption   concerns responding to external pressures that are mainly influential on incremental and adaptive shifts in behaviour and operations.

Re-orientation   impacts on redefining the organisation or its system and engenders knowledge and support in nature.

Re-creation   involves reactive change, transforming the organisation or its system. The alignment and impact of ambiguity relate to the complexity and needs of the change processes outlined. For example, change that in nature is tuning for an organisation (where incremental and other less complicated ways of working are at hand) requires less sophistication and information to support reform. This is compared with re-orientation and re-creation, which compel more novel and unique information about and opportunities for new ways of working that may not be readily recognisable to organisations.

The change management process needs to address these key levels of response, as the environment is dynamic, driven by research, technology, consumer demand, ageing populations and health economics. Associated to this is a matrix of change drivers: environmental factors, risk and safety dynamics, and significant and finite resourcing.

Several studies identify important skills and competencies that enhance leaders' capacity and effectiveness in managing problems of ambiguity and change management processes:

Problem-finding   involves the identification of the right problem through judgement, intuition and logic and then recognition of the opportunities available.

Map-building   is the ability to generate one or more conceptualisation approaches to a situation by relating organisational and personal values and identities to situational demands.

Janusian thinking   (from the Greek god Janus, who faces two directions at once) involves constructively joining contradictory beliefs through mapping a direction that compensates for poorly structured issues with creative thinking.

Controlling and not controlling   is judgement application: knowing which things can be influenced and when.

Humour   diffuses stress and encourages creativity, reassuring and fusing tense and hostile situations.

Charisma   is the provision of enthusiasm, commitment and confidence to the problem-solving situation. (McCaskey, 1988)

These skills and competencies align with research undertaken by Hodgson & White (2003) in terms of effective skills for leadership, and strategy in handling ambiguity and the feelings of uncertainty. In order to overcome fear of failure, the high levels of uncertainty experienced by leaders and managers in modern organisations should be addressed and the need for them to experiment and take risks, along with associated reconditioning in their organisations and their agendas, stressed.

Leaders effective in the management of ambiguity in organisations are good at helping others to find energy and fun through the introduction of experimentation in new approaches to confronting situations. Simple and clear questions and communication are features of dynamic and responsive organisations. This relates not only to problem identification and generation of alternatives but also to the process and effectiveness of implementation. Achieving balanced focus is necessary; it should not be too narrow and blinded to the possibilities but should be able to hold and retain clear understanding of a few key tasks. Mastery of inner sense involves combining skills in management of rational and factual activity with use and confidence of instinct, experience and intuition.

Evaluating health services

The effectiveness of goals, objectives and tasks in health organisations needs evaluation, to appraise the outcomes of leadership of change, development and problem-solving, and to progressively and iteratively consider the strengths and weaknesses of the efforts made. An evaluation logic model is useful in informing the evaluation of problem-solving in the context of ambiguous situations and in focusing targets of knowledge and information. Use of an evaluation logic model gives context, structure and mechanisms in grounding thinking and review, thereby reducing ambiguity.

There are several forms and approaches in such models, but one that is useful comes originally from a system evaluation developed in the 1970s by Carol Weiss (1998; see Figure 7.1). The model highlights three core components useful in evaluation of programs and structures in health organisations. The first relates to inputs, processes and outputs in health organisations' clinical and non-clinical operations. Focus gives clarity to issues associated with resourcing, systems and approaches to organisation of direct and indirect care, and differentiation of outputs from those processes.

The second component relates to outcomes of care and services. Outcomes are the results that may or may not have been intended from the service, activity or care provided. Ambiguity regarding resources and processes affects the success of outcomes.

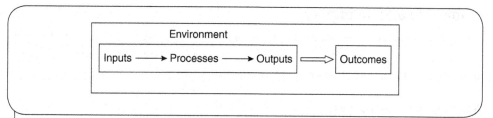

Figure 7.1 Evaluation logic model. Adapted from W. K. Kellogg Foundation. (2004). *Logic model development guide* (p. 11). Retrieved from United States Environmental Protection Agency website: http://www.epa.gov/evaluate/pdf/eval-guides/logic-model-development-guide.pdf.

Finally, healthcare organisations operate in complicated and sophisticated environments (for example, ownership, stakeholder, regulatory, economic and research and development environments). Environments are multifaceted; therefore, a high degree of complexity is found within them.

Leadership and ambiguity

Communication

Eisenberg (1984) highlights important subtleties in interpretation and flexibility associated with leadership of ambiguity, particularly as it relates to communication in organisations. While leaders often strive for clarity and open communication in organisations, Eisenberg cautions against an overemphasis on such clarity. A degree of ambiguity in development and communication of strategy actually supports development of an environment for change. Where ambiguity exists, there is opportunity to encourage multiple viewpoints or opinions, to create debate and discernment. Opportunities to foster agreement on abstract issues without limiting interpretation provide for contribution and goal focus in thinking and problem-solving. Many organisations articulate goals and objectives with a degree of ambiguity in them to allow them the freedom to alter plans and operations over time.

Managing ambiguity

In large healthcare systems, particularly with development agendas related to networking and aggregation of impact, sometimes, simplistic assumptions of problems or standardisation may be limiting. Best (2012) discusses the unexpected nature of complex political, economic and scientific environments and makes a case for a degree of discretion and judgement in ambiguous situations. The power and expertise of the managers in an organisation can help solve complex situations by working within the ambiguity. Therefore, ambiguity may be an effective management strategy to bring about complex change.

Leadership and ambiguity

Key qualities and activities that leaders can bring to health organisations to sensitively manage ambiguity include personal characteristics and processes that support discernment, and development of strategic planning and decision-making processes.

Priorities and effectiveness

Leaders contribute through evolving and articulating mind maps of strategies to handle ambiguous situations and problems. Key leadership behaviours include direction-setting, role-acting and role-modelling, while important discernment and action processes include situation awareness, communication, knowledge, agility, trust, framing, needful interrelating, adjusting and ongoing management of ambiguity itself (Baran & Scott, 2010).

Information and direction articulation

Health organisations collect significant amounts of data. In scoping direction and leading for resolution in messy and complex problems, healthcare leaders need to align situational and decision-making analysis opportunities with useful and focused information.

Framing

Framing involves the deliberate use of conscious and less conscious skills within a sense of perception so as to appraise an event in a way that enables individuals and teams to understand what might be taking place beyond the limits of their current knowledge. It provides insight into the meaning and significance of the situation in order to make sense of it.

ς
hoice of the language used
be an issue to make it adopt
ositive or a more negative
nce

Framing is a valuable strategy for leaders involved in the discernment and development of change and problem-solving in organisations. Considerable work on the usefulness and techniques of framing have been developed by Bolman and Deal (2008), who set out four keys frames for perspective in organisations:

Structural frames   focus on the organisation and its structure.

Human resource frames   give perspectives on the people and relationships in the organisation.

Political frames   consider power and the tensions of competition in the organisation.

Symbolic frames   look at meaning in the organisation through examination of its rituals, stories and culture.

making
•d of giving meaning to
s and activities

Sense-making

Sense-making is a useful illustrative mechanism for understanding and articulating complexity in situations and activities, and it can generate emerging maps, or pictures, that can be built upon with information, option development and strategic decision-making to produce engaging agendas for action. There are three core activities in sense-making: exploring the wider system, creating a map of the current system and acting to change the system to learn more about it (Ancona, 2012).

Summary

- Healthcare organisations operate in complex internal and external environments, and their situations foster ambiguous situations in structures, processes, roles and directions.
- Awareness, identification, management and minimisation of, and engagement with, ambiguity are critical parts of effective leadership in healthcare organisations.
- Framing, articulating and communicating about ambiguous situations within health organisations are important for strategic direction-setting and decision-making processes.
- Healthcare leaders are responsible for bringing individual traits, characteristics and skills to the management of ambiguity for matching the nature and complexity of ambiguous situations to the processes and methods designed to manage them.

Reflective questions

1 Discuss the relationship between uncertainty, clarity and ambiguity.

2 Identify ambiguous situations that might have a negative impact on healthcare organisations.

3 Identify situations in which working with ambiguity can provide positive or useful opportunities for healthcare organisations.

4 What issues or situations might bring ambiguity into the role and function of a health professional's job?

5 What problems can arise for individuals and organisations from role ambiguity?

Self-analysis questions

Consider an ambiguous situation in a healthcare organisation. List two or three contributions that a healthcare leader could make to bring clarity and resolution to the situation. Then list two or three identification and conceptualisation approaches that could be used to bring context, structure and meaning to the situation. What experience and skills would you personally need to take on a leadership or management role in the situation?

References

Ancona, D. (2012). Sensemaking: Framing and action in the unknown. In S. Snook, S. Nohria & R. Khurana (Eds), *The handbook for teaching leadership* (pp. 3–19). Thousand Oaks, CA: Sage.

Baran, B. E. & Scott, C. W. (2010). Organizing ambiguity: A grounded theory of leadership and sensemaking within dangerous contexts. *Military Psychology, 22*(Suppl. 1), S42–S69. doi: 10.1080/08995601003644262

Best, J. (2012). Bureaucratic ambiguity. *Economy and Society, 41,* 84–106. doi: 10.1080/03085147.2011.637333

Bolman, L. G. & Deal, T. E. (2008). *Artistry, choice and leadership* (4th ed.). San Francisco, CA: Jossey-Bass.

Eisenberg, E. M. (1984). Ambiguity as strategy in organizational communication. *Communication Monographs, 51,* 227–242. doi: 10.1080/03637758409390197

Hodgson, P. V. & White, R. P. (2003). Leadership, learning, ambiguity, and uncertainty and their significance to dynamic organizations. In R. S. Peterson & E. A. Mannix (Eds), *Leading and managing people in the dynamic organization* (pp. 185–199). Mahwah, NJ: Lawrence Erlbaum.

Leatt, P. & Porter, J. (2003). Where are the healthcare leaders? The need for investment in leadership development. *Healthcare Papers*, 4(1), 14–31. doi: 10.12927/hcpap.2003.16891

McCaskey, M. B. (1988). The challenge of managing ambiguity and change. In L. R. Pondy, R. J. Boland & H. Thomas (Eds), *Managing ambiguity and change* (pp. 1–30). London, United Kingdom: Wiley.

Nadler, D. A. & Tushman, M. L. (1995). Types of organization change: From incremental improvement to discontinuous transformation. In D. A. Nadler, R. B. Shaw & A. E. Walten (Eds), *Discontinuous change: Leading organization transformation* (pp. 15–34). San Francisco, CA: Jossey-Bass.

Pfeffer, J. (1977). The ambiguity of leadership. *Academy of Management Review*, 2(1), 104–112. doi: 10.5465/AMR.1977.4409175

Rizzo, J. R., House, R. J. & Lirtzman, S. I. (1970). Role conflict and ambiguity in complex organizations. *Administrative Science Quarterly*, 15(2), 150–163. doi: 10.2307/2391486

Tarrant, T. & Sabo, C. E. (2010). Role conflict, role ambiguity, and job satisfaction in nurse executives. *Nursing Administration Quarterly*, 34(1), 72–82. doi: 10.1097/NAQ.0b013e3181c95eb5

Weiss, C. H. (1998). *Evaluation: Methods for studying programs and policies* (2nd ed.). Upper Saddle River, NJ: Prentice Hall.

W. K. Kellogg Foundation. (2004). *Logic model development guide*. Retrieved from United States Environmental Protection Agency website: http://www.epa.gov/evaluate/pdf/eval-guides/logic-model-development-guide.pdf

8

Leadership and critical reflective practice

Lorraine Venturato

Learning objectives

How do I:
- improve my ability to reflect on my own practice?
- use a critical reflection approach?
- reflect *for* action, reflect *in* action and reflect *on* action?
- enhance my leadership abilities through reflective practice?
- choose a reflective technique that works for me?

Introduction

Humberto Maturana (1998) claims that 'to know with full confidence is the enemy of reflection. Reflection is when what we claim to know has the ability to step back and take another look'. Reflection is not a new concept in the health sciences. Contemporary conceptions of reflective practice are underpinned by the works of John Dewey (1910, 1916, 1933, 1938), Carl Rogers (1951, 1969), Paulo Freire (1995) and Donald Schön (1983, 1987). Today, reflection is a core component of healthcare education and is evident in the governing codes and guidelines that underpin professional practice in many health disciplines in Australasia. References to reflection appear in each health discipline's code of professional practice or code of conduct, and effective and purposeful reflection is seen to be a core component of proficiency and ongoing professional development. Despite this, students, practitioners and healthcare leaders often struggle with reflection and critical reflective practice.

This chapter explores what is meant by reflection and critical reflective practice, how to adopt a critically reflective attitude and foster reflective skills in leadership, and how leaders can use critical reflection to support growth and change at personal, team and organisational levels.

Definitions

Why should we reflect?

We are familiar with the idea of reflection at its broadest level: looking in a mirror, we can see our image reflected back at us. This kind of reflection is passive, requiring little effort from us. Despite this passivity, a mirrored reflection invites us to do more than merely recognise our own image.

Firstly, gazing upon our reflected image invites a more critical inspection and active engagement. When we look in a mirror, our gaze often carries implied questions: Is my face clean? Is my hair messy or tidy? Should I grow a moustache? That is, we actively engage in a cognitive process built around a question and answer dialogue with ourselves. Secondly, it is often these questions that direct us to the mirror in the first place: looking in the mirror does not occur by accident but is an intentional activity. Finally, the mirror may also reflect our location or the context in which we find ourselves: the pictures on the wall behind us, the person standing beside us or the vase of flowers on the shelf can all indicate if we are in our private bathroom or in a public store.

Professional reflection shares some of these elements. It is intentional and active, it involves thinking and questioning, and it may help us to look at the broader context of our experiences. Indeed, the term reflection is often used interchangeably with thinking, but reflection is more than just sitting around thinking about our experiences (Rolfe, 2014). **Reflection** is defined as an intentional, active cognitive process of interpreting (understanding) and giving meaning to an experience by considering and critically assessing the content and process, and by critiquing our assumptions and practices (Dewey, 1933; Mezirow, 1991). Schön (1983) identifies three broad elements of reflection, and these appear in most definitions of reflection today: reflection involves an active intellectual engagement, it entails exploring experiences or problems, and it results in a subsequent change in perspective or practices, or generates new insights.

Definitions of critical reflection and critical reflective practice extend this to consider the broader social, political and moral context in which such experiences occur. **Critical reflection** goes beyond reflection to include an awareness and challenge to the hidden assumptions of practitioners and leaders, as well as the broader social and political context. It often has an association with deconstructing long-held beliefs or habitual practices. **Critical reflective practice** moves critical reflection beyond consideration of a specific problem or incident.

Reflection
An intentional cognitive process thought and contemplation rega issue and its relationship to one' practice, beliefs, values or behav

Critical reflection
Reflection that includes an awar of and challenge to the hidden assumptions of the practitioner a leader, as well as the broader soc political context

Critical reflective practice
Critical reflection that occurs on ongoing basis and is seen as a w practising or leading

As an everyday practice, critical reflection occurs on an ongoing basis and features as the practitioner's and leader's way of practising or leading. Walker, Cooke, Henderson and Creedy (2013, p. 505) suggest that critical reflective practice engages one 'in the construction rather than the reproduction of knowledge'.

Types of reflection

One way of thinking about reflection is by considering where in the process of practice the reflection occurs; this is known as a temporal dimension of reflection, because it relates to the timing of the reflective process. Schön (1992) identifies three types of reflection based on temporal considerations: reflection *for* action, reflection *in* action and reflection *on* action. Reflection for action, or anticipatory reflection, occurs before an action. Here, a leader may consider ways of dealing with a situation prior to doing anything about it. While there is some debate and confusion around reflection on action and reflection in action (Usher & Bryant, 1997), in general, reflection in action is conceptualised as thinking on your feet, often occurring rapidly in the midst of an activity, while reflecting on action entails looking back at actions, processes and outcomes after the activity or event.

Hatton and Smith (1995) propose a hierarchical framework as a way of making distinctions between types of reflection. They identify four levels of reflection in writing: descriptive information, which describes events without any reflection; descriptive reflection, which describes events and attempts to provide some justification or explanation, with evidence of alternative viewpoints; dialogic reflection, which involves distancing from the events to explore the experience, is analytical and/or integrates alternative perspectives and factors, and recognises inconsistencies while providing a rationale or critique; and critical reflection, which situates events and actions within multiple perspectives, recognising the influence of numerous historical and sociopolitical contexts.

Pollard (2002, 2005) identifies seven characteristics of reflective teaching that fit equally well with characteristics of critical reflective practice:

- It is concerned 'with aims and consequences, as well as means and technical efficiency' (Pollard, 2002, p. 12). This situates critical reflection not just in everyday practice, but also in the broader sociopolitical and moral context.
- It is 'a cyclical or spiral process' in which practice is continuously monitored, evaluated and revised (Pollard, 2002, p. 12). Critical reflection is not a one-off event, but a continuous and embedded way of practising – a critical reflective practice.
- It requires a degree of competence in evidence-informed inquiry; thus it is a key element of experiential learning in continuing professional development and evidence-based practice (Stewart, 2012), and it supports the higher-order thinking skills that constitute clinical reasoning (Donaghy & Morss, 2000).

- It requires 'open-mindedness, responsibility and whole-heartedness' (Pollard, 2002, p. 13; see also Dewey, 1933). Critical reflection encompasses inquisitiveness and openness to other ways of thinking and doing. This does not imply a naivety or blind acceptance; rather, it implies curiosity and lack of defensiveness in thinking and questioning.
- It requires judgement. Critical reflection and critical reflective practice draw on experience, practice, evidence and context in order to evaluate and innovate.
- It entails dialogue, which may be with colleagues (Pollard, 2002) or internal with oneself, and is essential, as it serves as a trigger for learning and thinking (Snyder, 2014).
- It entails creative mediation: negotiation between opposing or conflicting ways of thinking or acting, and movement towards a resolution in terms of thought or action.

Perhaps an eighth defining characteristic of critical reflective practice lies in a focus on action and activity (Bradbury-Jones, Coleman, Davies, Ellison & Leigh, 2010), which differentiates it from just thinking about something (Rolfe, 2014). Its focus on activity and its continuous, or cyclical, nature make reflection a practice rather than a one-off or occasional event, often in response to a critical incident. Reflective practice is active and continuous – a way of being, or, as Rolfe (2014) suggests, a way of doing.

Reflective practice is experiential in nature; that is, we get better at it the more we do it and the more experience we have to build on (Wainwright, Shepard, Harman & Stephens, 2010). Therefore, reflective practice is a key element in experiential learning (Tate, 2004), contributing to the progression from novice to expert clinicians and leaders (Stewart, 2012). It is also a key element in professional development and adult learning, and a central feature of professional practice.

Part of the strength of critical reflective practice lies in the premise that self-reflective and self-initiated learning involving both feelings and cognition is the most lasting and pervasive learning. Independence, self-reliance, creativity and personal growth are all facilitated when self-criticism and self-evaluation are strong and evaluation by others is of secondary importance.

Because of its active, continuous and experiential learning components, critical reflective practice is also identified as an important way of integrating theory and practice (Binding, Morck & Moules, 2010; Plack, Dunfee, Rinsflesch & Driscoll, 2008; Wainwright et al., 2010), and it can help us to understand and resolve contradictions in expectations and actual practice (Johns, 2006). Therefore, critical reflective practice facilitates the integration of new theory and practice with previous beliefs and practices (see Figure 8.1).

Critical reflective practice is also closely linked to critical thinking (Brookfield, 1998), higher-order thinking (Mezirow, 1991) and critical awareness. These skills facilitate examination of attitudes, values, beliefs and goals (self-awareness),

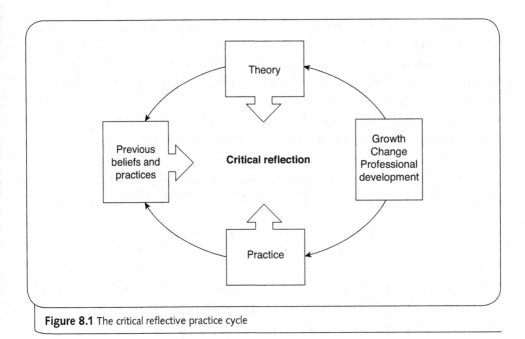

Figure 8.1 The critical reflective practice cycle

appreciation of the perspectives of others, awareness of alternative positions, and evaluation and sense-making of one's own position (Plack et al., 2008), as well as consideration of broader policies, social and political circumstances, and moral obligations.

Leadership and critical reflective practice

Critical reflective practice is an important aspect of professional practice and leadership in contemporary healthcare environments. The rationale for its importance draws on the links between learning and self-awareness and the ability to be innovative and to manage and cope with change (Horton-Deutsch, Young & Nelson, 2010).

Benefits of critical reflective practice

Critically reflective leaders are self-aware and thoughtful, and they critically question and evaluate their leadership in a continuous and active cycle of development and learning. They have moral purpose, build relationships and are able to integrate theory and practice with past experiences in order to lead through change at personal and organisational levels. The key benefits of critical reflective practice are further discussed below.

Self-awareness

This is an essential element in leadership development and growth (Vitello-Cicciu, Glass, Weatherford, Seymour-Route & Gemme, 2014) and in enhanced learning in practice (Bradbury-Jones et al., 2010). Self-awareness supports recognition of our strengths and limitations, and assists us to deal with challenges and relationships with others and to maintain a sense of openness (Bradbury-Jones et al., 2010; Enterkin, Robb & McLaren, 2013; Horton-Deutsch et al., 2010; Snyder, 2014; Vitello-Cicciu et al., 2014).

Transferable learning

Critical reflective practice can offer insights into our previous experiences that may help us to understand and make sense of future experiences and facilitate future learning (Lee, 2009).

Understanding

Critical reflective practice can help leaders to clarify career goals and identify career development needs at personal and team levels (Enterkin et al., 2013). Opportunities for career development are central to staff empowerment, which is intrinsic to retention and change (Snyder, 2014).

Exploration

Critical reflective practice is also associated with a wider, contextualised viewpoint. Social and organisational contexts must factor in to reflective leaders' strategic thinking in developing supportive networks and engaging in change activities at organisational or political levels (Enterkin et al., 2013).

Adaptability

Understanding and working with change are parts of daily practice in contemporary healthcare settings for both leaders and clinicians. Adaptability requires self-awareness and a broad understanding of the context in which change occurs (Horton-Deutsch et al., 2010). Critical reflective practice is transformative, and 'reflective leaders model an adaptive capacity, manage conflict, and … [enable others] to embrace the future and share in the creation of it' (Horton-Deutsch, 2013, p. 4).

Innovation

Critical reflection can expand thinking about further developments and new ways of thinking and acting, and can develop and drive innovation (Lee, 2009).

Critical reflective practice and career-planning

I was invited to speak to a group of first-year nursing students on my career and on career-planning in general. My initial thought was that there wasn't a lot of planning involved! On reflection, I recognised that there were pivotal moments and considered choices underpinned by careful and critical reflection.

When I finally spoke with the students, I described my growing realisation that the career I thought I wanted before I studied as a nurse was, in fact, not the one presenting itself to me in reality. When I entered nursing, I thought I wanted a career in intensive care or emergency or maybe to travel to exotic lands doing medical aid work. With each practicum, I grew more aware of situations that triggered a response in me – ways of working that were most satisfying.

For example, during a much sought after practicum in a busy emergency department, I realised that having patients in and out so quickly was not satisfying. I recognised over future practicums that I liked areas where I got to know patients' names, preferences, family. It didn't necessarily matter if it was an oncology, rehabilitation, palliative care or long-term care facility; there were significant connections to be made, and the therapeutic relationship was central.

I also realised I enjoyed working with people who were dealing with 'big' issues. I realised that I had a million questions and that I enjoyed seeking answers in a systematic way. Thinking like this led me to a career I could never have foreseen, but one that fits me well. My advice to the students that day was to stay open to possibilities, to think about what they most connected with and to reflect on their experiences; that's how you build a career.

The relationship between reflection and leadership

Like reflection, leadership itself is a complex concept – it often includes a combination of personal qualities and attributes, context, actions and behaviours – and is frequently discussed in terms of leadership styles, such as transformative, authoritarian or democratic. Critical reflective leadership may be embedded in different styles of leadership, though it may be more evident and compatible with particular leadership styles, such as transformative or congruent leadership (Latimer, 2011).

Warwick and Swaffield (2006) note that reflection contributes to 'good' leadership in much the same way as it contributes to 'good' practice. They highlight the value of reflection in leadership in relation to facilitating clear aims, goals and directions underpinned by values; being able to build relationships, collaborations and engagement in dialogue; and being able to understand and facilitate change through a process of monitoring, evaluating, reflecting and revising. The link between 'good' leadership and reflection lies in the capacity of self-awareness and self-regulation, as well as in enhancing relationships and empowering others (Enterkin et al., 2013; Vitello-Cicciu et al., 2014), thereby improving emotional intelligence and, ultimately, communication, teamwork, goal-setting and attainment, and effective change management.

Strategies for developing critical reflection

Numerous strategies for developing reflective skills are available to clinicians and healthcare leaders.

Reflective writing

Reflective writing is one of the main strategies identified and is often considered essential in integrating concepts, context and experience (Binding et al., 2010; Jasper, 1999). Reflective writing may take many forms, including diaries, journals and, increasingly, personal blogs (Latimer, 2011). It is one of three reflective activities identified by Stewart (2012), along with reflective thinking and reflective practice. In reality, however, reflective thinking and writing may both support reflective practice. Reflective writing is most often seen in educational settings and is one way in which reflective thinking and practice are taught and assessed in health professional training programs.

Supervision and mentorship

Clinical supervision and mentorship are also important strategies for developing critical reflective practice. Latimer (2011) says that clinical supervision is particularly useful in this regard when timely clarification and advice are required, when the student is learning and may benefit from expert guidance and mentorship, and when there is a significant emotional toll; in the last case, a mentor or supervisor may provide the emotional distance required for critical reflection.

Learning circles and group reflection

Learning circles and group reflection are other ways to support and develop critical reflective practice (Enterkin et al., 2013; Lee, 2009; Snyder, 2014; Walker, Henderson, Cooke & Creedy, 2011; Walker et al., 2013). Group reflection methods support shared learning and peer support, and can minimise isolation (Enterkin et al., 2013), while learning circles can promote individual and organisational growth and change (Walker et al., 2013). Learning circles may also be useful in work-integrated environments where negotiation, communication and relationship-building are key elements. Group reflection can assist in identifying and exploring problems and issues in the workplace, can generate new insights and can develop action plans (Walker et al., 2011). It is also useful in uncovering the voice of the other and supporting listening and empathy in novice reflective practitioners.

Critical questioning

Critically reflective students, clinicians and leaders ask tough questions. Critical questioning revolves around identifying and resolving problems and issues through a process of question and answer (Snyder, 2014). What is the issue? Why do certain problems exist? Why did this occur? How can this be resolved? Who benefits? Whose voices are heard and not heard? Bradbury-Jones et al. (2010) suggest that questions should also include subjective questions on thoughts and feelings: How did I feel? Why did I feel like that? What was I thinking? What were the consequences of my feelings and thinking? Such questions can be useful prompts for novice practitioners and new leaders as they learn to integrate critical reflection into their everyday practices, establishing it as a part of the inner dialogue necessary to develop new roles.

Creativity and arts-based approaches

Creativity and arts-based approaches are also useful in developing critical reflective practice. Arts-based approaches include arts-based learning, research and knowledge translation (practice change), while creative thinking is closely aligned with change and innovation (Latimer, 2011). Creativity and creative thinking challenge the status quo and generate new possibilities for practice and leadership. Thorsen and DeVore (2013) refer to this as imaginative thinking and associate it with the highest level of reflective thinking in LaBoskey's (1994) continuum of reflective practice. An example of arts-based learning being used to support and develop critical reflection is presented in Snyder's (2014) work, which details the use of film to stimulate discussion and reflection. Such an approach is particularly useful when experience is limited, as it can expose novice practitioners and leaders to previously unencountered situations.

A cautionary note

While reflection is widely espoused in healthcare as an important underpinning strategy for learning and change, it is not without its critics (Mackintosh, 1998; Rolfe, 2014). One of the critiques of reflection is whether it can be taught or is a predisposition. Jasper (1999) and others (Stewart, 2012; Wainwright et al., 2010) argue that reflection and reflective writing skills can be taught, while Rolfe (2014) contends, following Dewey's (1916) and Schön's (1987) argument, that reflection as experiential learning is essentially unteachable. This argument is largely based on the differences between teaching and learning, and in particular teaching about learning. Rolfe's (2014) argument is that while reflective practice is unteachable it can be learned through experience and practice. Despite this, many studies recommend intentional instruction and explicit, purposeful development of reflective capabilities as part of professional preparation for practice in health disciplines (see, for example, Wainwright et al., 2010).

Secondly, some authors point out that critical reflective practice needs time (Wainwright et al., 2010). Sufficient time to reflect, to listen and to have the space to question is often lacking in today's busy, complex healthcare environments.

A third critique argues that reflection is often difficult and may not come easily. The focus on reflective writing in education may challenge those who reflect best through oral traditions and storytelling, and who struggle to write, losing key elements when confronted with the need to construct reflections in writing. Despite this criticism, writing can force us to be clearer in reflection, and being able to think and communicate clearly in writing is a part of professional life (Jasper, 1999). Reflective writing offers potential to develop not just reflective ability but also writing skills – an important skill combination in healthcare environments.

Critical reflective leaders establish critical reflection as a daily way of doing; it is who they are as leaders. Critically reflective practice is not automatic; nor is it always easy. It is, however, an important skill and attribute of successful and sustainable healthcare leadership in the 21st century.

Summary

- Reflection is a way of thinking and doing that for practitioners and leaders combines theory and practice to facilitate learning and development. Critical reflective practice is a core element of professional practice in healthcare.
- Critical reflective practice is associated with critical thinking and experiential learning.
- There are several different models and ways of thinking about reflection; among these are reflection for action, reflection in action and reflection on action.
- Critically reflective leaders are self-aware and thoughtful, and they critically question all aspects of their practice in a continuous process of development, evaluation and learning that underpins change and growth.
- Strategies that promote critical reflection in leadership include reflective writing, clinical supervision and mentorship, learning circles and group reflection, critical questioning techniques and creativity and arts-based approaches.

Reflective questions

1 What is reflection?

2 How does critical reflection differ from reflection in general?

3 What is meant by the term critical reflective practice?

4 How do principles of critical reflective practice apply to leadership in healthcare?

5 Why is critical reflective practice important to the work of professionals?

Self-analysis questions

Think about your current practice and leadership style. What do you think are your strengths and challenges in relation to critical reflective practice? How might you apply some of the critical reflection strategies identified in this chapter to develop your leadership potential?

References

Binding, L., Morck, A. C. & Moules, N. J. (2010). Learning to see the other: A vehicle of reflection. *Nurse Education Today, 30*(6), 591–594. doi: 10.1016/j.nedt.2009.12.014

Bradbury-Jones, C., Coleman, D., Davies, H., Ellison, K. & Leigh, C. (2010). Raised emotions: A critique of the Peshkin approach to reflection. *Nurse Education Today, 30*, 568–572. doi: 10.1016/j.nedt.2009.12.002

Brookfield, S. (1998). Critically reflective practice. *Journal of Continuing Education in the Health Professions, 18*(4), 197–205.

Dewey, J. (1910). *How we think*. Boston, MA: DC Heath.

——. (1916). *Democracy and education: An introduction to the philosophy of education*. New York, NY: MacMillan.

——. (1933). *How we think: A restatement of the relation of reflective thinking to the educative process*. Boston, MA: DC Heath.

——. (1938). *Experience and education*. Indianapolis, IN: Kappa Delta Pi.

Donaghy, M. & Morss, K. (2000). Guided reflection: A framework to facilitate and assess reflective practice within the discipline of physiotherapy. *Physiotherapy Theory and Practice, 16*, 3–14.

Enterkin, J., Robb, E. & McLaren, S. (2013). Clinical leadership for high quality care: Developing future ward leaders. *Journal of Nursing Management, 21*, 206–216. doi: 10.1111/j.1365 -2834.2012.01408.x

Freire, P. (1995). *Pedagogy of hope: Reliving pedagogy of the oppressed*. New York, NY: Continuum.

Hatton, N. & Smith, D. (1995). Reflection in teacher education: Towards definition and implementation. *Teaching and Teacher Education, 11*(1), 33–49. doi: 10.1016/0742-051X(94)00012-U

Horton-Deutsch, S. (2013). Thinking it through: The path to reflective leadership. *American Nurse Today, 8*(2). Retrieved from http://www.americannursetoday.com

Horton-Deutsch, S., Young, P. K. & Nelson, K. A. (2010). Becoming a nurse faculty leader: Facing challenges through reflecting, persevering and relating in new ways. *Journal of Nursing Management, 18*, 487–493. doi: 10.1111/j.1365-2834.2010.01075.x

Jasper, M. (1999). Nurses' perceptions of the value of written reflection. *Nurse Education Today, 19*(6), 452–463. doi: 10.1054/nedt.1999.0328

Johns, C. (2006). *Engaging reflection in practice: A narrative approach*. Oxford, United Kingdom: Blackwell.

LaBoskey, V. K. (1994). *Development of reflective practice: A study of preservice teachers*. New York, NY: Teachers College.

Latimer, S. (2011). Reflection. In D. Stanley (Ed.), *Clinical leadership: Innovation into action* (pp. 265–276). Melbourne: Palgrave Macmillan.

Lee, N. J. (2009). Using group reflection in an action research study. *Nurse Researcher, 16*(2), 30–42. doi: 10.7748/nr2009.01.16.2.30.c6760

Mackintosh, C. (1998). Reflection: A flawed strategy for the nursing profession. *Nurse Education Today, 18*(7), 553–557. doi: 10.1016/S0260-6917(98)80005-1

Maturana, H. R. (1998). *The biology of cognition and the biology of love: Implications for health care*. Presentation to Faculty of Nursing, University of Calgary, Calgary, Canada.

Mezirow, J. (1991). *Transformative dimensions of adult learning*. San Francisco, CA: Jossey-Bass.

Plack, M. M., Dunfee, H., Rindflesch, A. & Driscoll, M. (2008). Virtual action learning sets: A model for facilitating reflection in the clinical setting. *Journal of Physical Therapy Education, 22*(3), 33–42.

Pollard, A. (2002). (With J. Collins, M. Maddock, N. Simco, S. Swaffield, J. Warin & P. Warwick). *Reflective teaching: Effective and evidence-informed professional practice*. London, United Kingdom: Continuum.

——. (2005). (With J. Collins, M. Maddock, N. Simco, S. Swaffield, J. Warin & P. Warwick). *Reflective teaching* (2nd ed.). London, United Kingdom: Continuum.

Rogers, C. (1951). *Client-centered therapy: Its current practice, implications, and theory*. Boston, MA: Houghton Mifflin.

——. (1969). *Freedom to learn: A view of what education might become*. Columbus, OH: Charles Merill.

Rolfe, G. (2014). Rethinking reflective education: What would Dewey have done? *Nurse Education Today, 34*(8), 1179–1183. doi: 10.1016/j.nedt.2014.03.006

Schön, D. A. (1983). *The reflective practitioner: How professionals think in action.* New York, NY: Basic Books.

———. (1987). *Educating the reflective practitioner: Towards a new design for teaching and learning in the professions.* San Francisco, CA: Jossey-Bass.

———. (1992). The theory of inquiry: Dewey's legacy to education. *Curriculum Inquiry, 2*(2), 119–139.

Snyder, M. (2014). Emancipatory knowing: Empowering nursing students towards reflection and action. *Journal of Nursing Education, 53*(2), 65–69. doi: 10.3928/01484834-20140107-01

Stewart, J. (2012). Reflecting on reflecting: Increasing health and social care students' engagement and enthusiasm for reflection. *Reflective Practice: International and Multidisciplinary Perspectives, 13*(5), 719–733. doi: 10.1080/14623943.2012.670627

Tate, S. (2004). Using critical reflection as a teaching tool. In S. Tate & M. Sills (Eds), *The development of critical reflection in health professionals* (Occasional Paper no. 4, pp. 8–17). Retrieved from http://www.hsaparchive.org.uk/lenses/occasionalpapers/col10004/m10127.html

Thorsen, C. A. & DeVore, S. (2013). Analyzing reflection on/for action: A new approach. *Reflective Practice, 14*(1), 88–103. doi: 10.1080/14623943.2012.732948

Usher, R. & Bryant, I. (1997). *Adult education and the postmodern challenge: Learning beyond the limits.* London, United Kingdom: Routledge.

Vitello-Cicciu, J. M., Glass, B., Weatherford, B., Seymour-Route, P. & Gemme, D. (2014). The effectiveness of a leadership development program on self-awareness in practice. *The Journal of Nursing Administration, 44*(3), 170–174. doi: 10.1097/NNA.0000000000000046

Wainwright, S. F., Shepard, K. F., Harman, L. B. & Stephens, J. (2010). Novice and experienced physical therapists clinicians: A comparison of how reflection is used to inform the clinical decision-making process. *Physical Therapy, 90*(1), 75–88. doi: 10.2522/ptj.20090077

Walker, R., Cooke, M., Henderson, A. & Creedy, D. (2013). Using a critical reflection process to create an effective learning community in the workplace. *Nurse Education Today, 33*(5), 504–511. doi: 10.1016/j.nedt.2012.03.001

Walker, R., Henderson, A., Cooke, M. & Creedy, D. (2011). Impact of a learning circle intervention across academic and service contexts on developing a learning culture. *Nurse Education Today, 31*(4), 378–382. doi: 10.1016/j.nedt.2010.07.010

Warwick, P. & Swaffield, S. (2006). Articulating and connecting frameworks of reflective practice and leadership: Perspectives from 'fast track' trainee teachers. *Reflective Practice: International and Multidisciplinary Perspectives, 7*(2), 247–263. doi: 10.1080/14623940600688704

Part 3

Engages Others

9

Communication leadership

Mark Keough

Learning objectives

How do I:
- use the basic principles of communication theory to improve my communication?
- understand communication as a process in a health services context?
- identify the barriers to effective communication, particularly in health services?
- develop skills to improve the use of communication in team-based health services settings?
- adapt to evolving communication practices, including electronic communication?

Introduction

Critical to successful engagement with any organisation is a strong basic understanding of the important elements affecting good communication. There are many dimensions to the study of communication, both generally and in health service settings, in the 21st century. This chapter considers the foundational concepts, with references that will help students to discover more about communication in organisational, social and cultural settings.

Many believe that even the definition of communication is worth questioning. As a notion it is so discursive and diverse that any definition other than the most simple becomes so complex as to cease being useful (Newman, 1960).

Communication, knowledge and learning are all inextricably linked. Not all our daily communication is merely functional. Increasingly, communication contains significant amounts of information, some of it important and some of it not so important. The information transmitted has become so great in volume that there is a need for better information science to absorb what is important for now, store what is important for later and discard or archive what is not important at all. This classification process requires considerable skill, and everyone is engaged in analysing large numbers of incoming communications daily, if not hourly or minute by minute.

Definitions

Communication between people is so fundamental to life that it is somewhat surprising that it is only since the Second World War that it has been a significant domain of academic study. This was fuelled by the extensive advances in the technology of human communication that took place in the late 19th century and the 20th century, and it has been accelerated even further by the **globalising** effects of the internet and the world wide web since the 1990s. The study of communication has become the cornerstone of any review of socialised human endeavour, including our use of media, organisational behaviour and human, family and interpersonal relations.

> **Communication**
> A two-way exchange of informa through writing, speaking or an medium
>
> **Globalisation**
> The process through which an organisation develops a presenc influence in more than one coun

Until the 20th century, the focus of study was the art of communication rather than the process of communication. The art of communication can be observed through language, visual representation, drama and music. After the Second World War, the Bell Laboratories, a division of the Bell Telephone Company, proposed the first model of communication (Shannon & Weaver, 1949). Not surprisingly, it was the development of radio and telephone communication technologies that gave rise to the model. The basic model proved too simplistic for most people and was progressively developed from a simple process to describe communication using telephony to a model applicable in the much broader realm of human social relations. In the early 1960s, based on the work of David Berlo (1960), the model was expanded and clarified to what is now widely accepted as the basic model of communication: that of source, message, channel and receiver.

Understanding of communication and its impact has grown rapidly in recent years, beginning with the modernist premise that preceded the growth in advertising communications in the 1960s. The idea that 'the medium is the message' was promoted by Marshall McLuhan (1964) and has been further developed in modern understanding that communication can be initiated by the inanimate. For example, the structure of an organisation, the architecture or a building, the clothing people wear (such as blue or pink uniforms or white coats) are all media for a message. And the media may be the message. This is further complicated by notions of identity and ideas about self. Self-awareness as people, which preferences personalities contain, even mood: all form part of the source of messages that are sent.

Essential elements of communication

Sender

The **sender** of human communication (usually but not always a person) retains the belief that whatever techniques they employ, their message and the information contained therein are always received in the detail and context with which it was intended. Messages rely heavily on language, and of course the language used must be understood. When sending a message it is important to ensure that the language used is simple, clear and to the point. Messages constructed carefully will have the best chance of being understood. Think about a simple request like 'I would like you to make a cup of coffee for me, please'. When messages are clear they contain a reference to the source ('I' and 'for me'), the subject ('you'), the object ('a cup of coffee') and an emotive adjunct to the phrase to support the desired behaviour ('please').

> on or system initiating a
> cation

When messages are ambiguous, receivers may start to look for other meanings than that which was originally intended. For example, if the message was simply 'I would like a cup of coffee', the receiver may assume it has nothing to do with them, because the subject ('you') is not identified. Of course, if the sender said, *'Fais-moi un café, s'il te plaît'*, they would be assuming the subject could speak French. Language and its careful construction, tone and use are often critical to communication.

Emotion

When messages are loaded with emotion, such as anger or happiness, the meaning can also become unclear. In fact, an angry or happy message will most likely convey the emotion rather than the message itself: emotion can cloud a message to the point where no part of the message is retained save for the emotional impact. How people send a message – the language, tone and medium – is critical to what message will be received.

Distortion

Ambiguity is only one of the possible distortions that result in a message being lost or a communication being ineffective. Message **distortion**, or noise, can have several causes. Sometimes it is accidental, but sometimes a deliberate and disruptive act by the receiver or a third-party stakeholder with an interest in skewing the message.

> ion
> e in something's usual, original,
> r intended meaning, condition

A distortion effect can occur in a workplace when a communication between one person and another, or one person and many other people, becomes skewed by external interference. If communication is to be clear, understood and acted upon, sources of distortion must be eliminated or minimised. A critical skill in communication leadership is establishing an intuitive alert mechanism for distortion.

Feedback

One way in which it is possible to test if a message is getting through is by asking for **feedback** from the receiver. Feedback is essential if the sender is to achieve confirmation that a message is heard and understood. Without feedback, even in the most straightforward of personal communications, the sender can have no idea whether the message has been received, let alone understood.

> **Feedback**
> An indication of the reaction of receiver

Non-verbal communication

A smile, a happy disposition, an open stance or a warm handshake or greeting immediately indicates a positive disposition between a communication sender and receiver. Folded arms, clenched teeth, hands covering the face and an agitated disposition have the opposite effect. Non-verbal acts can communicate vividly or undermine all attempts to communicate with equal and stunning effect. More subtle clues lie in interpersonal behaviours, such as the use of eye contact and shuffling in one's seat, or perhaps in the choice of clothing for a particular situation. Any of these factors can enhance or detract from the effectiveness of communication. Good communicators pay a lot of attention to non-verbal cues; understanding them in their cultural, social and workplace contexts is critical to successful communication (Dwyer & Boyd, 2003).

A bad 'noise' bleed

Any health service is full of competing communications. Noisy waiting rooms, workstations, corridors, cleaners and machines are everywhere. I experienced the distractions caused by noise and competing conversations on a recent overseas visit.

I was at an expensive and important health conference, seeing a number of world-renowned speakers all in one day. The talks were held in adjacent rooms separated by quite thin walls designed to be just thick enough to be unable to hear the speech next door. It was a poor venue for such a gathering. Unfortunately, the rooms were often crowded, and for those standing at the rear or edge of a room, the experience was spoiled by the 'bleed' of noise from the adjacent room. The intended communication became a cacophony of conflicting sounds, and it was difficult to focus on the presentation at hand. It also didn't help that the public address system kept failing in one of the rooms.

Receiver

The situation of the **receiver** of a message or group of messages is completely dependent on their reading comprehension, listening or perceiving skills – that is, their situational

> **Receiver**
> The person or system who perce communication

awareness. If the receiver is not aware or listening, they will not receive the message. Given that they are not the initiator of the message, it is highly likely that the sender may need to first gain their attention. With a telephone call this is relatively simple: the sender dials a number, the phone rings, and the receiver answers. Most cultural protocols would include some identifying language and confirmation that the receiver is ready to listen.

When this is translated into a workplace situation it can be either simpler or more complicated. For example, we should assume that in the earlier example someone would not ask another person to make them a cup of coffee unless the subject could hear the request and there was some idea or evidence that they were listening or taking it in. In other situations, such as a speech or instructions to a group, it is difficult to guarantee that an individual in the receiving group is alert and listening. In more complex situations, the true message may be so couched in neutral or inoffensive language, in order not to offend members of an audience, that comprehension of the actual request becomes very difficult. If the receiver is not skilled, capable or ready to receive a message, the communication will be lost.

Healthcare and communication

Communication in health services settings can be broadly grouped into three streams: administrative (financial, human resources and organisational), clinical (medical and interprofessional) and client (patient and family). This chapter focuses on the second two; many good texts about organisations are available which describe the nature and importance of sound administrative communications, while special skills and structures are needed to lead clinical and client communications successfully.

Formal and informal communication

In health management settings, understanding when a communication should be formal or informal is critical. For new team leaders, it can be embarrassing to have written a formal memorandum-style email to a team member and colleague and afterwards discover that a personal conversation would have been more appropriate. An important part of managers' and leaders' armoury is a consistent set of formal and informal protocols for communication.

Upward communications (reports, proposals, requests for approval) are often formal. Most managers respect, however, that subordinates may need to talk over an idea in an informal setting. Downward communications (procedures, requests, memorandums, meeting minutes) are also often formal, whereas peer or sideways communications are more likely to be informal in most instances, except where a structured communication is called for due to an administrative requirement or clinical situation.

Clinical communication

In any health service context, strong communication skills can literally be a matter of life and death. The lore of human health experience is littered with examples and anecdotes of situations in which poor communication led to a terrible health outcome, escalating illness or even causing unnecessary loss of life (see, for example, Mid Staffordshire NHS Foundation Trust Public Inquiry, 2013). A challenging issue in healthcare is the unintended silo effect of having experts from many differently focused fields of healthcare advising on a single situation without first communicating with each other. This can and has led to many unfortunate outcomes in which information was conveyed without the correct context and a tragic result occurred.

Structured communication

New developments derived from experiences of the US military have led to a popular model for structured communication in clinical practice: the formalising of communication protocols for situations in which information and context must be conveyed with as much accuracy as possible – for example, the clinical handover of information from one daily rostered shift to the next or from one health service location to the next. The ISBAR model is one such framework and is commonly in use in many health settings. Figure 9.1 describes the protocols involved and the core questions required to establish the critical clinical information. It is not only useful in clinical settings but can be used to manage any organisational communication in which the use of a formal protocol is likely to be well known and understood. Whenever communication is of a critical nature and distortion must be minimised, following this structured method will assist in ensuring clarity.

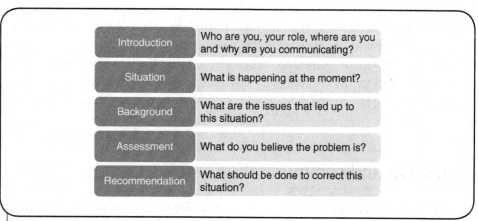

Figure 9.1 The ISBAR model. ISBAR. (2011). NSW Ministry of Health / New South Wales and South Australian Department of Health (Version 1.0) [Mobile application software]. Retrieved from https://itunes.apple.com.

Electronic communication

In any study of communication at this time in history we cannot ignore the impact of communication technology and the way it has changed society through a form of communicative action (Habermas, 1987). Mobile communication technology in particular has 'taken on the full figure of the discursive action: it has inserted itself into the daily needs of the projective selves who carry and operate it' (Keough, 2011, p. 519).

While the principles of good communication and attributes of poor communication apply universally, there are some important characteristics of electronic communication worthy of special note. Every time we communicate electronically there are three important and common aspects that are often overlooked. Firstly, non-verbal markers are severely discounted. Online communication is mostly written and often brief. We make the mistaken assumption that the receiver can see the wink in our eye or the 'tongue in our cheek'. Secondly, many people falsely believe electronic communication is more anonymous than verbal or personal communication and sometimes write a little too courageously only to later regret the message's tone. Finally, we believe that the only person reading an electronic communication is the person to whom it was directed.

All people in organisations rely heavily on emails to communicate, which makes writing an effective email a fundamental skill. An effective email will ensure that receivers understand the message quickly and will generate a faster and more effective response. Ineffective emails are more often than not ignored.

When writing an email, especially when it is aimed at work colleagues, it is important to start with the key message, using the best fit for language level and tone, having taken time to understand the audience. When the purpose of an email is clear from the start, it will be opened and read, so a good subject header is a critical first component. Then, the most important information should be positioned at the top of the email, in the opening paragraph. There should be one piece of information in each paragraph. If the email is longer than one screen page, it is advisable to use simple subheadings to divide the information. Understanding the audience involves knowing what position the receiver holds, whether they will understand the chosen terminology and whether a message being sent to more than one person should be the same for all recipients or tailored for different people. It is important to use plain language, avoiding jargon and complicated wording, to make sure the key message is understood.

Leadership and communication

Communicating within teams is both challenging and rewarding, as we seek to establish successful and functional groups with a shared purpose. Team communications are critical when the outcome of a service can be achieved only by a number of people working together. These complex situations are common in all health services.

Active listening

Active listening is a key skill in health service teams. It means listening with focus and intent. Some methods for putting active listening into action are discussed below.

Firstly, ask rather than tell, by using open questions, which encourage others to express their views. Open questions invite the provision of information, such as, 'Jenny, I would like your opinion on this'. Closed questions are designed to narrow the focus of the answers given and are often used to qualify information in a situation, leading to a yes or no answer. They are helpful in some situations – for example, 'Are you allergic to peanuts?' – but can stifle conversation and limit onward discovery.

It is also important to try to suspend judgement and consider matters from other people's perspectives, without filtering what is heard through a narrow viewpoint. This is quite a skill, but it is always helpful to quietly ask 'If I were in their shoes, how would I feel about this?' in order to maintain a sense of accurate context for the information being received.

Ensuring genuine interest in understanding the other person is vital. Take time to actively check understanding by reflecting and paraphrasing before responding. Listen for the true message the person is trying to convey. This can be enhanced by taking careful notice of tone, body language and situational context.

The results of active listening are usually more beneficial than those of a passive approach. Conversations become more two-way, and the participants feel more engaged.

Difficult conversations

Holding regular difficult conversations can help avoid workplace tension and reduce the likelihood of a crisis, leading to healthier and more productive relationships at work. Difficult conversations may take place one-to-one or during team sessions. When a difficult conversation becomes necessary, before starting it is important to think about the most suitable place and time for it to occur. Grabbing someone on their way to lunch in the corridor is not a good idea, and in some cases a witness may be required.

In order for a difficult conversation to be successful, the facts of the situation need to be checked and corroborated. It is important to ensure that the other person or audience understands the problem and the expectations and desired outcomes. During the conversation, it is best to keep to the main point without bringing up other issues. This helps to ensure that trust is kept intact, which is most important to a beneficial outcome. No matter what occurs with the receiving party, the initiator of the conversation must be respectful and keep their emotions in check.

When tackling difficult conversations, 'I' messages should be used when the issue is more complex or is ongoing. Such messages have four parts. Firstly, the person's problem-causing behaviour is described in an objective, non-blaming way. Secondly, the phrase 'the effects are' is used to help the person understand the consequences of the behaviour. Then, the manager describes how the behaviour makes them feel; a simple 'I feel' avoids a direct accusation. Finally, such phrases as 'I'd prefer' are used, rather than 'you should', to identify the preferred behaviour. For example, 'When you raised your voice in front of my peers, it was uncalled for in that setting, and I felt really stupid. I'd rather you had pulled me aside to speak about this in private'.

It is useful when tackling difficult conversations to use plain language to avoid feelings being misunderstood. For example, saying 'I'm angry' could mean a person is either furious or just irritated. It can be misread. If there is uncertainty in a situation, of course, it is important to say so.

Electronic communication

A challenge for health service managers exists in the way tools for electronic communication blur boundaries between personal and professional life. Social networking tools, like email, tend to engender the feeling of anonymity, often encouraging us to write our emotional responses to an issue or occurrence with the feeling that we are in a safe 'social' situation among friends and family. However, social networking tools come with the permanence of writing, the forensic accuracy of a time and date stamp, and occasionally an escalation in audience numbers from local to global.

The responsibility of employees and managers to carefully and responsibly navigate this area is not helped when clear legislation, policies and procedures have lagged well behind social and organisational practice. Clear local organisational policies and procedures are essential for health services settings.

· ·

Communication and learning

The communication revolution of the late 20th and early 21st centuries is truly remarkable and for the most part has initiated a great leap forwards for all humankind. Online webs of communication have dramatically impacted on learning: imagine a world without search engines such as Google. What can be known and authenticated from online information is astonishing; internet tools save lives, speed learning and make knowledge truly global. Provided there exists the privilege of access to these global learning networks, there is no excuse for ignorance or decisions based on significantly out of date information.

There are many ways to learn more about the expanding domains of communication, but leaders in health services settings may consider the work of Etienne Wenger (1998a, 1998b) in his definition of **communities of practice and interest**. This body of thinking offers managers and leaders a framework for understanding how modern organisations function, communicate and learn. It offers a useful way of understanding the role of mature communication in an organisation, supporting improvement in service quality, and client and employee satisfaction.

·nity of practice and interest
of people who share a concern
ɔn for something they do and
ᵣn how to do it better as they
regularly (Wenger 1998a,

All communication in this age is learning communication, and all communication networks create new societal benefits. Although, as Castells (2013) cautions, too much control over communication networks may lead to unintended and unfortunate consequences, stifling innovation and creativity, through communication skills and technologies, the future of positive society and working relationships is surely in everyone's interests.

Summary

- Communication consists of a five-step process: source, sender, message, channel and receiver.
- Team-based communication is not helped by the common professional and administrative silos in health services.
- Communication in health settings is helped by structures and protocols such as the ISBAR model, particularly in sensitive areas.
- Poor communication practices can lead to harmful outcomes in health services, including unnecessary loss of life.
- Health service managers face increasing challenges in managing communications, due to the diversity and universality of electronic communication.

Reflective questions

1 Is communication an art or a process?
2 What types of distortions are common in health services communication?
3 What technologies are present in health services settings?
4 When is it better to communicate with patients and clients electronically and when must it be face-to-face? Explain why.
5 Why are non-verbal signals important in communication?

Self-analysis questions

Reflect on what makes a leader a good communicator, considering particular aspects of leadership that you think most affect communications – for example, self-assurance or confidence. Is it important to be organised with structured protocols or is flexibility and a listening ear more critical? The ability to listen and identify with a wide range of people is desirable, but is it critical in a health service setting? Is being reflective and considered more important than being timely and decisive?

Consider your leadership strengths and how they naturally support good communication. Then ask some trusted friends whether they agree with your analysis.

References

Berlo, D. K. (1960). *The process of communication: An introduction to theory and practice*. New York, NY: Holt, Rinehart & Winston.

Castells, M. (2013). *Communication power*. Oxford, United Kingdom: Oxford University.

Dwyer, J. & Boyd, A. (2003). *The business communication handbook*. Sydney: Prentice Hall.

Habermas, J. (1987). *The theory of communicative action: Vol. 2. Lifeworld and system: A critique of functionalist reason*. Cambridge, United Kingdom: Polity.

ISBAR. (2011). NSW Ministry of Health / New South Wales and South Australian Department of Health (Version 1.0) [Mobile application software]. Retrieved from https://itunes.apple.com

Keough, M. (2011). *Toward learning utility: The evolution of online learning as a network utility in industry settings*. Adelaide: University of South Australia.

McLuhan, M. (1964). *Understanding media: The extensions of man*. London, United Kingdom: Routledge & Kegan Paul.

Mid Staffordshire NHS Foundation Trust Public Inquiry. (2013). *Report of the Mid Staffordshire NHS Foundation Trust Public Inquiry: Executive summary* [Chaired by R. Francis QC]. Retrieved from Gov.uk website: https://www.gov.uk/government/uploads/system/uploads/attachment_data/file/279124/0947.pdf

Newman, J. B. (1960). A rationale for a definition of communication. *Journal of Communication* 10(3): 115–124. doi: 10.1111/j.1460-2466.1960.tb00530.x

Shannon, C. E. & Weaver, W. (1949). *The mathematical theory of communication.* Urbana, IL University of Illinois.

Wenger, E. (1998a). Communities of practice: Learning as a social system. *Systems Thinker,* 9(5): 2–3.

——. (1998b). *Communities of practice: Learning, meaning, and identity.* Cambridge, United Kingdom: Cambridge University.

10

Leading interprofessional teams

Katrina Radford and Janna Anneke Fitzgerald

Learning objectives

How do I:
- understand the place that interprofessional teams have in healthcare organisations?
- analyse the enablers and barriers to leading interprofessional teams?
- apply principles of successful leadership of interprofessional teams to enhance my teamwork skills?
- work with the benefits and challenges associated with hybrid roles in leading interprofessional teams?

Introduction

Leadership is an elusive concept. Key authors cannot agree on the characteristics of leaders, but all agree that leadership is about relationships and evolves over time. For example, Rost and Barker (2000, p. 3) state that 'leadership is an influence relationship among leaders and followers who intend real changes and outcomes that reflect a shared purpose'. Meanwhile, Landsdale (2002, p. 56) suggests that 'effective leaders enable people to move in the same direction, toward the same destinations, at the same speed, but not because they have been forced to, but because they want to'. This raises the question of how we get people to want to go in the same direction and at the same pace. In the health services this is particularly challenging because of the multidisciplinary nature of the key stakeholders. It requires appropriate leadership of interprofessional teams.

The increased complexity of patient needs has driven the necessity of interprofessional teamwork in health services (Bridges, Davidson, Odegard, Maki &

Tomkowiak, 2011). Consequently, the importance of such teams within a health context is increasingly being accepted (Bajnok, Puddester, MacDonald, Archibald & Kuhl, 2012). While working in interprofessional teams is challenging, it also has benefits. Healthcare professionals working in interprofessional teams have reported that the system produces greater patient satisfaction and outcomes, reduced healthcare costs and improved job satisfaction (Baggs & Schmitt, 1997; Clarke & Hassmiller, 2013; Hendel, Fish & Berger, 2007; Zwarenstein, Reeves & Perrier, 2005).

This chapter stresses the importance of leading interprofessional teams and presents some suggestions for how collaborative teams can work together effectively to achieve common goals. By the end of this chapter, students will have an understanding of the place that interprofessional teams have in healthcare organisations today, as well as the benefits and challenges of such a collaborative approach to healthcare.

Definitions

Professional identity refers to the way in which each profession categorises itself and differentiates itself from other professions (Schein, 1978). A professional's identity is built from three aspects: the way a person sees others, the way others see the person and the way the person sees themselves (Fitzgerald, 2002). When our professional identity is threatened, we tend to fall back on stereotypical and (usually negative) social categorisations of our profession and that of others, which can cause conflict if we are working within a team of professionals from varying fields. During conflict, team dynamics can become toxic and may require increased time investment (Bajnok et al., 2012). However, an

> **Professional identity**
> A categorisation and differentiat
> profession
>
> **Interprofessional team**
> A group of professionals from di
> disciplines working collaborative
> integrated team to draw on indi
> and collective skills and experier

investment in an **interprofessional team**, by appropriate management of the team, is rewarding. It creates efficiencies within an organisation and ultimately improves care delivery.

Working with a variety of different professionals in a team allows sharing of expertise and perspectives to meet the common goal of providing quality care to patients within a healthcare setting. This form of teamwork is commonly known as interprofessional collaborative practice and involves 'health professionals working collaboratively in integrated teams to draw on individual and collective skills and experiences across disciplines' (Clarke & Hassmiller, 2013, p. 334). An example of the types of professions that could make up an interprofessional health team is provided in Figure 10.1.

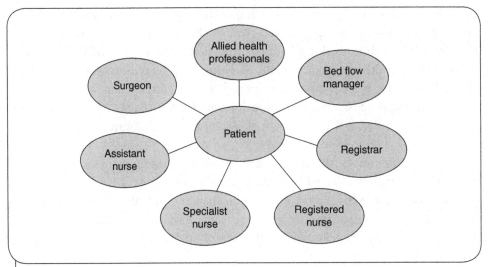

Figure 10.1 Example of an interprofessional team within an acute care setting. Adapted from N. Gopee & J. Galloway (2009). *Leadership and management in healthcare*. Thousand Oaks, CA: Sage.

Teams with professional boundaries

There are many terms used within healthcare to indicate the context within which health professionals work together. Similarly, there are many models for the facilitation of team-work proposed in the literature. In addition to these models, leaders need to consider the impact that the role of each team member has on team effectiveness and interactions. Three models identified by Mumma and Nelson (2002) are multidisciplinary, interdisciplinary and transdisciplinary teams, which are discussed below.

Multidisciplinary teams

Multidisciplinary teams have discipline-specific goals. There are clear boundaries between disciplines, and effective communication is essential for success and to ensure that crossover of workloads does not occur. This model involves each discipline working within the parameters of its profession to provide appropriate patient-centred care.

Interdisciplinary teams

In contrast to multidisciplinary teams, **interdisciplinary teams** collaborate to identify patient goals and use an expanded problem-solving model that goes beyond discipline-specific boundaries in order to maximise patient outcomes. This model involves working together to achieve common outcomes and may mean holding

sciplinary team
of professionals from different
s working collaboratively with
iplinary boundaries

sciplinary team
of professionals from
disciplines working closely
to achieve common
s through regular meetings
collaborative patient care
and not bound by discipline-
boundaries

regular patient-centred meetings with representatives from a variety of disciplines in order to maximise patient outcomes through a collaborative patient care approach.

Transdisciplinary teams

Transdisciplinary teams tend to work across boundaries between disciplines and have the flexibility to minimise duplication of effort. However, this model takes the most work to manage in terms of effective communication and teamwork.

> **Transdisciplinary team**
> A group of professionals from di
> disciplines working collaborative
> boundaries with flexibility betwo
> disciplines to minimise duplicatic

···

Teams with role-related boundaries

In addition to interprofessional teams that are delineated by professional boundaries there are teams that are delineated by their role – for example, clinical leaders, managers and practitioners (or clinicians). These roles can exist within and across professions, making leading this type of interprofessional team more challenging. For example, the principal concerns of practitioners and those of managers are distinct (Edwards, Kornacki & Silversin, 2002; Edwards, Marshall, McLellan & Abbasi, 2003), as is evident in Table 10.1.

Table 10.1 Principal concerns of clinicians and managers

Clinicians	Managers
Patient or client outcomes	Patient experience
Individual patients or clients	Population or organisation
Optimum care for each patient or client	Managing competing claims
Professional autonomy	Public accountability
Self-regulation	Systems
Evidenced-based practice	Fair allocation of resources
Personal responsibility	Delegation
Role clarity	Role ambiguity
Explicit knowledge	Tacit knowledge

Source: Adapted from N. Edwards, M. Kornacki & J. Silversin (2002). Unhappy doctors: What are the causes and what can be done? *British Medical Journal, 324*(7341), 835–838. doi: 10.1136/bmj.324.7341.835; N. Edwards, M. Marshall, A. McLellan & K. Abbasi (2003). Doctors and managers: A problem without a solution? *British Medical Journal, 326*(7390), 609–610. doi: 10.1136/bmj.326.7390.609; A. Fitzgerald (2002). Doctors and nurses working together: A mixed method study into the construction and changing of professional identities. (Doctoral dissertation, University of Western Sydney). Available from http://uwsprod.uws.dgicloud.com/islandora/object/uws%3A789.

There are deep differences in clinicians' and managers' backgrounds, as well as varying concerns, which give rise to 'unavoidable conflict between the reductionist approach to medicine and the messy political and complex world of policy' (Edwards et al., 2002, p. 837). For example, practitioners' work is rooted in biological sciences, based on cause-and-effect relationships and has a strong academic focus. Clinicians are responsible for their own individual patients and enact professional discretion in treatment decisions; they tend to think operationally, work to short timeframes and function in a professional culture. In contrast, managers draw from economic, financial, social and behavioural sciences, which operate in a more qualitative paradigm. Their focuses are groups and populations, and they tend to base their decisions on rational or legal policy. Managers think strategically, plan for distant time horizons and work well in teams. They function in a task-and-role culture (Parkin, 2009). Consequently, because of the differences in the paradigms in which they work, practitioners and managers may not always agree with each other on core matters.

For leaders, it becomes important to consider the frame of reference that their team members may be using in order to lead effective interprofessional teams. To try to respond to these differences in reference points, organisations have begun to embed the hybrid clinical manager role into practice. Hybrid clinical managers in a healthcare environment are medical doctors who work in a dual clinical and managerial role in order to bridge the differences between managers and practitioners (Kippist, 2013). They are discussed further below.

Leadership of interprofessional teams

Resource deficiencies, changing expectations of clients and tightened funding outcomes have caused the leadership of interprofessional teams to become more important and prevalent in the health sector globally. In the United Kingdom, the practice has long been advocated for its ability to support clients with complex needs (Trivedi et al., 2013). Similarly, within Australia, hospitals are increasingly pushing for interprofessional teams in order to maximise productivity (Novak & Judah, 2011). Yet leading these teams can be a difficult and challenging experience, especially as communication styles differ, and leadership styles need to be flexible in order to support such diverse teams.

Successful team dynamics are achieved when members see their role as important to the team and when there is between team members open communication, existence of autonomy and equality of resources (Morrison, 2007). Further, a blending of professional cultures is necessary, which includes sharing skills and knowledge to improve the quality of patient care (Bridges et al., 2011).

To be successful, leaders of interprofessional teams must demonstrate **integrated care**, which involves training

ted care

approach involving training
cation, open communication
ual respect (Interprofessional
n Collaborative Expert Panel,

and education, open communication and mutual respect (Interprofessional Education Collaborative Expert Panel, 2011). In addition, Clarke and Hassmiller (2013) propose four key competencies for successful interprofessional collaborative practice: understanding and demonstrating values and ethics of interprofessional practice throughout the organisation and unit, espousing clear roles and responsibilities for each team member, providing clear interprofessional communication and encouraging effective teams and teamwork. The following list contains important guidelines for leaders of interprofessional teams:

- Identify key stakeholders and know who matters most.
- When problem-solving, be sure to examine the diversity within the team in order to provide varying perspectives for members, meaning decisions will be more widely accepted.
- Understand how team members respond to conflict and expectations.
- Work towards understanding and valuing the benefit of individuals' differences and appreciating all contributions.
- Avoid assumptions that all professional groups act and respond in the same ways.
- Avoid labelling.
- Recognise similarities between team members.
- Treat resistance as a form of communication.
- Seek out different experiences from the majority and from those who matter most.
- Pay close attention to verbal and non-verbal communication.
- Ask for clarification to avoid assumptions.
- Assist those in minority groups to be successful by including them in informal networking within the team culture.

Working within an interprofessional team is not easy and requires strong leadership to be successful. This is because working in a team calls for cooperation, understanding and the use of effective communication (Burzotta & Noble, 2011). Strong leadership of such a team requires the following values and traits to be established by the leader within the team before collaboration begins: responsibility, accountability, coordination, communication, cooperation, assertiveness, autonomy, and mutual trust and respect (Bridges et al., 2011; Burzotta & Noble, 2011; Clarke & Hassmiller, 2013). Development of the softer skills of management is also needed to be an effective interprofessional team leader.

Management of interprofessional teams

The successful management of collaborative teams involves addressing some key challenges, which include managing knowledge held by team members about other team members' disciplines, personal values and beliefs, professional identity, perceptions of occupational esteem and workload (Reese & Sontag, 2001).

Understanding the professional identity of team members is critical to the management of interprofessional teams, as it cannot be assumed that team members will respond to management in similar ways. Deconstructing professional identities is sometimes useful in trying to understand interprofessional team difficulties. This can be achieved by categorising and analysing how each professional discipline views its professional autonomy, authority and sovereignty. Some idea of these views can be gained by discovering how team members see their roles and tasks (occupational or professional), how they define their role (ambiguous or clear), what kind of knowledge they enact (tacit, intuitive or explicit, scientific) and the nature of their work (dirty or clean). In addition, the manner and aptness in which professionals are rewarded are also useful identity constructs (Fitzgerald, 2002).

Poor team dynamics can be a result of poor communication styles within the team, lack of time investment in team development and poor understanding of other professional roles and codes of conduct (Burzotta & Noble, 2011). Working interprofessionally can also mean problems are identified by different team members through different means and at different times.

The complexities of interprofessional teams

In a small Australian metropolitan residential aged care facility, Paul, the clinical care manager, was charged with leading a team to redesign the processes around patient care plan reviews to ensure all parties were consulted in a timely fashion. To help, Paul put together a team of registered nurses, personal care workers, clinical managers, the local general practitioner, clients and family representatives.

The first meeting was attended by 90 per cent of the team members, with the notable absence of the general practitioner and the registered nurse, who were both unable to attend. At this meeting it was agreed that care plans should be reviewed every three months for each client, as per the current arrangement. However, to assist the timely review of these plans, each party involved should provide a written report with their input to the lead clinician two days prior to the care plan meeting. This would speed up the process of providing feedback and reviewing the care plan, thus allowing the facility to keep on top of the regular reviews.

Upon hearing of this decision, the general practitioner and registered nurse felt that a written report was unnecessary, as they currently fed into the care plan on the floor; writing a report would increase their workload. Paul was left to reconsider the purpose and outcomes of the first team meeting.

It took a further six meetings, at which not all representatives were ever present at the same time, for the approach to be successfully redesigned. However, by the end of the process, Paul felt dismayed at the complexities and challenges he had encountered in leading an interprofessional team.

Hybrid clinical managers

Healthcare organisations are driven by the need for cost reductions and organisational efficiencies; this is known commonly as the business of health, and it responds to organisational targets such as cost reduction and performance measures driven by the current economic and political climate. As a result, the business of health has had an increasingly large influence over the practice of health in recent years, and practitioners have expressed resentment towards health service managers because they perceive that they, more than clinical need, drive the structural and operational changes implemented in healthcare organisations. From the practitioners' perspective, managers have limited practitioners' autonomy and control over their clinical practice (Fulop & Day, 2010; Spurgeon, Clark & Ham, 2011). In contrast, managers may feel that change is warranted based on the social, political, historical and economic needs of the environment within which they are operating. As mentioned earlier, the hybrid clinical manager's role was introduced to engage practitioners with management objectives so they could better contribute to the significant changes in healthcare service delivery.

The rationale behind the development of the hybrid clinical manager role was two-fold: firstly, practitioners use more resources than any other group within healthcare organisations, and secondly, they make up the most powerful group within healthcare organisations. Consequently, developing a hybrid clinical manager role means, theoretically, that these managers would be able to engage practitioners more effectively.

The clinical manager role has occupational and performance targets, and organisational change agendas may oppose clinical professional values. At the intersection of professional values and organisational objectives there is potential for individuals to experience conflict and tension (Kippist, 2013), and this increases the complexity of working within interprofessional teams as well as leading them within a healthcare environment.

Summary

- Interprofessional teams are defined as 'health professionals working collaboratively in integrated teams to draw on individual and collective skills and experiences across disciplines' (Clarke & Hassmiller, 2013, p. 334).
- Principles of successful interprofessional teams include effective communication, existence of autonomy, equality of resources, blending of professional cultures, integrated care and mutual respect.
- Leading interprofessional teams is a difficult and challenging experience, especially as communication styles differ, and leadership styles need to be flexible in order to support such diverse teams.
- There are enablers and barriers to leading interprofessional teams.

Reflective questions

1. Why are interprofessional teams important in healthcare organisations today?
2. How is leading interprofessional teams different from leading other teams?
3. List three different models of interprofessional teams that could be used in healthcare organisations.
4. How can team member roles affect team dynamics?
5. Why are interprofessional teams hard to manage?

Self-analysis question

What is your understanding of the differences between the values and the beliefs of team members, and how much do these affect your leadership?

References

Baggs, J. & Schmitt, M. H. (1997). Nurses' and resident physicians' perceptions of the process of collaboration in the MICU. *Research in Nursing and Health, 20*(1), 71–80. doi: 10.1002/(SICI)1098-240X(199702)20:13.0.CO;2-R

Bajnok, I., Puddester, D., MacDonald, C. J., Archibald, D. & Kuhl, D. (2012). Building positive relationships in health care: Evaluation of the teams of interprofessional staff interprofessional education program. *Contemporary Nurse, 42*(1), 76–89. doi: 10.5172/conu.2012.42.1.76

Bridges, D., Davidson, R. A., Odegard, P. S., Maki, I. V. & Tomkowiak, J. (2011). Interprofessional collaboration: Three best practice models of interprofessional education. *Medical Education Online, 16*(6035). doi: 10.3402/meo.v16i0.6035

Burzotta, L. & Noble, H. (2011). The dimensions of interprofessional practice. *British Journal of Nursing, 20*(5), 310–315. doi: 10.12968/bjon.2011.20.5.310

Clarke, P. & Hassmiller, S. (2013). Nursing leadership: Interprofessional education and practice. *Nursing Science Quarterly, 26*(4), 333–336. doi: 10.1177/0894318413500313

Edwards, N., Kornacki, M. & Silversin, J. (2002). Unhappy doctors: What are the causes and what can be done? *British Medical Journal, 324*(7341), 835–838. doi: 10.1136/bmj.324.7341.835

Edwards, N., Marshall, M., McLellan, A. & Abbasi, K. (2003). Doctors and managers: A problem without a solution? *British Medical Journal, 326*(7390), 609–610. doi: 10.1136/bmj.326.7390.609

Fitzgerald, A. (2002). *Doctors and nurses working together: A mixed method study into the construction and changing of professional identities* (Doctoral dissertation, University of Western Sydney). Available from http://uwsprod.uws.dgicloud.com/islandora/object/uws%3A789

Fulop, L. & Day, G. E. (2010). From leader to leadership: Clinician managers and where to next? *Australian Health Review, 34*(3), 344–351. doi: 10.1071/AH09763

Gopee, N. & Galloway, J. (2009). *Leadership and management in healthcare.* Thousand Oaks, CA: Sage.

Hendel, T., Fish, M. & Berger, O. (2007). Nurse/physician conflict management mode choices: Implications for improved collaborative practice. *Nurse Administrative Quarterly, 31*(3), 244–253.

Interprofessional Education Collaborative Expert Panel. (2011). *Core competencies for interprofessional collaborative practice: Report of an expert panel.* Washington, DC: Author.

Kippist, L. (2013). *Where is the leadership in the doctor-manager role in Australian hospitals?* Paper presented at the 27th Australian and New Zealand Academy of Management Conference: Managing on the Edge, Hobart.

Landsdale, B. M. (2002). *Cultivating inspired leaders.* Hartford, CT: Kumarian.

Morrison, S. (2007). Working together: Why bother with collaboration? *Work Based Learning in Primary Care, 5,* 65–70.

Mumma, C. M. & Nelson, A. (2002). Theory and practice models for rehabilitation nursing. In S. P. Hoeman, *Rehabilitation nursing: Process, application and outcomes* (pp. 20–36). St Louis, MO: Mosby.

Novak, J. & Judah, A. (2011). *Towards a health productivity reform agenda for Australia* [Report]. Retrieved from the Australian Centre for Health Research website: http://www.achr.com.au/pdfs/Health_Productivity_Reform_Agenda_v3.pdf

Parkin, P. (2009). *Managing change in health care.* Thousand Oaks, CA: Sage.

Reese, D. J. & Sontag, M. A. (2001). Successful interprofessional collaboration on the hospice team. *Health and Social Work, 26*(3), 167–175. doi: 10.1093/hsw/26.3.167

Rost, J. C. & Barker, R. A. (2000). Leadership education in colleges: Toward a 21st century paradigm. *Journal of Leadership Studies, 7*(1), 3–12. doi: 10.1177/107179190000700102

Schein, E. H. (1978). *Career dynamics: Matching individual and organizational needs.* Reading, MA: Addison-Wesley.

Spurgeon, P., Clark, J. & Ham, C. (2011). *Medical leadership: From the dark side to centre stage.* Oxford, United Kingdom: Radcliffe.

Trivedi, D., Goodman, C., Gage, H., Baron, N., Scheibl, F., Illiffe, S. … Drennan, V. (2013). The effectiveness of inter-professional working for older people living in the community: A systematic review. *Health and Social Care in the Community, 21*(2), 113–128. doi: 10.1111/j.1365-2524.2012.01067.x

Zwarenstein, M., Reeves, S. & Perrier, L. (2005). Effectiveness of pre-licensure interprofessional education and post-licensure collaborative interventions. *Journal of Interprofessional Care, 19*(Suppl 1), 148–165. doi: 10.1080/13561820500082800

11

Clinical governance

Cathy Balding

Learning objectives

How do I:
- understand the origins of clinical governance?
- ensure my organisation has the key components of clinical governance?
- make the connection between corporate governance and clinical governance?
- explain responsive regulation?
- develop skills to lead clinical governance in my organisation?

Introduction

The past two decades have seen the rise of clinical governance, firstly as a concept and ultimately as a system. Increased knowledge of the scope of iatrogenic harm to consumers coupled with public inquiries into poor care around the world has driven the development of governance of clinical care as a component of corporate governance. Despite this growing awareness and activity, various studies suggest we still do not have the processes in place for consistently safe, high-quality care for consumers. Compared with other high-risk industries, healthcare appears to have a high tolerance for ambiguity in processes, outcomes and roles (Spear & Schmidhofer, 2005). Accreditation, although now more focused on the quality of clinical care, is still seen as an administrative burden by many, with most health services subject to a rolling schedule of requirements and visits from a range of accreditation providers. It appears that the adverse event rate for overnight stay patients in public and private hospitals has plateaued at around 10 per cent (Australian Institute of Health and Welfare, 2013). These are not easy issues for governing bodies and executives to address within a funding environment focused more on efficiency than quality and safety (Balding, 2008).

Over time, governments, consumers, boards, managers and clinicians have realised the value, and necessity, of addressing clinical care with the same focus that financial and business issues receive from corporate governance. 'If clinical governance is to be successful it must be underpinned by the same strengths as corporate governance: it must be rigorous in its application, organisation-wide in its emphasis, accountable in its delivery, developmental in its thrust, and positive in its connotations' (Scally & Donaldson, 1998, p. 62).

The Australasian approach has evolved within a complex and rapidly growing healthcare industry comprising multiple stakeholders with varying perspectives on how quality care should be assured. We have moved from an environment in which individual professional expertise, skill and goodwill largely determined the quality of care towards a more accountable and systems-driven approach. Health professionals are now more responsible for the skills and expertise they bring to their care and are expected to work in partnership with consumers and to a set of governance requirements. Within this context, the need for strong, committed leadership at all levels of the health system is obvious, and it is necessary for this leadership to be built on robust governance systems that support healthcare staff to do what they are trained to do – provide safe, quality experiences for their consumers.

History

Genesis

Every year, millions of people interact safely with healthcare systems and receive good-quality care. But things can, and do, go wrong. Healthcare is a complex and high-risk industry, with many steps and people involved (Plsek & Greenhalgh, 2001). Add to this the explosion of new technologies, medications and medical devices and the constant growth in knowledge and research, and it is no surprise that we struggle to contain risk to consumers. It is also challenging to implement a systems-based approach within an individualised craft production environment encompassing many health professional subcultures. The complexity and challenges of assuring quality consumer experiences become obvious when we add limitless demand and expectation, along with the vagaries of state and federal politics and funding (Balding, 2008).

Clinical governance puts a system of monitoring and accountability around the historical individualism of healthcare. There are many definitions of clinical governance, but ultimately it must be defined within the broader context of corporate governance. The Australian Stock Exchange Corporate

> **Clinical governance**
> 'The set of relationships and responsibilities established by a health service organisation between its executive, workforce and stakeholders (including consumers)' to support quality care (Australian Commission on Safety and Quality in Health 2012a, p. 6)

te governance
ework of rules, relationships,
nd processes within and
authority is exercised and
d in corporations' (Australian
of Company Directors,
?)

governance framework
, roles, relationships, systems
esses that support safe, quality
in an organisation

Governance Principles describe **corporate governance** as 'the framework of rules, relationships, systems and processes within and by which authority is exercised and controlled in corporations' (Australian Institute of Company Directors, 2011, p. 2). Clinical governance is a subset of corporate governance, inasmuch as a **clinical governance framework** sets out the 'rules, roles, relationships, systems and processes' that support safe, quality care within an organisation.

Why do we need clinical governance? There is a long history of quality improvement programs in Australian and New Zealand healthcare organisations, stretching back before the Australian Council on Healthcare Standards made organisation-wide quality programs a formal requirement for accreditation in 1986. Health professionals have traditionally pursued high standards through data collection, professional associations and education programs. In the decades prior to the 1974 introduction of accreditation in Australia, many health services had developed some form of improvement, variously motivated by government initiatives, clinically driven audit programs and individual clinical improvement champions. And before the introduction of clinical governance in Australia in the early 2000s, many improvement approaches had been adopted to improve these systems' weaknesses, with some systems implemented from other industries with varying success. Quality programs evolved slowly, limited by a lack of focus, data and resources and minimal attention paid to this aspect of the professional role in clinical education (Balding, 2008).

There remained large variations in care practices and processes, and when things went wrong, resulting in patient harm, there were few mechanisms for identifying, discussing and learning from suboptimal care, with blame and shame being the most likely outcomes. Fear of legal consequences and a hospital culture that blamed error on human failing ensured that healthcare was slow to acknowledge and learn from mistakes. This culture, the lack of reliable data and the heavy reliance on individuals to provide consistently good care masked many clinical and systems inadequacies (Spear & Schmidhofer, 2005).

Turning point

The first large-scale Australian study of hospital-acquired adverse events provided much-needed focus and clarity. The 1995 Quality in Australian Health Care Study revealed that 16.6 per cent of reviewed admissions were associated with an adverse event, with 51 per cent of these considered preventable (Wilson et al., 1995). The study results were presented in federal parliament, and for the first time the safety of the healthcare provided in hospitals joined healthcare access and efficiency as public and political issues. Australia responded in 2000 by setting up the Australian Council for Safety and Quality in Health Care, charged with developing Australia's first national approach to system-wide quality issues (Wilson & Van Der Weyden, 2005). New Zealand instituted national certification of health and aged care services in 2001, and in 2010, to lead a national safety and quality approach, the New Zealand Health Quality & Safety Commission (2013) was established.

Just as health professionals were coming to terms with the problems identified by the Australian data, and with other studies from around the world showing similar results, the statistics were given a startlingly human face by a series of public inquiries into safety and quality of care in hospitals, firstly in the United Kingdom, with the Bristol Royal Infirmary case (United Kingdom Department of Health, 2001), and then in a number of Australian hospitals (Dunbar, Reddy, Beresford, Ramsey & Lord, 2007). The United Kingdom's National Health Service introduced clinical governance after the Bristol inquiry in 1998 and subsequently built a whole reform program around it, defining it as 'a system through which NHS organisations are accountable for continuously improving the quality of their services and safeguarding high standards of care by creating an environment in which excellence in clinical care will flourish' (Scally & Donaldson, 1998, p. 62).

Australia has also had its share of public inquiries, with investigations into Camden and Campbelltown hospitals in New South Wales, Canberra hospital in the Australian Capital Territory, King Edward Memorial hospital in Western Australia and Bundaberg hospital in Queensland. Each review arose after internal mechanisms failed to resolve perceived issues and whistleblowers alerted politicians directly. 'None of the substantiated problems had been uncovered or previously resolved by extensive accreditation or national safety and quality processes; in each instance, the problems were exacerbated by a poor institutional culture of self-regulation, error reporting or investigation' (Faunce & Bolsin, 2004, p. 44).

Publicly reported reviews of care in the United Kingdom, Australia and other countries provided impetus for the development of clinical governance to underpin and strengthen traditional quality improvement programs. Each Australian jurisdiction and New Zealand district health board defined a purpose and approach, with most including common issues such as the management of complaints, clinical risk, medical credentialing and evidence-based care. These continue to be central components of all clinical governance frameworks. In addition, some early national approaches were achieved, such as an Australian medication collaborative that agreed on a national generic medication chart.

Despite the introduction of clinical governance in the United Kingdom in 1998, a decade on, through the Mid Staffordshire inquiry, the National Health Service found itself embroiled in another major public inquiry which embodied the issues of all previous inquiries at a level previously unseen. The chair of the inquiry, Robert Francis (2013, p. 1), summarised the issues raised as 'a story of appalling and unnecessary suffering of hundreds of people [over three to four years] ... failed by a system which ignored the warning signs and put corporate self interest and cost control ahead of patients and their safety'. Consistent organisational and management issues have been identified from analysis of the series of public inquiries held around the world; these are listed below:

- culture of blame and inattention
- focus on meeting external key performance indicators and targets at the expense of internal standards of care
- lack of leadership of, clear lines of accountability for, and reporting on the quality and safety of the services provided
- insufficient consideration of patients and their families
- tolerance of substandard care
- ineffective credentialing, training and support for staff
- preoccupation with corporate matters at the expense of focus on clinical care
- ineffective reporting and action relating to clinical care. (Mid Staffordshire NHS Foundation Trust Public Inquiry, 2013; Walshe & Shortell, 2004)

The Mid Staffordshire inquiry's recommendations are consistent with those from all similar public inquiries. While each inquiry addresses its own context, the common actions required for change are clear: leadership of safety and quality from the top of the organisation, engagement of patients and families in care, rigorous implementation and monitoring of basic care standards, and support for staff to provide quality care and robust, transparent reporting and action (Travaglia, Hughes & Braithwaite, 2011). Clinicians, consumers and their families have played a key role in blowing the whistle on substandard care, and in some cases this has resulted in the executives involved losing or leaving their jobs.

Above all, the combination of studies into adverse events and public inquiries into poor care have reinforced the knowledge that reliance on well-trained and well-intentioned individuals trying hard is not enough to guarantee consistently good care in a complex environment such as healthcare.

The Mid Staffordshire NHS Foundation Trust Public Inquiry

The Mid Staffordshire hospitals underwent two public inquiries investigating poor care during the period from 2005 to 2009. The case represents perhaps the best example in healthcare of what can happen without a system of leadership, accountability and monitoring. It caught international attention in a way that many other public inquiries have not, possibly because it was about the denial of basic standards of care.

At these hospitals, elderly and vulnerable patients were left unwashed, unfed and without fluids. Some were left in excrement-stained sheets and beds. Patients who could not eat or drink without help did not receive it. Medicines were prescribed but not given.

How could this happen in a modern hospital in 21st-century England? The chair of the inquiry, Robert Francis, was clear: it happened because of a complete breakdown of

continued ›

continued ›

clinical governance. According to Francis, the hospital trust board did not listen sufficiently to its patients and staff or ensure the correction of deficiencies that were brought to their attention. It failed to tackle a culture involving tolerance of poor standards and disengagement from managerial and leadership responsibilities. The board and executive were preoccupied with achieving access and budget targets rather than focusing on the standard of care they were providing. The hospitals met their external compliance requirements, but these were focused more on corporate than on clinical matters (Mid Staffordshire NHS Foundation Trust Public Inquiry, 2013).

Evolution

Clinical governance has changed in response to these lessons. What began as a focus on risk and credentialing by governments, boards and executives has evolved over the past two decades into a complete system that supports governing bodies to address clinical safety and quality with the same rigour as corporate governance.

The challenge for boards is the associated requirement that they have the same knowledge of clinical quality matters as they do of financial matters. Boards must be satisfied that there is sufficient focus on staff accountability and responsibility for quality and safety throughout the organisation. This requires chief executive officers and senior managers to implement and report on a planned and systematic organisational approach to monitoring, managing and improving safety and quality.

Implementation

Clinical governance is a system within the existing corporate governance system. Ultimately, the board of a healthcare facility or service is accountable for the clinical care provided by the organisation and requires organisation-wide clinical governance that provides feedback on the quality of care that is delivered, the prevention of unacceptable events and the management of clinical and non-clinical risks. Clinical governance is essential to ensure that accreditation will be maintained and that the organisation will survive and prosper over the long term. In addition, insurance may not cover negligence if adequate clinical governance is not in place (Australian Institute of Company Directors, 2011).

International research suggests that hospitals with boards that are actively engaged in quality issues are more likely to have effective clinical governance programs in place, which enable better performance on indicators such as risk-adjusted mortality rates (Jiang, Lockee, Bass & Fraser, 2009). Some boards lack understanding of patient safety problems and receive inadequate information for sound decision-making (Bismark, Walter & Studdert, 2013). The establishment of clinical governance is challenging for many Australasian boards for a range of reasons, including concern about the technical competence required by directors to understand clinical matters, the independent contractor model of doctors in Australian hospitals and health services that separates medical and management functions, and resistance from clinicians and a fear of interfering with clinicians' business (Australian Institute of Company Directors, 2011).

Australian system

The introduction of clinical governance in Australia received a significant boost by the requirement from 2013 for health services to meet a national mandatory set of 10 safety and quality standards, the first two of which provide a governance platform for supporting safe, high-quality care in high-risk services.

The Australian Commission on Safety and Quality in Health Care (2014) developed these National Safety and Quality Health Service Standards in partnership with a wide range of stakeholders, and they have been endorsed by health ministers for use in health services across Australia. Accreditation to the standards came into effect on 1 January 2013 for hospitals (including inpatient mental health services), day procedure services and most public dental services.

Standard 1, which is concerned with 'governance for safety and quality in health service organisations', provides comprehensive information on the requirements of an effective health service governance system, incorporating 'the set of processes, customs, policy directives, laws and conventions affecting the way an organisation is directed, administered or controlled' (Australian Commission on Safety and Quality in Health Care, 2012a, p. 6).

The introduction to the standard says that 'health service organisation leaders implement governance systems to set, monitor and improve the performance of the organisation and communicate the importance of the patient experience and quality management to all members of the workforce. Clinicians and other members of the workforce use the governance systems' (Australian Commission on Safety and Quality in Health Care, 2012a, p. 7). They do this to create safe, quality consumer experiences. As an overview, Standard 1 requires the following conditions of health organisations:

- There is an integrated system of governance that actively manages patient safety and quality risks.
- The governance system sets out safety and quality policy, procedures and/or protocols, and assigns roles, responsibilities and accountabilities for patient safety and quality.
- The clinical workforce is guided by current best practice and uses clinical guidelines that are supported by the best available evidence.
- Managers and the clinical workforce have the right qualifications, skills and approach to provide safe, high-quality healthcare.
- Patient safety and quality incidents are recognised, reported and analysed, and this information is used to improve safety systems. (Australian Commission on Safety and Quality in Health Care, 2012a)

Standard 2, which is concerned with 'partnering with consumers' aims to ensure that health services are 'responsive to patient, carer and consumer input and needs' (Australian Commission on Safety and Quality in Health Care, 2012b, p. 6), based on the premise that the importance of health services partnering with patients, families, carers and consumers is recognised at a national and international level. According to the standard, significant benefits to clinical quality and outcomes, the experience of care and the business and operations of delivering care are created by such partnerships (Australian Commission on Safety and Quality in Health Care, 2012b).

Other sectors, such as primary, mental and community health and aged care, have developed their own approaches, usually emanating from accreditation requirements. These models may look different, but the components are essentially the same, and include the following requirements:

- The leadership plans, resource and implement a culture and systems for creating quality consumer experiences.
- There is a focus on learning from mistakes in a just way – that is, not blaming people for honest mistakes or systems failures, but holding people to account for errors arising from flouting rules and policies.
- Systems are in place to support consumer participation in their care and in improvement of the service more broadly.
- There is workforce development, support and guidance.
- There are compliance, risk and improvement systems to get the basics right and monitor and improve care.

Responsive regulation

The National Safety and Quality Health Service Standards form part of a broader national accreditation reform agenda, based on a responsive regulation approach to clinical governance. Responsive regulation is a hierarchical approach with mechanisms that range from persuasion to command and control, as shown in the following list:

Voluntarism   clinical protocols, new technology, personal monitoring, continuing education

Market mechanisms   competition, performance payments and contracts, consumer information

Self-regulation   voluntary accreditation, performance targets, benchmarking, peer review, open disclosure

Metaregulation   enforced self-regulation, mandated continuous improvement, incident-reporting and root cause analysis, external audit, protection for whistleblowers, published performance indicators, consumer complaints commissioner, funding agreements, clinical governance

Command and control   criminal or civil penalty, licence revocation or suspension, physician revalidation. (Healy & Dugdale, 2009)

Australian health professionals and services have traditionally practised a mix of voluntarism and self-regulation for the standard of care they provide. Each jurisdiction also uses market mechanisms, such as the requirement that health services report certain data (for example, infection rates) as part of performance contracts and payments (Healy & Dugdale, 2009).

With the advent of clinical governance, federal and jurisdictional governments have increased the use of metaregulation and command and control mechanisms. The national safety and quality standards, as mandatory requirements for accreditation of high-risk services, cover each level of the regulation hierarchy and bring command and control into play in a way not previously seen, as the mandatory nature of the standards requires each jurisdiction to employ a regulatory response to health services failing to meet the standards, based on the level of risk to consumers. Continued and serious breaches of the standards may incur financial penalties and result in services being temporarily closed. Licence removal or service closures are last resorts (Healy & Dugdale, 2009).

Leadership and clinical governance

In the same way that they govern the finances of the health service, boards and executives must have a plan for the safety and quality of care and services they intend to provide for their consumers. Boards who effectively enact their clinical governance role work with their executives and staff to ensure a suite of safety and quality measures is in place that reports on progress with the plan. Board directors have a responsibility to ascertain to their satisfaction that consumers are central to the business of the organisation, that staff are supported to provide high-quality care and services and that systems and reporting are resourced and effective (Australian Institute of Company Directors, 2011).

Crafting and assigning these accountabilities in a meaningful and sustainable way requires managers at all levels of the organisation to embed the clinical governance program in day-to-day care and service provision (Balding, 2011). Clinician leadership, in particular, has been found to be a key success factor in improvement programs, which require the executive to establish sustainable organisational roles and processes to facilitate clinician involvement (Akins & Cole, 2005; Ham, 2003).

It is therefore up to the chief executive officer and senior executives to translate the strategic quality plans and governance systems into operational plans and strategies for implementation by managers and clinical leaders. Those on the frontline of care create the consumer experience, but the operationalisation must be led from the executive team through line management.

Summary

- Clinical governance is a key component of the governance of any health service and should be given the same priority as corporate governance.
- Clinical governance supports accountabilities for the safety and quality of care at each level of a health service.
- The key components of clinical governance relate to risk management, quality improvement, evidence-based care, a skilled clinical workforce and learning from clinical incidents.
- Responsive regulation in this context is a hierarchy of approaches to regulate the safety and quality of healthcare, from persuasion to command and control.
- Leading clinical governance requires the board and executive to develop a clear vision for safe, quality care in the organisation, to implement governance systems to support staff to achieve it and to closely monitor and drive progress.

Reflective questions

1 Why does a modern healthcare system need clinical governance?

2 Why did clinical governance not develop naturally as part of corporate governance in health services?

3 What would happen in your health service if the clinical governance system was terminated?

4 Who is responsible for the safety and quality of care in a health service?

5 Who is ultimately accountable for the quality of the care provided in a health service?

Self-analysis questions

A local hospital has advertised for a new board member, who will also be a member of the board's clinical governance subcommittee. Write a one-paragraph application outlining the clinical governance skills, knowledge and values that you currently hold. Following this, write one paragraph describing the gaps in your knowledge and experience and how you will fill them.

References

Akins, R. & Cole, B. (2005). Barriers to implementation of patient safety systems in healthcare institutions: Leadership and policy implications. *Journal of Patient Safety*, *1*(1), 9–16. doi: 10.1097/01209203-200503000-00005

Australian Commission on Safety and Quality in Health Care. (2012a). *Safety and quality improvement guide standard 1: Governance for safety and quality in health service organisations* (Safety and Quality Improvement Guide). Retrieved from http://www. safetyandquality.gov.au/wp-content/uploads/2012/10/Standard1_Oct_2012_WEB1.pdf

——. (2012b). *Safety and quality improvement guide standard 2: Partnering with consumers* (Safety and Quality Improvement Guide). Retrieved from http://www.safetyandquality.gov. au/wp-content/uploads/2012/10/Standard2_Oct_2012_WEB.pdf

——. (2014). *Accreditation and the NSQHS standards.* Retrieved from http://www.
safetyandquality.gov.au/our-work/accreditation-and-the-nsqhs-standards

Australian Institute of Company Directors. (2011). *The board's role in clinical governance.*
Available from http://www.companydirectors.com.au/Director-Resource-Centre/
Publications/Book-Store/PUB59

Australian Institute of Health and Welfare. (2013). *Australia's hospital performance: Adverse
events treated in hospitals.* Retrieved from www.aihw.gov.au/haag11-12/adverse-events

Balding, C. (2008). From quality assurance to clinical governance. *Australian Health Review,*
32(3), 383–391. doi: 10.1071/AH080383

——. (2011). *The strategic quality manager: A handbook for navigating quality management
roles in health and aged care.* Melbourne: Arcade.

Bismark, M., Walter, S. & Studdert, D. (2013). The role of boards in clinical governance: Activities
and attitudes among members of public health service boards in Victoria. *Australian Health
Review, 37*(5), 682–687. doi: 10.1071/AH13125

Dunbar, J., Reddy, P., Beresford, B., Ramsey, W. & Lord, R. (2007). In the wake of hospital
inquiries: Impact on staff and safety. *Medical Journal of Australia, 186*(2), 80–83. Retrieved
from https://www.mja.com.au

Faunce, T. A. & Bolsin, S. N. C. (2004). Three Australian whistleblowing sagas: Lessons for
internal and external regulation. *Medical Journal of Australia, 181*(1), 44–47. Retrieved from
https://www.mja.com.au

Francis, R. (2013). *Press statement.* Retrieved from Mid Staffordshire NHS Foundation Trust
Public Inquiry website: http://www.midstaffspublicinquiry.com/sites/default/files/report/
Chairman%27s%20statement.pdf

Ham, C. (2003). Improving the performance of health services: The role of clinical leadership.
Lancet, 361(9373), 1978–1980. doi: 10.1016/S0140-6736(03)13593-3

Healy, J. & Dugdale, P. (2009). Regulatory strategies for safer patient health care. In J. Healy &
P. Dugdale (Eds), *Patient safety first: Responsive regulation in health care* (pp. 1–23). Crows
Nest: Allen & Unwin.

Jiang, H. J., Lockee, C., Bass, K. & Fraser, I. (2009). Board oversight of quality: Any differences
in process of care and mortality? *Journal of Healthcare Management, 54*, 15–29. Retrieved
from http://www.wsha.org

Mid Staffordshire NHS Foundation Trust Public Inquiry. (2013). *Report of the Mid Staffordshire
NHS Foundation Trust Public Inquiry: Executive summary* (Chaired by R. Francis QC).
Retrieved from Gov.uk website: https://www.gov.uk/government/uploads/system/uploads/
attachment_data/file/279124/0947.pdf

New Zealand Health Quality & Safety Commission. (2013). *Annual report 2012–13.*
Retrieved from http://www.hqsc.govt.nz/assets/General-PR-files-images/Annual-report
-Nov-2013.pdf

Plsek, P. & Greenhalgh, T. (2001). The challenge of complexity in health care. *British Medical
Journal, 323*, 625–628. doi: 10.1136/bmj.323.7313.625

Scally, D. & Donaldson, L. (1998). Clinical governance and the drive for quality improvement in
the new NHS in England. *British Medical Journal, 317*, 61–65. doi: 10.1136/bmj.317.7150.61

Spear, S. & Schmidhofer, M. (2005). Ambiguity and workarounds as contributors to medical
error. *Annals of Internal Medicine, 142*(8), 627–630. doi: 10.7326/0003-4819-142-8
-200504190-00011

Travaglia, J., Hughes, C. & Braithwaite, J. (2011). Learning from disasters to improve patient safety: Applying the generic disaster pathway to health system errors. *Quality and Safety in Health Care*, *20*(1), 1–8. doi: 10.1136/bmjqs.2009.038885

United Kingdom Department of Health. (2001). *The report of the public inquiry into children's heart surgery at the Bristol Royal Infirmary 1984–1995: Learning from Bristol*. London, United Kingdom: Stationery Office.

Walshe, K. & Shortell, S. (2004). When things go wrong: How health care organizations deal with major failures. *Health Affairs*, *23*(3), 103–111. doi: 10.1377/hlthaff.23.3.103

Wilson, R., Runciman, W., Gibberd, R., Harrison, B., Newby, L. & Hamilton, J. (1995). The Quality in Australian Health Care Study. *Medical Journal of Australia*, *163*(9), 458–471.

Wilson, R. & Van Der Weyden, M. (2005). The safety of Australian healthcare: 10 years after QAHCS. *Medical Journal of Australia*, *182*(6), 260–261.

12

Partnering with stakeholders

Sharon Brownie and Audrey Holmes

Learning objectives

How do I:
- understand definitions, rationale, key concepts and public policy associated with stakeholder partnerships in healthcare settings?
- identify stakeholder groups essential to quality health service delivery?
- use the success factors associated with effective partnerships?
- evaluate real-world situations, undertake a stakeholder analysis and recommend key points for stakeholder engagement?
- reflect on the skills associated with developing, formalising and maintaining effective stakeholder partnerships?

Introduction

This chapter outlines how partnering with stakeholders is important for quality health service management and healthcare delivery, and highlights common patterns that drive partnership-based public policy. It also provides an introduction to concepts associated with partnering in health services, defining key terms and discussing the managerial skills or competencies required to engage with stakeholders and implement partnership-based policy. The interests of key stakeholders within the health sector are identified and discussed, and important steps are outlined for a manager undertaking a stakeholder analysis. Finally, the chapter explores the factors essential to successful partnerships and the competencies managers need to successfully develop and maintain stakeholder partnerships.

Definitions

The roots of contemporary whole-of-government and partnership-based public policies are evident in economic development theory dating back 25 years or more

(Brownie, 2007). During the 1990s, a number of leading economic development theorists wrote of networked and associational approaches as being essential for local development and economic success (Cooke & Morgan, 1998; Morgan, 1997; Morgan & Nauwelaers, 1999). In 2001, the Organisation for Economic Co-operation and Development (2001) noted that governments across most of its member countries worked in partnerships involving the public, provider and not-for-profit sectors, plus partners from the wider community.

Today, partnership-based public policy is found in all government health and social services. **Partnership** models are promoted as the ideal ways in which to manage **stakeholder** relationships (Friend, 2006). They have the potential to achieve an **alchemical effect**, which occurs when stakeholders can achieve more working together than they can working individually (Nelson & Zadek, 2000). Examples of this can be found in slogans launching major government strategies, such as the Western Australian Mental Health Commission's (2014) strategic plan Mental Health 2020: Making It Personal and Everybody's Business.

Partnership
A group of two or more organis‹ working collaboratively to pursu‹ achieve common goals and obje‹

Stakeholder
'Anybody who can affect or is a‹ by an organisation, strategy or ‹ (Morphy, n.d., para. 2)

Alchemical effect
'Participants seek to achieve mc‹ the sum of their individual parts‹ creating leverage and synergy b‹ and between key components c‹ partnership' (Nelson & Zadek, 2‹ p. 15)

Importance of stakeholder partnerships

Health service demand is rising because of factors such as ageing populations, rising levels of chronic and non-communicable disease, environmental health concerns and public expectations of longer and healthier lives. Human and financial resources are limited. **Collaboration**, in the form of collaborative partnerships, is recognised as an effective means of addressing complex healthcare problems and issues of service coordination and healthcare demand (Beatty, Harris & Barnes, 2010; Brownie, Thomas, McAllister & Groves, 2014; Conway et al., 2006; Daley, 2009).

The need for improved coordination of services is a central theme driving current health service reform (National Health and Hospitals Reform Commission, 2009; Brownie et al., 2014). The term **wicked problems** is used to describe difficult health and social problems that are hard to define, unstable, without a clear solution, and socially and politically complex. In order to be resolved, they require significant changes in individual and population behaviours (Australian Public Service Commission, 2007; Head & Alford, 2013; Termeer, Dewulf, Breeman & Stiller, 2013).

Collaboration
'A process through which parties see different aspects of a proble‹ constructively explore their diffe‹ and search for solutions that go beyond their own limited vision [‹ or resources] of what is possible' 1989, p. 5)

Wicked problems
Difficulties that 'have many interdependencies and are often multi-causal' and cause issues as are 'highly resistant to resolution‹ (Australian Public Service Comm‹ 2007, pp. iii, 3)

It is widely accepted that improvement in these issues requires the cooperation and input of multiple parties. This means that delivery of improved healthcare depends on the capacity and willingness of different partners to work together (National Health and Hospitals Reform Commission, 2009; McMurray, 2006). Partnering with stakeholders has a number of benefits, including increased and streamlined access to services, cost efficiencies and avoidance of duplication. By working together, partners can also develop creative solutions to difficult barriers or obstacles. Partnerships are means by which policies and programs can be more flexible and health services more responsive to community and health service user needs (Laffin & Liddle, 2006; Taylor & Thompson, 2011).

Nests of wellness

Providing consistent access to high-quality, timely and affordable care is particularly challenging in rural communities. Innovative collaborative partnerships can overcome demographic and geographic barriers to provide health and social services.

A general practitioner in a remote New Zealand community was nationally recognised for his leadership, vision and advocacy in healthcare, including his work in developing a low-cost health clinic to make basic healthcare accessible in an area where access was difficult, working in partnership with schools and other stakeholders to establish a full-time school-based health clinic and establishing a 'well home' initiative in which run-down homes were repaired on the basis that wellness begins in warm, safe homes. Even though these initiatives were a result of individual passion, vision and drive, they depended on the development of interagency and cross-sector relationships and partnerships for implementation and ongoing success.

Similarly, in Western Australia, the WA Cystic Fibrosis Model of Care was developed to deliver services across the continuum of care to people with cystic fibrosis nearer to their homes. It incorporated a number of service components, including co-care, self-management, transition from paediatric to adult services, and outreach. These factors depended on well-developed partnerships between public, private and non-government organisation services to provide care and support to people with cystic fibrosis and their families across urban and rural areas. Central to this partnership were consumers and their families, with continuous liaison ensuring that care was delivered to the right people at the right time and in the right place.

Stakeholder groups in healthcare

Consumers

A key stakeholder partnership in any health system is between healthcare professionals, or service providers, and the people who use health services. The terminology describing users of health services varies and includes patients, clients, service users and consumers. For the purpose of this chapter we refer to health service users as consumers.

Meaningful partnerships with consumers within a model of patient-centred care are now an expected aspect of quality health services (NHS Choices, 2012). An effective partnership allows the consumer to become active in their own care and participate in decision-making processes. However, for these partnerships to be truly collaborative, consumers may need to be educated and supported into a more active role (Doss, DePascal & Hadley, 2011).

Establishing and maintaining a partnership between health professionals and consumers takes time and effort on both sides (Doss et al., 2011). Effective and appropriate communication is essential. Like any partnership, collaboration must be based on shared understanding, trust and respect. Considerations include incorporating consumer perspectives, knowledge and values into planning and delivering care; sharing information openly and in a way that encourages participation; and supporting consumers and their families or caregivers to participate as much or as little as they wish (Conway et al., 2006). Meaningful partnerships also involve inviting consumer collaboration on the development and implementation of health policy and programs, as well as service design and delivery. This can encourage quality improvement and can be effective at local, national and global levels (Crawford et al., 2002; Kotter, Schaefer, Scherer & Blozik, 2013). Committed providers develop ways for consumers and families to be involved at different levels and offer relevant training and support for individual consumers (Conway et al., 2006).

Families and caregivers

The health status of many consumers is often maintained through extensive support from family members and other caregivers (Barrow & Harrison, 2005). Partnering with consumers requires partnership with families and other caregivers (Crawford et al., 2002), and such collaborative partnerships can be particularly important for vulnerable and dependent consumers, such as children or the elderly, and those with chronic or other health problems that require high use of health services. Family and caregiver involvement is also important for consumers from vulnerable populations, such as those living with mental illness or intellectual disability (Wallcraft et al., 2011). These partnerships can be complex, due to challenges such as when both the consumer and the caregiver age; often, there is no alternative family member able to provide care as the carer becomes increasingly in need of supporting health services (Walker & Ward, 2013; Yorke, 2013). Key components of successful partnerships with families and caregivers include mutual respect and consideration, good communication, sharing information and joint decision-making.

Well-developed partnerships between healthcare professionals and families and caregivers result in significant improvements in health outcomes and events. For example, a systematic review by Kuhlthau et al. (2011) found that partnerships between health professionals and the families of children with special needs are associated with improved health outcomes, including better access, communication and efficiency. Partnering with family and caregivers can increase understanding of the individual consumer's needs, develop knowledge of their specific health concerns and provide a basis for shared participation in care and decision-making. In addition, families have unique knowledge about the consumer; they understand the consumer's personal and social context and how their health concerns impact their daily life. They can assist the consumer in communicating with health professionals and assist the health professional in communicating with the consumer. This means the consumer is better supported throughout their healthcare experience.

Research collaborators

Compared with medical research, health services research is a relatively new science. Traditionally, research in hospitals was the domain of academic clinicians, and research tended to have a clinical focus. Increasingly, the focus has shifted to health service and health outcomes research (Dimick & Greenberg, 2014). The phrase 'better research – better healthcare' is now well known (Evans, Thornton, Chalmers & Glasziou, 2011), and commitment to patient wellbeing and safety has become paramount (Kronick, 2014). Against this backdrop, partnerships among academic researchers, health service providers and policy-makers are increasingly active.

Commonly identified areas for health service research include prevention of hospital-acquired infections, reduction of medication error rates, strategies for reducing harm in labour and delivery, prevention of falls and improving safety in nursing homes, and other areas of patient dissatisfaction or hospital error. This is driven by 'a requirement for a strong clinical evidence base to ensure patient safety and effective practice across biomedical, complementary and integrative health care settings' (Adams, Sommers & Robinson, 2013, p. 1).

Whole-of-government collaborators

Collaborative interagency partnerships are increasingly important in addressing healthcare complexity and entwined health and social issues (Head & Alford, 2013). Slogans such as 'Mental Health Is Everybody's Business' highlight the need for collaboration and service coordination across all government departments, including health, housing, police, social welfare and more. Recent Australian health reforms are based on the understanding that well-coordinated, integrated continuity of care is central to effective health systems, especially for those serving consumers with multiple, ongoing and complex conditions (National Health and Hospitals Reform Commission, 2009; National Health Workforce Taskforce, 2010).

While the mandate for whole-of-government partnerships and collaboration is clear, implementing such partnerships is complex and challenging (Australian Public Service Commission, 2007; Brownie et al., 2014). Structural reform can provide part of the solution, but success also depends on fundamental changes in the way in which health professionals form working partnerships to deliver services.

Success factors in stakeholder partnerships

The success of a partnership depends on several factors: strong leadership, a clearly defined purpose with realistic goals and objectives, and a high level of participation and input from all partners are central to success.

Good, timely communication is particularly important for the success of a partnership. Channels or mechanisms for communication need to reflect the different internal structures and information needs of each partner. To reach all partners, communication may therefore need to be in multiple forms or styles. A strategically focused communication plan is an essential tool, as it ensures that information flows within and between partnering organisations as well as to and from stakeholders outside the partnership.

Trust and respect are also important factors for successful partnerships (Daley, 2009). Within a partnership they allow partners to work alongside one another towards common goals, encourage input and participation, and facilitate sharing of resources and responsibilities. A genuine partnership is based on an understanding that each partner has something to contribute and implies that the risks and benefits are shared. Trust and respect between partners allow partnering organisations to gain from the partnership without compromising partnership goals. To achieve this, all partners must be committed to reciprocity, equity and recognition of the independence of partner organisations (Zafar-Ullah, Newell, Ahmed, Hyder & Islam, 2006).

A partnership structure must be robust and have the flexibility to adapt to meet changing needs as the partnership progresses. The frequency of interactions between partners and clear definition of roles and expectations, both internal and external, are central to a partnership's success (Beatty et al., 2010). All partners must work to establish a shared understanding of the underlying purpose of the partnership, and all parties must be committed to the partnership. Partnership structures need to be transparent and to allow shared planning, implementation and evaluation; the partnership also needs sufficient human and financial resources (Taylor & Thompson, 2011). Partners must understand how to jointly make decisions within the partnership structure (Grudinschi et al., 2013).

Management and stakeholder partnerships

The concept of stakeholder partnerships is easy to talk about but difficult to put into action; 'partnerships are sometimes compared to a "black box": inputs and outputs are visible, but the mechanisms enabling the transformation from input to output are not' (Organisation for Economic Co-operation and Development, 2001, p. 18). On their own, traditional management competencies are not sufficient to respond to increased interagency collaboration and partnership with stakeholders.

In his book *Getting agencies to work together: The practice and theory of managerial craftsmanship*, Eugene Bardach (1998) outlines how managers need to develop individual and organisational interagency collaborative capacity, described as 'managerial craftsman-ship'. This concept has been expanded by other writers, with Friend (2006, p. 270) describing how managers need to engage in 'responsible scheming' – for example, map-ping changing structures and relationship patterns among stakeholders and partnering agencies. Getting things done when you are not in charge and being able to influence when you do not have authority are additional competencies necessary for effective stakeholder engagement. This is because power held through a role in one organisation may not be relevant in a partnership context (Bellman, 2001; Cohen & Bradford, 2005; Middleton, 2007).

The range of skills needed by health service managers is outlined by Termeer et al. (2013), who identify four characteristics managers need to address complex or wicked problems specifically:

Reflexivity   capability to deal with multiple issues

Resilience   capability to adjust in demanding and changing circumstances

Responsiveness   capability to respond to changing expectations and agendas

Revitalisation   capability to unblock stagnations.

Another good skill for managers to have is cultural intelligence: being able to work across geographic and cultural boundaries, with different age groups and with people of differ-ent ethnicities and beliefs (Middleton, 2014).

A good manager recognises the impact stakeholders can have in helping or hinder-ing service development and delivery. They understand that knowing their stakehold-ers and establishing sound communication plans increase the chance of successfully

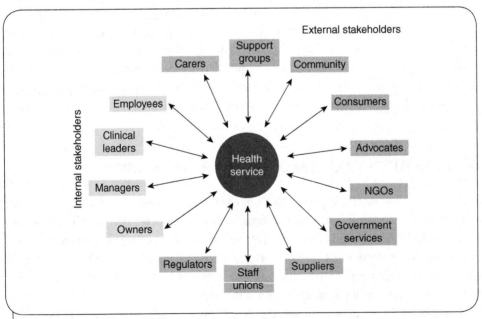

Figure 12.1 Internal and external stakeholders

achieving their objectives. Stakeholder analysis and management are therefore key tools for managers. Morphy (n.d.) recommends a systematic four-step approach to identifying and engaging with stakeholders: stakeholder identification, stakeholder analysis, communication-planning and engagement.

When identifying stakeholders, it helps to think about whether they are internal or external stakeholders (see Figure 12.1). Specific strategies may be needed to gain the interest, involvement and commitment of different stakeholders (Debono, Travaglia, Sarrami-Foroushani & Braithwaite, 2013). One size does not fit all, so it is important to consider the needs and characteristics of each stakeholder.

Health service managers need to get to know the specific interests of each stakeholder group, including the ability of each stakeholder to influence the organisation. A simple guide for stakeholder analysis is to ask the following questions: What are they most interested in? What are their biggest concerns? Who can they influence and what is their potential impact? What do we need to do to get their support?

Leadership and stakeholder partnerships

Leadership roles in collaborative partnerships differ from traditional organisational leadership roles (Nowell & Harrison, 2011). Partnerships are centred on cooperation between organisations and often aim to address complex problems. Different sectors (such as health, social services and education) or different stakeholder groups (such as government, service providers and the community) may need to be involved. This means that different cultures, needs and points of view must be considered and aligned.

Leadership within a partnership draws together stakeholders with different levels of resources and expertise. Leaders need to keep the big picture in mind and ensure the focus remains on the shared vision or goals. Leaders must be able to clearly communicate these goals, work to direct partnership resources and action, and obtain any necessary support from outside the partnership. Effective leaders should also understand sharing of power, whereby all partners can influence goals and outcomes by contributing expertise. This power-sharing helps to foster joint ownership and collective responsibility (Alexander et al., 2001).

Leadership within a partnership can be neutral, with leaders having few ties to partner organisations and no agenda outside the partnership goals. This allows all partners to have an equal voice and representation, irrespective of differences in available resources or standing in the community. Leadership can also use a distributed model, in which all partners participate, or an equity-based model, which assumes all partners' views are respected but that influence depends on each partner's financial support of the partnership. To be effective and ensure stakeholder engagement, leaders of partnerships need to develop a unique set of skills, including strong interpersonal and communication skills, to encourage input and participation across all partners.

Summary

- Partnering with stakeholders is essential for quality health service delivery.
- Partnership success factors include strong leadership, a clearly defined purpose with realistic goals and objectives, and a high level of participation with input from all partners.
- Identifying key stakeholders in the health service, department or organisation is essential, as is determining the various interests of these stakeholders and how best to interact with them.
- Leaders and managers must possess reflexivity, resilience, responsiveness, revitalisation and cultural intelligence skills and attitudes to work well with stakeholders.

Reflective questions

1 Who are the stakeholders of importance to your role as a health service manager, and can you describe their priority issues and concerns?

2 How much do you know about your stakeholders, their level of influence and their potential impact on the viability and effectiveness of your service? Do you have the knowledge to complete a simple stakeholder analysis worksheet?

3 Consider ways in which you can find out about your stakeholder concerns and interests and reflect these in your practice.

4 Can you think of a time when you were working on an issue with a stakeholder but using different terminology to refer to the same concept? How did it impact on the achievement of your mutual goals? How did you work through it?

5 Can you think of a time when your relationship with a key stakeholder has gone badly wrong? What were the contributing factors, and how did you respond to and salvage the situation?

Self-analysis questions

As a health service manager, how satisfied are you with the level and quality of your engagement with both internal and external stakeholders? When considering your skills in stakeholder identification, analysis and engagement, which areas of competency improvement are you able to identify, and how will you address these?

References

Adams, J., Sommers, E. & Robinson, N. (2013). Public health and health services research in integrative medicine: An emerging, essential focus. *European Journal of Integrative Medicine*, 5(1), 1–3. doi: 10.1016/j.eujim.2012.11.004

Alexander, J. A., Comfort, M.E., Weiner, B. J., & Bogue, R. (2001). Leadership in collaborative community health partnerships. *Nonprofit Management and Leadership*, 12(2), 159–175. Retrieved from http://tamarackcommunity.ca/downloads/CCI_downloads/cl_comhealthpartners.pdf

Australian Public Service Commission. (2007). *Tackling wicked problems: A public policy perspective* (Contemporary Government Challenges) [Discussion document]. Retrieved from http://www.apsc.gov.au/__data/assets/pdf_file/0005/6386/wickedproblems.pdf

Bardach, E. (1998). *Getting agencies to work together: The practice and theory of managerial craftsmanship*. Washington, DC: Brookings Institution.

Barrow, S. & Harrison, R. A. (2005). Unsung heroes who put their lives at risk? Informal caring, health and neighbourhood attachment. *Journal of Public Health, 27*(3), 292–297. doi: 10.1093/pubmed/fdi038

Beatty, K., Harris, J. K. & Barnes, P. A. (2010). The role of interorganizational partnerships in health services provision among rural, suburban, and urban local health departments. *The Journal of Rural Health, 26*(3), 248–258. doi: 10.1111/j.1748-0361.2010.00285.x

Bellman, G. (2001). *Getting things done when you are not in charge*. New York, NY: Berret-Koehler.

Brownie, S. (2007). *From policy to practice: The New Zealand experience in implementation partnership-based local development policy* (Doctoral dissertation, Charles Sturt University). Available from www.researchgate.net

Brownie, S., Thomas, J., McAllister, L. & Groves, M. (2014). Australian health reforms: Enhancing interprofessional practice and competency within the health workforce. *Journal of Interprofessional Care, 28*(3), 252–253. doi: 10.3109/13561820.2014.881790

Cohen, A. R. & Bradford, D. L. (2005). *Influence without authority*. Hoboken, NJ: Wiley.

Conway, J., Johnson, B., Edgman-Levitan, S., Schlucter, J., Ford, D., SodomkaP. & Simmons, L. (2006). *Partnering with patients and families to design a patient- and family-centered health care system: A roadmap for the future; A work in progress* [Report]. Retrieved from Institute for Patient- and Family-Centered Care website: http://www.ipfcc.org/pdf/Roadmap.pdf

Cooke, P. & Morgan, K. (1998). *The associational economy: Firms, regions, and innovation*. Oxford, United Kingdom: Oxford University.

Crawford, M. J., Rutter, D., Manley, C., Weaver, T., Bhui, K., Fulop, N. & Tyrer, P. (2002). Systematic review of involving patients in the planning and development of health care. *British Medical Journal, 325*(1263). doi: 10.1136/bmj.325.7375.1263

Daley, D. M. (2009). Interdisciplinary problems and agency boundaries: Exploring effective cross-agency collaboration. *Journal of Public Administration Research & Theory, 19*(3), 477–493. doi: 10.1093/jopart/mun020

Debono, D., Travaglia, J., Sarrami-Foroushani, P. & Braithwaite, J. (2013). *Consumer engagement in the agency for clinical innovation (ACI): Key stakeholder perspectives*. Retrieved from NSW Agency for Clinical Innovation website: http://www.aci.health.nsw.gov.au/__data/assets/pdf_file/0008/195830/ACI-AIHI_Community_Engagement_Research_Study.pdf

Dimick, J. B. & Greenberg, C. C. (2014). An introduction to health services research. In J. B. Dimick & C. C. Greenberg. *Success in academic surgery* (pp. 3–8). London, United Kingdom: Springer.

Doss, S., DePascal, P. & Hadley, K. (2011). Patient-nurse partnerships. *Nephrology Nursing Journal, 38*, 115–126.

Evans, I., Thornton, H., Chalmers, I. & Glasziou, P. (2011). *Testing treatments: Better research for better health care*. London, United Kingdom: Pinter & Martin.

Friend, J. (2006). Partnership meets politics: Managing within the maze. *International Journal of Public Sector Management, 19*(3), 261–277. doi: 10.1108/09513550610658222

Gray, B. (1989). *Collaborating: Finding common ground for multiparty problems*. San Francisco, CA: Jossey-Bass.

Grudinschi, D., Kaljunen, L., Hokkanen, T., Hallikas, J., Sintonen, S. & Puustinen, A. (2013). Management challenges in cross-sector collaboration: Elderly care case study. *The Innovation Journal, 18*(2), 1–22.

Head, B. W. & Alford, J. (2013). Wicked problems: Implications for public policy and management. *Administration & Society, 20*(10), 1–29. doi: 10.1177/0095399713481601

Kotter, T., Schaefer, F. A., Scherer, M. & Blozik, E. (2013). Involving patients in quality indicator development: A systematic review. *Patient Preference and Adherence, 7*, 259–268. doi: 10.2147/PPA.S39803

Kronick, R. (2014). Patient safety: The agency for health care research and quality's ongoing commitment. *Journal of Nursing Care Quality, 29*(3), 195–199.

Kuhlthau, K. A., Bloom, S., Van Cleave, J., Knapp, A. A., Romm, D., Klatka, C. J. … Perrin, J. M. (2011). Evidence for family-centered care for children with special health care needs: A systematic review. *Academic Paediatrics, 11*(2), 136–143. doi: 10.1016/j.acap.2010.12.014

Laffin, M. & Liddle, J. (2006). New perspectives on partnership (special issue). *International Journal of Public Sector Management, 19*(3), 224–227.

McMurray, R. (2006). From partition to partnership: Managing collaboration within a curative framework for NHS care. *International Journal of Public Sector Management, 19*(3), 238–249. doi: 10.1108/09513550610658204

Middleton, J. (2007). *Beyond authority: Leadership in a changing world.* New York, NY: Palgrave McMillan.

——. (2014). *Cultural intelligence: CQ: The competitive edge for leaders crossing borders.* London, United Kingdom: Bloomsbury.

Morgan, K. (1997). The learning region: Institutions, innovation and regional renewal. *Regional Studies, 31*, 491–503. doi: 10.1080/00343409750132289

Morgan, K. & Nauwelaers, C. (1999). *Regional innovation strategies: The challenge for less-favoured regions.* London, United Kingdom: Stationery Office.

Morphy, T. (n.d.). *Stakeholder definition.* Retrieved from http://www.stakeholdermap.com/stakeholder-definition.html

National Health and Hospitals Reform Commission. (2009). *A healthier future for all Australians: Final report of the national health and hospitals reform commission* (Chaired by Dr C. Bennett) [Commission report]. Retrieved from http://www.health.gov.au/internet/nhhrc/publishing.nsf/Content/1AFDEAF1FB76A1D8CA257600000B5BE2/$File/Final_Report_of_the%20nhhrc_June_2009.pdf

National Health Workforce Taskforce. (2010). *Final report: Acute aged care interface workforce competencies project, education and training.* Melbourne: Author.

Nelson, J. & Zadek, S. (2000). *Partnership alchemy: New social partnerships in Europe* [Report]. Retrieved from Simon Zadek website: http://www.zadek.net/wp-content/uploads/2011/04/Copenhagen-Centre_Partnership_Alchemy_New-Social-Partnerships-in-Europe_2000.pdf

NHS Choices. (2012, December 18). *New NHS planning guidance puts patient first.* Retrieved from http://www.nhs.uk/news/2012/12December/Pages/New-NHS-planning-guidance-puts-patient-first.aspx

Nowell, B. & Harrison, L. M. (2011). Leading change through collaborative partnerships: A profile of leadership and capacity among local public health leaders. *Journal of Prevention & Intervention in the Community, 39*(1), 19–34. doi: 10.1080/10852352.2011.530162

Organisation for Economic Co-operation and Development. (2001). *Local partnerships for better governance*. Paris, France: Author.

Taylor, K. P. & Thompson, S. (2011). Closing the (service) gap: Exploring partnerships between Aboriginal and mainstream health services. *Australian Health Review, 35*(3), 297–308. doi: 10.1071/AH10936

Termeer, C., Dewulf, A., Breeman, G. & Stiller, S. J. (2013). Governance capabilities for dealing wisely with wicked problems. *Administration & Society*, (January). doi: 10.1177/0095399712469195

Walker, C. & Ward, C. (2013). Growing older together: Ageing and people with learning disabilities and their family carers. *Tizard Learning Disability Review, 18*(3), 112–119. doi: 10.1108/TLDR-02-2013-0018

Wallcraft, J., Amering, M., Freidin, J., Davar, B., Froggatt, D., Jafri, H. … Herrman, H. (2011). Partnerships for better mental health worldwide: WPA recommendations on best practices in working with service users and family carers. *World Psychiatry, 10*(3), 229–236.

Western Australia Mental Health Commission. (2014). *Mental Health 2020: Making it personal and everybody's business* (Strategy document). Retrieved from http://www.mentalhealth. wa.gov.au/Libraries/pdf_docs/Mental_Health_Commission_strategic_plan_2020.sflb.ashx

Yorke, M. (2013). Some personal consequences for the carer. In C. Proot & M. Yorke, *Life to be lived: Challenges and choices for patients and carers in life-threatening illnesses* (pp. 65–72). Oxford, United Kingdom: Oxford University.

Zafar-Ullah, A. N., Newell, J. N., Ahmed, J. U., Hyder, M. K. A. & Islam, A. (2006). Government–NGO collaboration: The case of tuberculosis control in Bangladesh. *Health Policy and Planning, 21*(2), 143–155. doi: 10.1093/heapol/czj014

13

Power and political astuteness

Nicola McNeil

Learning objectives

How do I:
- understand the use of power in organisations?
- identify the main sources of power in organisations?
- critically analyse the positive and negative aspects of power and influence?
- understand how political processes operate in organisations?
- understand the consequences of political activities in organisations?
- enhance my skills in the various tactics that can be used to shape political outcomes in organisations?

Introduction

Politics is an inevitable feature of organisation life, particularly in large bureaucratic organisations such as hospitals. Political activities arise when there is a lack of consensus about how an organisation should be managed. They are typically employed in an attempt to reconcile these divergent interests, which may be the result of competition for resources within the organisation, the pursuit of personal goals by individuals or a high level of uncertainty within the organisation.

Traditionally, political activities have been concerned with obtaining, developing and exploiting power to influence others in order to achieve desired outcomes (Pfeffer, 1981). Consequently, decisions shaped by political activities are not always rational – they do not always produce optimum outcomes, as individuals seek to satisfy their own wants and needs, often at the expense of others (Kumar & Ghadially, 1989). However, more recently, organisational behaviourists have conceptualised organisational politics as the *perception* that an individual or group is using influence and tactics to serve their own personal agenda (Ferris & Kacmar, 1992). One person may consider a co-worker's behaviour to be a typical rational response, whereas another colleague may view the same behaviour as self-serving and highly political. Therefore, what is deemed to be political or normal behaviour ultimately depends on the opinion of the observer.

Definitions

At the core of any politics is the exercise of power and influence. Researchers argue that an understanding of power – where it comes from and how it can be used – is crucial to achieving both personal and organisational goals (Runde & Flanagan, 2007). There are several ways of viewing the idea of **power**: it can be seen as a characteristic that an individual possesses or as something that is generated by social relations. However, power is most commonly defined as the ability to change another's behaviour or to influence others: holders of power generally exert their power to attain an outcome they desire (Astley & Sachdeva, 1984). That is, a person has power over another when they are able to get them to do something they would not otherwise have done (Dahl, 1957).

> **Power**
> An agent's ability to influence th

Relationships of power exist where there is a perceived dependency between two or more people in an organisation. For example, a manager may appear to control vital information or resources that are needed by others in the organisation. This need for information or resources creates a dependency on the manager, which in turn leads to the manager having power over the others.

Authority

Power is not the same as **authority**. Pfeffer (1978) argues that authority is a unique manifestation of power. He suggests that authority stems from an individual's place in the hierarchy; therefore, authority is attached to a position in the hierarchy, rather than to an individual. So position-holders within an organisation can use the authority vested in their position to make decisions and shape outcomes.

> **Authority**
> A unique manifestation of powe
> attached to a position in the hier
> rather than to an individual (Pfe
> 1978)

There are a few important points to note about authority. Firstly, subordinates typically comply with the instructions of their supervisors or managers because they recognise that the authority they hold is legitimate. Secondly, authority is reflected in the organisational hierarchy and is devolved down the chain of command of an organisation, with more authority being vested in positions at the top of the hierarchy. Power is not confined to positions of authority. For example, a nurse may exercise power over their supervisor: there may be a relationship of dependence between the two that results in the nurse being able to shape the behaviour of her supervisor. Thus, power can be exercised in any direction in the hierarchy – up, down or horizontally – that is, between units in the organisation.

Sources of power

French and Raven (1959) identify two main sources of individual power: power that is derived from the position an individual holds in the organisational hierarchy, or position power (which includes legitimate, reward and coercive power); and power that stems from an individual's characteristics, or their personal power (which includes expert and referent power).

Legitimate power

Legitimate power is derived from the authority vested in an individual by virtue of the position they hold within the organisation. The source of this power is based on the idea of legitimate authority, which is conferred on an individual who occupies a particular position. For example, a charge nurse will typically have legitimate power over subordinates, as part of their job description will require them to direct and monitor the behaviour of the nursing staff they supervise.

> **ate power**
> rived from the authority vested
> vidual by virtue of the position
> within the organisation

However, the effective exercise of this power relies upon the willingness of the subordinates to accept someone's authority over them (Giddens, 1997; Hardy & Clegg, 1996). For example, the power of a nurse manager to make a nurse change their working hours to suit a roster depends on the willingness of the nurse to agree to such an arrangement.

There are a few other interesting points to note about legitimate power. Firstly, an individual will surrender this source of power when they vacate the position. Secondly, legitimate power is limited in its scope, as it applies to work-related situations. For example, a chief executive officer would not have legitimate power over how an employee spent their leisure time or how they might spend their discretionary income.

Reward power

Reward power concerns the capacity to reward employees (or to withhold rewards or privileges). It is held by an individual who has the ability to confer promotions, financial rewards, leave or praise to employees. For example, the dean of a faculty of medicine holds reward power: they have the ability to allot bonuses to high-performing staff, award citations for high-quality teaching and research, and promote and provide opportunities to deserving staff.

> **power**
> acity to reward employees

In some respects, reward power is similar to legitimate power, in that the ability to reward individuals is tied to a position in the hierarchy; for example, a chief executive officer or general manager can offer rewards, but a co-worker cannot.

The use of reward power is an important element in understanding how to motivate employees. If the reward being offered is highly valued by employees, reward power will be strong. Conversely, reward power will be weakened when the rewards offered have little appeal for employees.

Coercive power

Coercive power results from the ability to rebuke employees for inappropriate behaviours and actions. Exercising this power can result in chastising, demoting or terminating the employment of subordinates. In certain circumstances it may be necessary to use coercive power to stem inappropriate, unethical or illegal behaviour of employees. For example, if an employee repeatedly refuses to follow health and safety protocols, which endangers not only themselves but patients and other co-workers, it may be appropriate for a supervisor to exert their coercive power to quash such behaviours.

> **Coercive power**
> Power resulting from the ability rebuke employees for inappropr behaviours and actions

Expert power

Expert power stems from a person's high level of knowledge and skill in a given area. When an individual demonstrates their expertise, their thoughts and recommendations will be given more credibility, and they are more likely to be trusted and respected by others. People may be persuaded to follow suggestions and instructions because they defer to a higher level of understanding.

> **Expert power**
> Power stemming from a person's level of knowledge and skill in a area

Marie Curie, who discovered the chemical elements radium and polonium and pioneered research into the treatment of tumours using radiation, had expert power. Her contributions to chemistry and medical research were recognised by the award of a Nobel Prize in both chemistry and physics. Prior to her death in 1934, Curie was able to use her expert power to attract funding and other resources to continue her important work, and she also changed the way other researchers conducted their studies (*Marie Curie – Biographical*, 2015).

Referent power

Referent power stems from a person's charisma, likeableness or appeal and the resultant influence this has on others. A prime example of referent power is the influence that celebrity endorsements have on our purchasing behaviour. For example, consider the recent growth in celebrity-branded fragrances, including perfumes by Beyoncé, David Beckham, Kim Kardashian, Britney Spears and Kylie

> **Referent power**
> Power stemming from a person's charisma, likeableness or appeal

Minogue. Consumers may strongly identify with these celebrities and be persuaded to purchase the perfumes they endorse.

In the work environment, an employee with charisma or appeal may find they have considerable influence over others who respect or wish to please them. The obvious danger of referent power is that someone who is affable or charismatic may acquire significant power in the organisation without having the requisite authority or knowledge to use this power effectively.

Use of power

While an individual may possess power, it does not necessarily mean that they will be able to influence the behaviour of others. Hickson, Hinings, Lee, Schneck and Pennings (1971) argue that the effective exercise of power is influenced by external factors, or contingencies, which can advance or impede the use of power by an individual or a department. Hickson and his colleagues identify uncertainty, substitutability and centrality as the main contingencies of power.

Uncertainty

Uncertainty refers to a lack of information about events that may impact on an organisation in the future. This may include scarcity of information about the availability of resources, changes to government regulations or laws, actions of competitors or viability of existing markets. Where there is uncertainty in the business environment, organisational planning becomes more difficult, as contingency plans must be made to address all possible eventualities. Pfeffer (1981) argues that the most valued skill within an organisation is the ability to protect organisational members from uncertainty.

> **_inty_**
> or no understanding of
> ge or information regarding a
> te or situation

Hickson et al. (1971) suggest, however, that it is the ability to cope with sources of uncertainty that generates power, rather than uncertainty itself. Pfeffer and Salancik (1978) build on this idea by explaining the link between an organisation's environment and its political processes. They argue that the environment poses uncertainty for an organisation in terms of constraints, contingencies and resources. This in turn produces a need for someone to cope with this uncertainty on behalf of the organisation. The ability to cope is translated into power within the organisation.

Therefore, Pfeffer and Salancik (1978) argue, there is a direct relationship between the distribution of environmental uncertainty and the distribution of power within an organisation. Those individuals or departments who can cope with such uncertainty garner power and influence within the organisation. The ability to manage uncertainty in turn creates certainty for others and creates power through the dependencies created.

Shifting power bases in modern healthcare

There is little doubt that many government-funded healthcare providers are under increasing pressure from government and other stakeholders to operate with maximum efficiency and accountability. This shift has had a significant impact on who manages hospitals, with a rise in non-clinical administrators assuming senior management positions and controlling much of the decision-making, policy development and budget allocations within hospitals.

However, a study by Amanda Goodall (2011) published in *Social Science & Medicine* suggests that hospitals perform better when doctors are in positions of leadership. Julian Le Grant (as cited in Brindle, 2011, July 20, para. 11), professor of social policy at the London School of Economics, attributes these findings to the fact that clinical managers 'command the respect of their colleagues, which is a fundamental problem where chief executives come in from outside'. This suggests that the expert power of clinicians is an important factor in influencing the behaviour of hospital staff.

Substitutability

The degree of control an individual or department has over valuable resources can also affect their power in an organisation. If they have complete control over a highly valued resource – whether it is an expensive piece of medical equipment, money or information – their power over others is heightened. However, if there are alternatives available to replace this important resource or an ability to access it from a different source, the power of the individual or department that holds the asset is diminished. This is referred to as **substitutability**. The dependence on the holder of the asset is reduced because a substitute asset can be found.

> **Substitutability**
> The capability of being replaced

Often, once an individual or department controls a critical resource within the organisation, it is unlikely that they will relinquish this control and dilute their power. For example, a medical college is unlikely to devolve control over the accreditation of hospitals or the training of specialists to third parties, because it would effectively reduce its power and standing.

Centrality

The final contingency that can affect the exercise of power is **centrality**. This concerns the association between the holder of power and the important activities of the organisation. For example, nursing staff are essential to the functioning of a hospital: without nursing staff, the hospital cannot admit, treat

> **Centrality**
> The position of the power-holder in relation to the important activities of the organisation

or discharge patients. Hospital management depend on nursing staff to deliver these key functions; therefore, nurses collectively hold a significant degree of power. However, maintenance staff may not hold the same degree of power over hospital management, because their role is not as central to the operation of a hospital. Moreover, some would argue that maintenance workers are more easily substituted compared to highly skilled nursing staff.

Influence tactics

Merely possessing the ability to alter people's behaviour is different from actually influencing their actions. The question of how the sources of power can be utilised to change behaviour brings us to a discussion of the notion of **influence**: conduct that attempts to modify someone else's attitudes or actions.

:e
e conduct (either positive or
that causes measurable results
5, which may or may not have
·nded, in respect to character,
:cesses and outcomes

Over the last 30 years, studies have identified various tactics that people may use to influence others. A summary of the most commonly identified tactics is presented in Table 13.1, drawing on the work of Kipnis, Schmidt and Wilkinson (1980). Tactics used to influence people can be classified in two broad categories: hard tactics and soft tactics (Kipnis & Schmidt, 1985). Hard tactics rely upon positional sources of power (legitimate, coercion and reward power) as a means to change attitudes and behaviours. Conversely, soft tactics draw on personal power. While hard tactics focus on ways to compel others to behave in a certain way, soft tactics aim for a more gentle means of persuasion.

Kipnis et al. (1980) surveyed over 700 managers and asked them to describe how they influenced their superiors, their co-workers and their subordinates and why they selected this particular approach. The authors found that to influence individuals managers often use different tactics depending on each individual's status within the organisation. For example, the tactic of forming coalitions was primarily used to influence the behaviour of subordinates, while the strategies of exchange and upward appeal were commonly used to influence superiors. Another study, by Falbe and Yukl (1992), examined the effectiveness of using one of multiple tactics to influence others. The researchers conclude that combinations of tactics are generally more effective than using a single tactic and that combinations of hard and soft tactics were more influential than combinations of only hard or only soft tactics.

Authority or sanctions

Authority or sanctions concerns the exercise of legitimate power to generate direct compliance with a request or instruction. The success of this tactic depends to a great extent on the degree of deference shown to this authority (Cialdini & Goldstein,

Table 13.1 Hard and soft influence tactics

Tactic	Description
Hard tactics	
Authority or sanctions	Using legitimate power to direct others' activities
Assertiveness	Placing pressure on others or making threats to shape their behaviour
Coalitions or networks	Developing an alliance and using the combined power of members to influence others
Upward appeal	Garnering the support and favour of others with position and personal power, and using these to influence others
Soft tactics	
Exchange	Pledging something that is valued in exchange for desired behaviours
Ingratiation	Deliberately establishing oneself in the favour or good graces of others
Rationality	Persuading others by using logic, clear evidence and reasoning

Source: Adapted from D. Kipnis, S. M. Schmidt & I. Wilkinson (1980). Intraorganizational influence tactics: Explorations in getting one's way. *Journal of Applied Psychology*, 65(4), 440–452. doi: 10.1037/0021-9010.65.4.440

2004). Some individuals willingly accept a higher degree of unequally distributed power throughout an organisation and will follow the instructions of those in power without question. Others may not be prepared to blindly follow the directions of those in power, and thus other tactics may have to be employed to influence their behaviour.

Assertiveness

Assertiveness involves the application of overt forms of legitimate and coercive power to shape behaviour. This can involve applying pressure on or coercing workers to comply or using reward power to modify the actions of others. This may include threatening an individual's job security or withholding rewards such as promotions or salary increases.

> **Assertiveness**
> The application of overt forms of legitimate and coercive power to behaviour

Coalitions or networks

Another tactic that can be employed to influence others is forming **coalitions** or building networks. A coalition involves assembling an informal group of individuals with a view to using the collective resources of the group members to influence people. These coalitions are likely to exert more influence than an individual acting alone (Cobb, 1991; Hogg & White, 1999; Mannix, 1993).

> **Coalition**
> An informal group of individuals use the collective resources of th members to influence people

Collective action tends to lend significance to an issue, as it indicates that many employees believe the issue is legitimate or support a particular course of action. Also, if people can identify with members of the group, they are more likely to accept the decisions or advice of the group. A study by Douglas and Ammeter (2004) found that belonging to a coalition increased employees' perceptions of the effectiveness of their manager and increased the influence of the manager over their subordinates.

Upward appeal

The final hard tactic is **upward appeal**, which is calling on people with significant positional or personal power for assistance in influencing others. This may involve engaging senior people within the organisational hierarchy or those with high levels of expertise both within and outside the organisation.

appeal people with significant l or personal power for e in influencing others **tion** erate act of trying to gain rom attempting to please or other person **lity** of logic, reliable evidence oned arguments to sway the attitudes and behaviours of **ge** on that people feel obligated to e favour', or give something en they have received a benefit tage (Cialdini, 2001)	## Ingratiation One soft tactic is **ingratiation**, which suggests that influence can be heightened by an individual's being amiable or creating the perception that they have much in common with the person they are trying to influence. Typical examples of ingratiation include admiration or vigorously supporting the views of others. However, some studies show that influence can be diminished when individuals exhibit high levels of ingratiation, as they may be perceived to be disingenuous and manipulative (Strutton, Pelton & Tanner, 1996). ## Rationality Another soft influence tactic is **rationality**, which relies on one's ability to use logic, reliable evidence and reasoned arguments to sway the opinions, attitudes and behaviours of others.

Exchange

Exchange may also be an effective tactic to influence others. It is based on the idea of reciprocity – the notion that people feel obligated to 'return the favour', or to give something back, when they have received a benefit or advantage (Cialdini, 2001). Influence can be exerted through building these exchange relationships and relying on the norm of reciprocity to shape behaviours.

Nurse A could use the exchange tactic to influence Nurse B to cover her shift by reminding Nurse B that she has covered Nurse B's shifts on three previous occasions. Nurse A is relying upon Nurse B to experience some obligation to return the favour and thus agree to cover the shift. Exchange tactics can also be used in senior management negotiations when deciding budget allocations or sharing information.

Increasing power

Political tactics are often used to achieve desired outcomes. However, as noted earlier, these tactics generally rely on individuals possessing some form of power over others. Therefore, the ability to influence the behaviour or attitudes of others is inherently linked to the size of the power base.

How can a person increase their power base? One approach is to create and foster dependencies. If an individual or a department possesses and controls important skills, knowledge, information or materials that are vital to the operation of the organisation, their power is augmented (Pfeffer, 1981). It is likely that those who need access to the resources are likely to acquiesce to any requests or demands made by their holders. Power would be further increased if the resources were scarce, or not substitutable. Another method of increasing power is to work to reduce any areas of uncertainty that the organisation may face. An individual can also increase their importance and power in an organisation by moving into the organisation's critical areas and addressing any problems that may exist therein (Hickson et al., 1971).

Summary

- Political activity is an increasingly important feature of organisational life.
- Political activity in organisations is the process by which individuals debate ideas, challenge assumptions and attempt to ensure that their interests are heard and protected. The ability to influence the behaviours, attitudes and opinions of others is critical to safeguarding such interests.
- The ability to influence others depends on the nature of the power held by an individual. Developing an appreciation of the nature of power and how individuals garner power is vital to understanding political activities within organisations.
- Implementing both hard and soft influence tactics being cognisant of the factors that may encumber the use of power and building strong power bases will contribute to the success of any political activities.

Reflective questions

1 What is power?

2 Discuss the claim that 'power is inherently tied to position in the hierarchy; only managers have power in organisations'.

3 What are the key contingencies that influence the exercise of power? Drawing on your experiences of work or being a student, provide an example of each contingency.

4 How can an individual increase their power within an organisation?

5 Many theorists argue that the basis of all influence can be traced back to the notion of reciprocity – that is, an obligation to return a favour. Can you think of a time when someone did something for you? Did you feel obligated to reciprocate? If that person asked you to do something for them, would you feel compelled to do it?

Self-analysis questions

Consider the following scenario. You are a graduate nurse just starting your first position at a suburban aged care facility. Your nurse manager has asked you to dispense to some residents medication that is not listed on their medication charts. When you question the nurse manager, she instructs you to 'do as she says'. What would you do in this situation? If you refuse to follow the order, what does this suggest about your deference to authority?

References

Astley, W. G. & Sachdeva, P. S. (1984). Structural sources of intra-organisational power: A theoretical synthesis. *Academy of Management Review*, 9(1), 104–113.

Brindle, D. (2011, July 20). Doctors are the best hospital managers, study reveals. *Guardian*. Retrieved from http://www.theguardian.com

Cialdini, R. B. (2001). Harnessing the science of persuasion. *Harvard Business Review*, (October), 72–79.

Cialdini, R. B. & Goldstein, N. J. (2004). Social influence: Compliance and conformity, *Annual Review of Psychology*, 55, 591–621. doi: 10.1146/annurev.psych.55.090902.142015

Cobb, A. T. (1991). Towards a study of organisational coalitions: Participant concerns and activities in a simulated organisational setting. *Human Relations*, 44(10), 1057–1079. doi: 10.1177/001872679104401003

Dahl, R. A. (1957). The concept of power. *Behavioral Science, 2*(3), 201–215. doi: 10.1002/bs.3830020303

Douglas, C. & Ammeter, A. P. (2004). An examination of leader political skill and its effect on ratings of leader effectiveness. *Leadership Quarterly, 15*(4), 537–550. doi: 10.1002/bs.3830020303

Falbe, C. M. & Yukl, G. (1992). Consequences for managers of using single influence tactics and combinations of tactics. *Academy of Management Journal, 35*(3), 638–652. doi: 10.2307/256490

Ferris, G. R. & Kacmar, M. K. (1992). Perceptions of organisational politics. *Journal of Management, 18*(1), 93–116. doi: 10.1177/014920639201800107

French, J. R. P. & Raven, B. H. (1959). The bases of social power. In D. Cartwright (Ed.), *Studies in social power* (pp. 150–167), Ann Arbor, MI: Institute for Social Research.

Giddens, A. (1997). *Sociology* (3rd ed.). Cambridge, United Kingdom: Polity.

Goodall, A. H. (2011). Physician-leaders and hospital performance: Is there an association? *Social Science & Medicine, 73*(4), 535–539. doi: 10.1016/j.socscimed.2011.06.025

Hardy, C. & Clegg, S. R. (1996). Some dare call it power. In S. R. Clegg, C. Hardy & W. R. Nord (Eds), *Handbook of organisational studies* (pp. 622–641). London, United Kingdom: Sage.

Hickson, D. J., Hinings, C. R., Lee, C. A., Schneck, R. E. & Pennings, J. M. (1971). A strategic contingencies theory of intra-organisational power. *Administrative Science Quarterly, 16*(2), 216–229. doi: 10.2307/2391831

Hogg, M. A. & White, K. M. (1999). The theory of planned behaviour: Self-identity, social identity and group norms. *British Journal of Social Psychology, 38*(3), 225–244. doi: 10.1348/014466699164149

Kipnis, D. & Schmidt, S. M. (1985). The language of persuasion. *Psychology Today*, (April), 40–46.

Kipnis, D., Schmidt, S. M. & Wilkinson, I. (1980). Intraorganizational influence tactics: Explorations in getting one's way. *Journal of Applied Psychology, 65*(4), 440–452. doi: 10.1037/0021-9010.65.4.440

Kumar, P. & Ghadially, R. (1989). Organizational politics and its effects on members of organizations. *Human Relations, 42*(4), 305–314. doi: 10.1177/001872678904200402

Mannix, E. A. (1993). Organizations as resource dilemmas: The effects of power balance on coalition formation in small groups. *Organizational Behavior and Human Decision Processes, 55*(1), 1–22. doi: 10.1006/obhd.1993.1021

Marie Curie – Biographical. (2015). Retrieved from http://www.nobelprize.org/

Pfeffer, J. (1978). The micropolitics of organisations. In M. W. Meyer (Ed.), *Environments and organisations* (pp. 29–50). San Fransisco, CA: Jossey-Bass.

——. (1981). *Power in organisations.* Marshfield, MA: Pitman.

Pfeffer, J. & Salancik, G. R. (1978). *The external control of organisations: A resource dependency perspective.* New York, NY: Harper & Row.

Runde, C. E. & Flanagan, T. A. (2007). *Becoming a competent leader: How you and your organisation can manage conflict effectively.* San Francisco, CA: Wiley.

Strutton, D., Pelton, L. E. & Tanner, J. (1996). Shall we gather together in the garden: The effect of ingratiatory behaviours on buyer trust in sales people. *Industrial Marketing Management, 25*(2), 151–162. doi: 10.1006/obhd.1993.1021

14

Influencing strategically

Mark Avery

Learning objectives

How do I:
- develop my skills in respect to influencing tactics and strategies?
- choose key influencing tactics and strategies that might be used in engaging internally in my organisation, as well as outside the organisation?
- understand the importance of influencing strategically as a leader?
- help my department and organisation achieve strategic goals through the use of influencing tactics and strategies?

Introduction

Everyone creates influence during their lives. This may be consciously or unconsciously, through communication, actions or behaviours. A person can be influential through who they are or what they do, such as through their creativity, dependency, vulnerability, position and example.

A critically important element of creating change, growth and renewal in health service organisations is the need for strong and effective leadership, of which influencing skills are an integral part. Healthcare organisations are complex entities with large numbers of internal and external stakeholders. Strategic influence is an important aspect of the leadership and management of these organisations, as leaders and managers rely on the ability to enhance the effectiveness of those working in all parts and levels of the organisations as well as those outside the organisations in the broader system. Healthcare managers can increase their impact and achievements through understanding and applying influence, and key aspects of healthcare leadership relate to the processes of influence.

When they influence to achieve strategic outcomes, leaders and managers work within and across two important areas: transformational change and negotiation. Links between these are important in healthcare leadership and management, as organisational power and personal influence are seen to influence outcomes (Lankshear, Kerr, Spence Laschinger & Wong, 2013).

This chapter explores the issues surrounding influence, particularly as it relates to leadership, management and organisations, as well as how a manager and leader can construct and develop influence to strategically affect projects, initiatives, teams, departments, facilities and organisations.

Definitions

Influence can relate to actions taken but can also be created through individuals or groups as well as in the presence of objects and environments. For example, in negotiating a contract for biomedical equipment acquisition, the health service procurement manager might undertake a competitive tender so as to apply pressure in the marketplace to maximise the benefit of price. Another example might be found in the existence of an extensive training program for new health graduates in a community health service, which may be a key reward factor creating interest in employment in the service.

Strategic influence supports healthcare leaders in influencing others as part of achieving specific and wider goals, objectives and plans for healthcare delivery. Influence is imparted to have impact on others in order to share ideas, concepts, opinions and actions.

> **Influence**
> Deliberate conduct (either positi[ve] [or] negative) that causes measurabl[e] or effects, which may or may no[t] been intended, in respect to cha[nge] aims, processes and outcomes
>
> **Strategic influence**
> Influence tactics and techniques [to] impact the thinking, reasoning, c[hoice] and outcomes of others with key arguments and perspectives to a[chieve] desired results

Using influence

Healthcare organisations and systems are large, complex and connected in different ways. The roles and effectiveness of leaders and managers in the health sector are critical to growth, development, efficiency, effectiveness, quality and safety. The collaborative and connected nature of healthcare, both within health organisations and externally, means that health mangers need to rationally and authentically influence specifically and widely to achieve objectives.

Effective use of influence can affect the behaviours of staff and others in the health system so as to achieve goals and objectives. It aids leaders and managers to engage with and make effective contributions to decision-making processes, as well as allowing them to harness and use their power to maximise engagement and involvement in strategic management processes. Finally, effective influence use helps leaders to be effective in health-related management, as it enables them to understand and manage the resources and constraints of clinical backgrounds experienced by healthcare managers (Spehar, Frich & Kjekshus, 2014).

The ability to work influence, strategy and leadership-enabling activities together forms a critical pathway towards strategic direction and achievement of outcomes. In healthcare, leaders seek to move teams, departments, units and organisations towards outcomes and seeks to change them in relation to the environments in which they work. Key strategic activities for managing organisations include identifying problems and goals, decision-making, planning, positioning, learning and reviewing. These activities are framed and managed through effective strategic leadership and management. Vital in these environments is the translation of ideas, directions and activities through internal and external strategic influence.

Targets

The agent of influence is the individual or group of people attempting to exert influence. In considering the strategic use of influence, the targets of the agent need particular consideration. The targets of influence are the people or groups that the agent is trying to influence. Targets can be people who are experiencing a problem, are engaged in the work of the organisation, are at risk or are in a position to make decisions and act. They can also be people and groups who are contributors to specific issues either through their actions or through their lack of actions.

It is important to remember that a manager's or leader's influence is not limited to their own direct areas of responsibility. Depending on the impact and outcomes that they are trying to effect, they may need to influence downwards, affecting those who work for them (subordinates) and over whom they have direct control and responsibility; upwards, seeking to affect those in higher positions of authority, power and responsibility; and laterally, to their peers – those with similar roles and responsibilities, powers and resources. Healthcare managers and leaders may also need to exert influence externally, in other organisations, in the community and with decision-makers in the healthcare system.

Negotiation

Positional authority or power is insufficient to sustain change in complex organisations with large numbers of internal and external stakeholders. Manning and Robertson (2003) report on two areas of influence tactics: strategist-opportunist and collaborator-battler. Strategist and opportunist tactics include those that use reasoning and partnership to effect change, with opportunistic leaders and managers capitalising on favour and exchange for influence. Collaboration tactics use partnering, and battler tactics use coercive and assertive tactics. Framing one's strategic influence style within one of these areas can be useful, because the impact of one's negotiations is supported by the types of influence strategies used. Consideration of the types of influencing tactics to be used when entering a negotiation can maximise outcomes.

Frameworks for influencing strategically

Tactics

Research and development of influence tactics, approaches and objectives were carried out between 1990 and 2000 by Gary Yukl from the University of Albany, New York. Yukl's formative work provides a sound understanding and expression of key knowledge about leaders' and managers' abilities to influence. The work has been criticised, as the results are difficult to replicate across industry sectors. Other authors have also extended Yukl's list of influencing tactics. However, the influencing tactics reported in the original research offer a useful way of considering how managers might develop their use of influence (Yukl & Chavez, 2002; Yukl & Falbe, 1990). This includes how they might influence others, identify tactics being used on them and frame complex responses when two or more approaches are necessary to achieve a strong influential effect.

Complex problems, situations and operations require a range of responses. In healthcare organisations, it is most likely that influence and influence strategy are not linear in nature or confined to a single approach, as different situations may require different approaches and strategies to bring about the desired outcomes. Over time, recognition of attributes and changes in personnel, or a change in the direction of goals and outcomes, may also require changes in influencing tactics. The following framework of 11 influencing tactics provides a guide for mapping individual approaches to influential leadership and management as well as tactics to support projects and operations (Yukl & Chavez, 2002; Yukl & Falbe, 1990).

Pressure

Pressure tactics support proposals or requests for help. Alignment is achieved through demands, intimidation, frequent requests or regular returning to the issue. Influence can be direct (such as sending emails or other communication requesting support and outlining consequences) or indirect (such as putting a project or service out to public procurement tendering to force competition).

Upward appeals

This approach is designed to leverage seniority in attaining compliance: senior management or a higher authority is invoked in order to persuade involvement or agreement from targets. To create such influence, the agent may only have to imply that senior managers would prefer the options being proposed.

Exchange

Exchange tactics involve offering rewards for compliance to a proposal. They can also involve connecting the current proposal to a past favour to be reciprocated.

Coalition

These tactics involve seeking the support or involvement of targets to work on an issue in partnership so as to persuade more targets to give support to the proposal.

Ingratiation

The agent causes the target to think favourably of them or creates an atmosphere of goodwill and connectivity as a prelude to asking for support for a proposal. The agent may activate a relationship or remind the target of a previous relationship or assistance as a mechanism for building connections in order to place the new proposal within that positive relationship.

Rational persuasion

With this approach, the agent provides a factual or evidence-based argument to highlight as the main focus the viability of the proposal to garner support.

Inspirational appeals

The agent appeals to values or ideals to increase the target's confidence in a proposal through the use of emotion, enthusiasm or excitement.

Consultation

The agent gains the target's involvement in the decision-making and planning for a project and thereby creates a situation of target engagement, through which they can work to ensure the target's further involvement.

Legitimation

This approach secures trust in a proposal by connecting it to policies, procedures, rules or other dependable sources inside and outside the organisation.

Apprisement

The agent explains the proposal in a way that shows how it will benefit the target: personal gain and value are highlighted as the results of the target's acceptance of the proposal.

Collaboration

Assistance is offered to the target in return for their acceptance of the proposal, and value alignments between the agent and the target are proposed in return for the distribution of influence to other targets.

Influencing from within a clinical team

The nurse unit manager on a busy oncology ward in a regional acute hospital suggests at a ward nursing unit team meeting that one staff member should take on the role of quality assurance team leader. Christine accepts the role for one year. While she has been involved in quality assurance and improvement activities in nursing services, her experience in the topic area needs to be developed, and she seeks support from the hospital's quality manager.

The ward's quality activities are geared towards reporting activity and indicators, as well as conducting audits on tasks and processes to measure performance against agreed standards. Christine is keen to expand the range of assurance and improvement activities. In this role, Christine acts as an internal consultant to the ward's nursing staff, as she has no formal power by virtue of a position or line management in the ward's hierarchical structure.

Six months into the role, Christine has noticed some key issues relating to how she can encourage, support and implement plans for the ward's quality program. Initially, she related ideas about how the quality management unit staff and senior nursing personnel in the hospital would appreciate, value and support various quality activities by nursing staff on the ward. This was enough motivation for engagement by the nurses on the ward to begin with, but after a time the approach waned in its effectiveness as nursing staff valued their local and immediate needs and ideas for action over what others across the hospital might want.

Christine tries some different approaches to re-ignite the staff's motivation and finds that the most effective methods of achieving sign-on and involvement are consultation, either on a one-to-one basis or through impromptu ward meetings with a small number of staff ('let's scrum down on this idea …'), and making suggestions and discussion at the fortnightly nursing team meetings.

Strategies

There are extensive studies and learning about different types of leadership approaches and its effectiveness. Key to effective and sustained futures for organisations is the use of transformational leadership (Burns, 1978; Northouse, 2007) where leaders engage in significant influence strategies and actions so as to move followers in organisations to accomplish more than what might usually expected of them. In transformational leadership leaders engage with followers and develop important and new connections that increase motivation for work to be done and achieved. To achieve these relationships within teams, units, department and organisations, leaders need significant connection to staff and they make this through influencing strategies.

The concept of strategic influence has been developed over several decades in defence strategy and international political influence spheres (Gough, 2003), where it includes components such as advocacy, diplomacy, public affairs and psychological operations. In considering influential strategy, managers and leaders can discover how they can harness their understanding and knowledge of the various influencing tactics and apply those systematically to support ideas and plans with stakeholders, decision-makers, colleagues and others in key roles or positions.

Important behaviours that managers utilise to strategically communicate with, and to affect the opinions and decisions of, others are found across three areas: the environment in which they are working, individuals and groups with whom they want to align their ideas and thoughts, and individuals and groups with whom they require engagement or connection. Within these three key action areas there are several approaches and behaviours that support successful influence.

Environment

The main vehicle for the use of influence strategies is recognition of an environment in which the manager wants to achieve impact. Healthcare services, systems and organisations are specialised, with their own languages, cultures, priorities, complexities and ways of working. Healthcare organisations tend to have strong cultures, and it requires considerable time and effort to bring about change within them. Similarly, influence strategies need to be proportional, with size and resources aligned to the nature of the issue, and targeted to the key levels or parts of the organisation.

Health services operate in a wide range of environments – economic, political, community, scientific and academic – which means that the most effective influence strategies are those that recognise and work in the environment of the setting. It is important to place the influencing strategy in the health environment context.

Alignment

Alignment-influencing strategies focus on the connection and appeal to targets that will maximise the chance of engagement and support. Relationship-building (coalition, ingratiation and collaboration approaches) is an important part of influential strategy. The main strategic goal is to make sound and strong connections with individuals and groups regarding the issues being addressed.

This approach is also important when agents are working with large groups or whole organisations. The development of a common vision and achieving agreement on that vision are critical steps in moving organisations in terms of goals, objectives and cultural change. Engendering reciprocal agreement and support for projects and initiatives in organisations is vital to sustained support and the unification of staff and other stakeholders in health organisations.

Engagement

The use of rational persuasion, ingratiation tactics or pressure tactics needs to be managed in the context of dialogue with individuals and groups, and bargaining and empowerment approaches should be presented and managed so that they are constructive in outcome. While it may be necessary to use coercive or pressure tactics to achieve goals, to ensure ongoing working relationships and sustained working environments, these must be managed so as to focus on problem-solving. An example might be the need to create a sense of urgency or understanding of threat in order to drive a change initiative. The object is to present threats, problems or poor outcomes that might occur if advice and suggestions (influence) are not followed, as opposed to creating destructive scenarios or environments that may inhibit further engagement and work between agents and targets.

Summary

- Influence can be exerted in any direction within an organisation: downwards, upwards and laterally.
- Managers and leaders may have influence that is internal and external to their own work unit.
- Knowledge of influence tactics can be useful in understanding how to create influence, how to identify when one is being influenced and how to use separate tactics to achieve the desired impact.
- Managers and leaders need to develop strategies for influence tactics to work effectively.

Reflective questions

1 When considering approaches to influencing strategically to gain support for a proposal, how could you set out an influence strategy plan?

2 What factors would you consider when deciding whether your influence strategies needed to be aimed downwards, upwards or laterally?

3 Differentiate between influence and strategic influence.

4 When planning to influence someone strategically, what criteria would you use to decide whether to create a formal strategic plan or to implement the tactics in an ad hoc manner?

5 Differentiate between coalition and collaboration influencing tactics.

Self-analysis questions

Consider the 11 influencing tactics discussed in this chapter. In your experience, which two do you most align with or use? What new skills or experience would you need to improve your use of those tactics? Which two tactics are your least preferred or used? What new skills or experience would you need to improve your use of those tactics?

References

Burns, J. M. (1978). *Leadership*. New York, NY: Harper & Row.

Gough, S. L. (2003). *The evolution of strategic influence* (Strategy Research Project). Carlisle Barracks, PA: US Army War College.

Lankshear, S., Kerr, M. S., Spence Laschinger, H. K. & Wong, C. A. (2013). Professional practice leadership roles: The role of organizational power and personal influence in creating a professional practice environment for nurses. *Health Care Management Review*, 38(4), 349–360. doi: 10.1097/HMR.0b013e31826fd517

Manning, T. & Robertson, B. (2003). Influencing and negotiating skills: Some research and reflections – part I: Influencing strategies and styles. *Industrial and Commercial Training*, 35(1), 11–15. doi: 10.1108/00197850310458180

Northouse, P. G. (2007). *Leadership: Theory and practice* (4th ed.). Thousand Oaks, CA: Sage.

Spehar, I., Frich, J. C. & Kjekshus, L. E. (2014). Clinicians in management: A qualitative study of managers' use of influence strategies in hospitals. *Health Services Research*, 14(251). doi: 10.1186/1472-6963-14-251

Yukl, G. & Chavez, C. (2002). Influence tactics and leader effectiveness. In L. L. Neider & C. A. Schiresheim (Eds), *Leadership* (pp. 139–165). Charlotte, NC: Information Age.

Yukl, G. & Falbe, C. M. (1990). Influence tactics and objectives in upward, downward, and lateral influence attempts. *Journal of Applied Psychology*, 75(2), 132–140.

15

Networking

John Rasa

Learning objectives

How do I:

- understand the purpose of networking and where it sits on the partnership continuum?
- use the three levels of networking?
- learn to appreciate the personal and organisational benefits of networking for leadership development?
- enhance my skills in networking?
- overcome the challenges to achieve the potential of intraorganisational and interorganisational networking?

Introduction

Networks, which are defined as groups or systems of interconnected people or things, can be formal and informal in nature and can be applied for different purposes. The capability to network can build influence in groups and organisations to support change or generate new ideas. The process of networking can be seen as a supportive system of sharing information and services among individuals, groups and organisations with a common interest. Networking can be applied at a personal level for career and leadership development, at an intraorganisational level for organisational development, and at an interorganisational level for research, knowledge management, process improvement and relationship development.

Definitions

Networking is a key leadership capability. Besides being a supportive system of sharing information, it can develop trust or sharing of turf between partners and is a useful strategy for individuals and organisations in the initial stages of working relationships. It is a useful skill in environmental scanning and managing change.

Advances in technology and the proliferation of mobile devices have changed the way we communicate with each other, and social networks challenge our notions of hierarchically ordered organisation and information flow. Social networks like Twitter are usurping the power of formal, hierarchical networks, and technology is disrupting structural boundaries within organisations (Baker, 2014).

The terms networking, collaborating, partnering and forming an alliance or coalition all involve working with someone else, or with others, in some kind of formal or informal relationship, to perform a task and achieve a shared goal. However, networking is positioned on a partnership continuum that moves from networking to coordinating to cooperating and finally to collaborating. Most partnerships are built on a clear purpose and value. They move up and down this continuum, which shows progression based on degree of commitment, change required, risk involved, levels of interdependence, power, trust and a willingness to share turf (Himmelman, 2001).

Coordination is one step up from networking on the partnership continuum and involves exchanging information for mutual benefit and altering activities for a common purpose. It requires more time and trust but does not include sharing the turf. **Cooperation**, which means working together to achieve a shared goal, is similar to coordination, but it also requires significant amounts of time, high levels of trust and significant sharing of turf. It may require complex organisational processes and agreements in order to achieve the expanded benefits of mutual action. Finally, **collaboration** involves all of the above plus a willingness to increase the capacity of another organisation for mutual benefit and a common purpose. It is defined as working together on a project or activity. It requires the highest levels of trust, considerable amounts of time and extensive sharing of turf. It involves sharing risks and rewards but can produce the greatest benefits.

According to Marinez-Moyano (2006), networking is a recursive process, in which two or more organisations work together to realise shared goals. This is more than the

---

King
...tive system of sharing
...on and services among
...ls, groups and organisations
...mmon interest

...ation
...ng information for mutual
...nd altering activities for a
...purpose

...ation
...together to achieve a shared

...ration
...together on a project or

Networking for improved services

Samantha and six of her university colleagues are living in the outer suburbs, 20 kilometres from the university, where rental accommodation is less expensive. Public transport is poorly coordinated, and parking in the city is too expensive. Samantha and her friends set up a networking coffee meeting at the start of semester with other affected students in the area to share information about bus and train timetables and explore options.

Having assessed the problems, Samantha and her friends coordinate a campaign to lobby the local council to examine better ways of planning bus and train timetables.

After months with little progress with the council on the timetabling issue, Samantha and her friends pool their information and resources, and cooperate with their local transport action group on a campaign involving social media and distributing leaflets at the local station in the morning.

After getting the attention of their local council, the students collaborate with the local transport action group to intensify the campaign. The students agree to ramp up the social media campaign with Facebook and Twitter, while members of the local transport action group agree to attend each monthly local council meeting to lobby council members armed with an improved timetable for bus scheduling generated by Samantha's student group. Samantha, her friends and the local transport action group agree to share the load of distributing pamphlets at the train station and local shopping centre.

The local council soon agrees to improve bus and train timetabling so that buses arrive five minutes before train departures and five minutes after train arrivals. Samantha and her friends share their success story on social media.

intersection of common goals seen in cooperative ventures; instead, it is a collective determination to reach an identical objective. This may be an endeavour that builds new understanding by sharing knowledge or learnings and achieving consensus. It could be the result of a collaborative trial of a new protocol to reduce variation in clinical practice, or changing processes of patient referral to improve access to care while enhancing cost performance.

Networking is widely seen by the health sector as a crucial way of sharing risk, boosting research productivity, discovering new therapies and ultimately reinventing the way healthcare is delivered. Public and private sector healthcare providers and academia are forming an array of partnerships and strategic networks to drive innovation. These require trust and openness in sharing resources and data, which at times can be challenging. De Long and Fahey (2000) maintain that the level of trust that exists in an organisation greatly influences the amount of knowledge that flows both between individuals and from individuals into the organisation's records.

An important development in strategic networking is the activity of co-creation. An example of this is the development of the Melbourne HealthPathways, in which four Victorian Medicare Locals and four Victorian health services (hospital networks) collaborated to develop web-based clinical pathways, using evidence-based practice and the latest research, to guide general practitioners to make appropriate clinical decisions when referring their patients to hospitals. The framework they used was based on the health pathways model stemming from the Canterbury Initiative in New Zealand (Timmins & Ham, 2013). The benefits of this co-creation collaboration and networking approach included identification of new opportunities and added credibility to the quality frameworks already in place. The network partners wanted research that was practical, with commonsense outcomes that people could understand, and that was normally achieved (Janamian, Jackson & Dunbar, 2014).

A further example of strategic networking is NHMRC Partnerships for Better Health, designed to create Partnership Projects to foster partnerships among decision-makers, policy-makers, managers, clinicians and researchers (National Health and Medical Research Council, 2013). This initiative provided funding to create new opportunities for researchers and policy-makers to work together for a mutual interest. This could include answering a specific research question to influence health and wellbeing through changes in the delivery, organisation, funding and access to health services.

As indicated earlier, networking often involves just the sharing of information or just keeping up to date in an area of common interest. It can have a narrow focus on information related to the introduction of a new procedure for handling patient feedback in a health service, or have a broader focus such as sharing updates on the introduction of major health reforms, like the reforms to primary healthcare in Australia and the introduction of casemix funding to Australian hospitals.

Networking can be a powerful way of sharing learning and ideas, building a sense of community and purpose, shaping new solutions to entrenched problems, tapping into hidden talent and knowledge, and providing space to innovate and embed change (Randall, 2013). On the other hand, networking can have a more active meaning, of engaging with colleagues attending a college professional development seminar or holding a cross-sectoral health-planning meeting to facilitate better coordination of services, or engaging online when updating profiles on LinkedIn, or adding to a professional interest group's blog. All of these activities can be described as different forms of active networking with varying levels of engagement.

Leadership and networking

Networking is primarily about relationship-building. It is, in fact, a leadership capability that involves building and maintaining genuinely helpful relationships with other people for mutual benefit. It is about creating a diversity of connections and win–win alliances with others through nurturing relationships that require some degree of trust. As a leadership capability, it can be learned and also nurtured with practice.

The ability of health managers or aspiring health leaders to develop networks, coalitions and partnerships is recognised as something worth developing in the leadership frameworks of the Australasian College of Health Service Management, Health Workforce Australia, the American College of Health Executives and the Canadian College of Health Leaders. Hence, conference and professional development events are likely to be structured to allow reasonable networking time.

Ibarra and Hunter (2007), in their work with emerging managers, discovered that there are three distinct but interdependent levels of networking, which are personal, operational and strategic. All three levels play an important role in developing managers to become leaders. Personal networking boosts personal leadership development, operational networking assists managers to meet current internal organisational responsibilities, and strategic networking opens managers' eyes to new organisational directions and the stakeholders they need to enlist to achieve their goals. While managers differ in how well they pursue operational and personal networking, almost all of them underutilise strategic networking. It appears the reasons are both attitudinal and behavioural. Managers often describe networking as somehow manipulative or insincere instead of being part of the role of a leader.

Often, the attitude of managers is that their comfort zone and interests lie in the strong command of the technical components or tasks of their jobs and in accomplishing their personal or their team's objectives. When challenged to move beyond their functional specialties and address strategic issues facing the organisation, many managers do not immediately grasp that this will involve relational activity, not analytical tasks. Nor do they easily understand that meetings and interactions with a diverse range of stakeholders are not distractions from their 'real work' but are actually part of what it is to be a leader (Ibarra & Hunter, 2007).

Personal networking

While effective personal networking can be more narrowly defined as being based on a genuine interest in assisting professional colleagues or significant others, networking is rapidly being recognised as a critical leadership skill impacting a manager's career and organisational effectiveness. Research indicates that as high-performing organisations try to develop their future leaders and assess the leaders they currently have, they will explicitly indicate that the abilities to manage relationships across boundaries and to sell ideas are critical leadership competencies (Ibarra & Hunter, 2007).

Personal networking is a technique for broadening a manager's professional knowledge beyond their usual work setting of acute, sub-acute or primary healthcare or aged care services. It enables managers to understand issues confronting other managers in allied organisations, both public and private, and to perhaps find common ground with managers outside their usual professional circles.

There are a number of avenues through which personal networking can be facilitated. At a one-to-one level, professional mentoring or coaching can play an important developmental role in establishing personal networks, by firstly gaining a broader understanding and secondly receiving important referrals to key individuals. Mentoring and personal networking can provide a safe space for a manager to undertake personal development and lay a real foundation for strategic networking.

Personal networking is mainly external, consisting of discretionary links to people who often share a common interest or provide possible career opportunities. Personal networks can represent useful referral potential and are an important first step for a manager in transitioning from being operational to strategic. It is part of the development of personal leadership to better understand one's inner self and open further avenues for communication.

However, to avoid the possibility of feeling that personal networking is ultimately time-wasting, a health manager needs to link their personal connections to organisational goals as part of a broader strategy. Leveraging a personal network through, say, a professional college relationship could assist a health manager interested in hospital performance, and sharing a common interest with a senior colleague could facilitate a move from a private sector role with a health insurer to a health department role overseeing public hospital performance. Linking the activity of personal network–building to career advancement, to developing one's knowledge of what constitutes efficient hospital performance, can benefit a health insurer to manage risk around hospital cost claims experience. The benefit of becoming a strategic networker within a health insurance company becomes clearer.

Personal networking can be either face-to-face or virtual. Increasingly, personal networking is facilitated through electronic means by the use of email, LinkedIn or internet blogs or groups, sometimes enabling personal networks to extend globally to colleagues in other countries. This is useful if health managers are wishing to extend their reach into other health systems, facilitate study tours or undertake international visits. International networking can also cast light on how other health systems have tackled health issues in quite a different manner. At a group level of personal networking, membership of professional associations, attendance at college-continuing professional development activities and keeping in touch with university alumni all assist health managers to gain new perspectives that allow them to advance in their careers.

However, quite often constraints for managers engaging in personal networking are time limitations and pressures of completing immediate work commitments. It is important that managers commit time to ensure personal networking opens up future career opportunities.

Reid Hoffman, the co-founder of LinkedIn, maintains that it is important for individuals to evaluate the type of business relationship they are in, so they know how to invest in each person. The more risky 'transactional relationships' require individuals to ensure a stream of short-term rewards for them so they constantly feel they are getting something out of the relationship. Hoffman argues that the more valuable and perhaps the more strategic relationships expect commensurate investment of time and energy over time by both parties ('How LinkedIn's boss links in', 2013).

Operational networking

Operational networking becomes important when a health manager needs to build good working relationships with the senior managers, work colleagues and staff who can help them get their job done more effectively. The purpose of operational networking is to ensure coordination and cooperation among people who have to know and trust one another in order to accomplish their immediate tasks. That isn't always easy, but it is relatively straightforward, because the task provides focus and a clear criterion for membership to the network. Either someone is integral to getting the job done, or they are not.

Generally, operational networking is internally focused, more concerned with sustaining cooperation within the existing network in the organisation than with building relationships to face unforeseen challenges outside the organisation. Operational networking can function within the work team, between departments or divisions in a larger organisation or even interprofessionally, in the case of multidisciplinary care teams delivering acute care or rehabilitation, or managing chronic disease in the primary healthcare setting. But as managers move into leadership roles, their network must become more externally focused and future-oriented.

Strategic networking

When health service managers begin the delicate transition from functional manager to organisational leader, they start to concern themselves with broad strategic and organisational issues. Lateral and vertical relationships with other functional or business unit managers outside the immediate control of the health service manager become important links, indicating how their own contribution fits into the organisational picture. Thus, strategic networking links 'the aspiring leader into a set of relationships and information sources that collectively embody the power to achieve personal and organisational goals' (Ibarra & Hunter, 2007, p. 43).

As an example, clinical directors, nurse unit managers or allied health department heads may be thrust into a clinical leadership role due to their organisational skills or because of seniority. The rise in managerialism in healthcare reflects organisational demand for efficiency and effectiveness in the delivery of healthcare services. The demand for innovation and continuous improvement in quality of health service delivery and the relentless push to improve productivity in the model of service delivery are about changing the behaviour of clinicians and patients. The clinical manager is well placed to influence these outcomes.

Leadership for successful innovation for the clinical manager often involves leadership skills like the exercise of political astuteness and the development of alignment and sometimes coalitions across different interests implicated by the innovation, in both formal and informal alliances. It involves mobilising existing relationships and developing new ones to encompass the range of practices involved in innovation, as well as seeking funding from the board or department of health (Storey & Holti, 2013).

It is important that the healthcare organisation provides the right environment for the clinical leader or manager to develop properly (Leggat & Balding, 2013). The health service organisation should facilitate networking training in areas like communications, leadership and organisation, human resources and financial systems, and policies and procedures. Networking skills are a capability that can be learned by the transitioning clinician.

The shift from clinician to clinical manager also involves a shift in mindset. Many managers need to change their attitudes about the necessity for networking. For the clinician, the mindset must shift from the highly valued individual patient focus to organisational objectives, from a narrower clinical focus to a broader organisational and strategic focus. This can often result in a challenge to their identity, from having personal clinical credibility to having a role in management of people and resources, in which they are less confident. The clinical manager will need organisational support to gain the required management credibility in this new role. At a personal leadership level, unless clinical managers shift their mindset about valuing their management role, they will not allocate sufficient time or effort to getting the job done.

The transition from clinician to manager can be greatly assisted by maintaining clinical networks and leveraging these to develop and support the building of necessary management skills. By encouraging the sharing of ideas around intractable clinical process problems, a clinical manager's management challenges can be more effectively addressed.

Organisations can support clinician managers by providing opportunities for internal networking with other managers and encouraging attendance at suitable external events. Developing clinical managers might accompany senior managers at networking events to enable role-modelling of appropriate networking behaviours, or organisations might suggest relevant external websites (for example, LinkedIn) that can assist in further developing personal networks. Organisations can also incorporate networking performance measures into assessment processes and appraise the clinical manager's skill in engaging with others. In these ways, the organisation sends a strong signal that it values networking capabilities.

The Australian Primary Care Collaboratives Program is an example of strategic networking. It used the Breakthrough Series collaborative methodology designed to help organisations close the gap in performance by creating a structure in which teams can easily learn from each other as well as from recognised experts in selected topic areas. General practices that participated in the program attended a series of learning workshops, undertook improvement and change activities in their health service and collected monthly data to track their progress. Learning workshops allowed participants to network, hear from topic area and quality improvement experts and actively share knowledge and experiences with their peers. The workshops enabled practice teams to test ideas and carry out change.

Interorganisational networking

Operating beside organisational members with diverse backgrounds, objectives and incentives needs a manager to work through networks that they require to compete for resources. Internally, the clinical manager will need to work closely with the hospital management team, comprising the directors of nursing, medical, finance and allied health services. They form part of a community of practice network, with expertise in leading and organising health professionals, managing finances and assessing operational performance within the organisation.

Externally, clinical managers may be part of an interorganisational community of practice network, in which groups of managers come together to learn, address organisational issues and, where possible, drive innovative practices or design alternative service models. These types of knowledge alliances are important ways for organisations to increase their learning in order to innovate and remain competitive (Ropes, 2009). Knowledge management in healthcare is emphasised in evidence-based medicine approaches and through collaborative efforts leading to the development of clinical pathways where context knowledge is essential (Yamazaki & Umemoto, 2010).

There are many examples of networks that have formed to facilitate interorganisational learning. For instance, Networking Health Victoria operated numerous networks of primary health organisations tasked with improving the coordination of primary healthcare services around chronic disease management. These networks came together to better coordinate after-hours primary care delivery, aged care, mental health services, telehealth services and health data collection, among many other areas. Networking Health Victoria provided insight into the interorganisational networking processes that were involved. The program operated on a facilitation model, relied on personal contacts and worked with its networks in a very structured manner. All network meetings strived to have content-rich agendas utilising data, critiques, analyses, 'Plan, Do, Study, Act' (or PDSA) cycles and follow-up activities. There was a strong sense of common purpose and expected outcomes from events and network meetings. Meetings were well documented, follow-up was always initiated, and organisational learning was subsequently shared.

Importantly, networking in the 21st century is ably assisted by systems of software, tools and technologies. Networking Health Victoria used client relationship management software from Salesforce to track key contacts and to support their networks. The software generates reports and dashboards of key metrics related to all activity with key stakeholders.

Intraorganisational networking

Research has demonstrated that at an operational level, an individual's productivity is inextricably linked to their networking capability (Ferreira & Du Plessis, 2009). Effective networkers within organisations reap rewards such as hastened career progression, capitalisation of leadership opportunities, greater job satisfaction and business success.

At an intraorganisational level, studies at Toyota have demonstrated the role of network knowledge resources in influencing an organisation's overall performance. In a sample of United States automotive suppliers selling to both Toyota and United States automakers, Pittaway, Robertson, Munir, Denyer and Neely (2004) found that greater knowledge-sharing on the part of Toyota resulted in a faster rate of learning within the suppliers' manufacturing operations devoted to the company. Indeed, from 1990 to 1996 suppliers reduced defects by 50 per cent for Toyota versus only 26 per cent for their largest United States customer (Dyer & Hatch, 2006).

Recent work on competitiveness has emphasised the importance of business networking for innovation. A systematic review of research by Pittaway et al. (2004) linking the networking behaviour of firms with their innovative capacity found that the principal benefits of networking include risk-sharing, obtaining access to new technologies and external knowledge, speeding products to market and pooling complementary skills. The evidence also shows that those firms which do not cooperate and do not formally or informally exchange knowledge limit their knowledge base in the long term and ultimately reduce their ability to enter exchange relationships. At an institutional level, national systems of innovation play an important role in the diffusion of innovation in terms of the way in which they shape networking activity. Evidence suggests that network relationships with suppliers, customers and intermediaries such as professional associations are important in affecting innovation performance and productivity (Pittaway et al., 2004).

Summary

- Networking is relationship-building and is a supportive system of sharing information among individuals, groups and organisations with a mutual interest.
- Networking is part of a partnership continuum that has its highest form in collaboration, involving high trust, time commitment and risk-sharing.
- Health service managers need to navigate three levels of networking: personal networking, operational networking and strategic networking.
- Networking is an important management capability that can build influence and be applied at a personal level for leadership development or at an intraorganisational level for organisational development and improvement.
- Networking can be applied at an interorganisational level for the purposes of research, knowledge management, process improvement and relationship development.

Reflective questions

1   Why is it important to understand the different forms of networking that are available?

2   Choose one of your organisation's goals or select a personal career goal. Can you map three personal connections you presently have and how, through networking, they might come to assist you in achieving that goal?

3   Reflect on the virtual networks that you currently use and explain why you choose to spend time connecting with other current or aspiring health managers through these media.

4   Based on your personal experience, which form of networking has contributed most to developing your leadership capabilities?

5   If you were given a problem to solve relating to the quality of care in a health organisation, which form of networking do you believe you would use, and why?

Self-analysis questions

List the personal networking activities that you regularly undertake. In what ways have they built your personal influence? What networking activities do you frequently undertake to share information that assists your personal leadership skill development? In what ways have they contributed to you being a better operational manager, a more strategic change agent in your organisation or a more innovative problem-solver? Can you see what you can do differently in the future to become more strategic in your networking?

References

Baker, M. N. (2014). *Peer to peer leadership: Why the network is the leader.* San Francisco, CA: Berrett-Koehler.

De Long, D. W. & Fahey, L. (2000). Diagnosing cultural barriers to knowledge management, *Academy of Management Executive, 14*(4), 113–119. doi: 10.5465/AME.2000.3979820

Dyer, J. H. & Hatch, N. W. (2006). Relation-specific capabilities and barriers to knowledge transfers: Creating advantage through network relationships. *Strategic Management Journal*, 27(8), 701–719. doi: 10.1002/smj.543

Ferreira, A. & Du Plessis, T. (2009). Effect of online social networking on employee productivity. *South African Journal of Information Management*, 11(1), 1–11. doi: 10.1002/smj.543

Himmelman, A. (2001). On coalitions and the transformation of power relations: Collaborative betterment and collaborative empowerment. *American Journal of Community Psychology*, 29(2), 277–284. doi: 10.1023/A:1010334831330

How LinkedIn's boss links in. (2013, February 28). *Business Management Daily*. Retrieved from http://www.businessmanagementdaily.com

Ibarra, H. & Hunter, M. (2007). How leaders create and use networks. *Harvard Business Review*, 85(1), 40–47.

Janamian, T., Jackson, C. L. & Dunbar, J. A. (2014). Co-creating value in research: Stakeholders' perspectives. *Medical Journal of Australia*, 201(3 Suppl), S44–S46. doi: 10.5694/mja14.00273

Leggat, S. G. & Balding, C. (2013). Achieving organisational competence for clinical leadership: The role of high performance work systems. *Journal of Health Organization and Management*, 27(3), 312–329. doi: 10.1108/JHOM-Jul-2012-0132

Marinez-Moyano, I. J. (2006). Exploring the dynamics of collaboration in interorganizational settings. In S. Schuman (Ed.), *Creating a culture of collaboration* (pp. 69–85). New York, NY: Jossey-Bass.

National Health and Medical Research Council. (2013). *NHMRC partnerships for better health*. Retrieved from https://www.nhmrc.gov.au/grants-funding/apply-funding/partnerships-better-health

Pittaway, L., Robertson, M., Munir, K., Denyer, D. & Neely, A. (2004). Networking and innovation: A systematic review of the evidence. *International Journal of Management Reviews*, 5(3–4), 137–168. doi: 10.1111/j.1460-8545.2004.00101.x

Randall, S. (2013). *Learning report: Leading networks in healthcare*. Retrieved from Health Foundation website: http://www.health.org.uk/public/cms/75/76/313/4003/Leading%20networks%20in%20healthcare.pdf%realName=yC2IOH.pdf

Ropes, D. (2009). Communities of practice: Powerful environments for interorganizational knowledge alliances? In C. Stam (Ed.), *Proceedings of the 1st European Conference on Intellectual Capital* (pp. 400–407). Reading, United Kingdom: Academic Conferences.

Storey, J. & Holti, R. (2013). *Towards a new model of leadership for the NHS* [Report]. Retrieved from NHS Leadership Academy website: http://www.leadershipacademy.nhs.uk/wp-content/uploads/2013/05/Towards-a-New-Model-of-Leadership-2013.pdf

Timmins, N. & Ham, C. (2013). *The quest for integrated health and social care: A case study in Canterbury, New Zealand* [Report]. Retrieved from King's Fund website: http://www.kingsfund.org.uk/sites/files/kf/field/field_publication_file/quest-integrated-care-new-zealand-timmins-ham-sept13.pdf

Yamazaki, T. & Umemoto, K. (2010). Knowledge management of healthcare by clinical-pathways. In S. Chu, W. Ritter & S. Hawamdeh (Eds), *Managing knowledge for global and collaborative innovations* (pp. 141–150). Singapore: World Scientific Publishing.

Part 4

Achieves Outcomes

16

Holding to account

Ged Williams and Linda Fraser

Learning objectives

How do I:

- understand the relationship between supervisor and subordinate and the implicit and explicit expectations of this relationship?
- clarify my manager's performance expectations of me and the broader expectations of managers to obtain the best performance from each individual?
- identify why some staff fall below expectations and determine the appropriate approaches to manage these issues?
- develop skills in using frameworks to guide my behaviour and actions in holding staff to account?
- adopt leadership styles that will be most effective in holding others to account?

Introduction

In contemporary healthcare services, managers are required to create environments in which competing forces place significant demands on the system as well as individuals to contribute to productivity. Each employee is held accountable and responsible for their part in contributing to this productivity.

Often, people feel that being held to account is something negative that usually happens to them when things go wrong, rather than something they can utilise to ensure success (Smith, 2014). Holding to account can be difficult if the perceptions of the supervisor and subordinate are at odds. It could reasonably be expected that a nurse manager would be aware of their supervisor's expectations and hold a shared perspective on performance accountabilities; however, this is not always the case. We cannot assume that people share the same understanding of what they are accountable for or the standards expected of them. Accountabilities need to be made explicit and clear.

Definitions

In business, government and healthcare, accountabilities may be legislated or described in high-level policy documents to inform senior leaders of their **accountabilities** and **responsibilities** (Australian Public Sector Commission, 2010; *Corporations Act 2001* [Cth]; *Financial Management and Accountabilities Act 1997* [Cth]; *Public Sector [Honesty and Accountability] Act 1995* [SA]). The chief executive officer may delegate accountabilities in a traditional hierarchical fashion to managers, who in turn will hold subordinates to account for responsibilities that are further delegated or directed.

> **Accountability**
> The requirement to account for actions and outcomes to a higher authority; cannot be delegated
>
> **Responsibility**
> The obligation of ensuring the required task is complete; can be delegated or shared; often used interchangeably with 'accountability'

Strategic accountability

At the strategic level of the health system, ministers and department leaders may have their accountabilities legislated through parliament (*National Health Act 1953* [Cth]; *Public Health Act 2010* [NSW]). These accountabilities are well documented, and expectations are clear and legally binding. The parliamentary process holds to account those in power for delivering on these accountabilities, and if the community is not satisfied with their performance, those in power may not be re-elected.

Publicly available external peer review is another way in which hospitals and health services are held to account. Health service accreditation through the Australian Council on Health Care Standards (http://www.achs.org.au), the Health Round Table (http://www.healthroundtable.org.) benchmarking groups and various medical college auditing procedures (Royal Australasian College of Physicians, n.d.) are some examples. These simple but effective external reviews can motivate chief executive officers and the organisations they administer to be accountable to an external standard set by a third party that acts on behalf of the community's interests.

Operational accountability

At the health service or departmental level, key accountabilities are often framed in an operational plan developed following a gap analysis between the current situation and the ultimate goal. In the operational plan, a list of priorities is developed and documented using the SMART format (see below) with specific individuals identified to be accountable for each element.

Individual accountability

Before accepting a task, the accountable officer should examine the accountability structure, specific expectations, allowable resources, authority to act, ability to negotiate or modify expectations (including timeframes) and consequences of success and failure.

Leadership and holding to account

Managers often try to be likeable, and they try to avoid tension, conflict and ongoing performance reviews. Accountability is particularly difficult if personal friendships cloud the professional relationships required at work. However, it is more important for managers to be respected rather than liked (Ehrler, 2005). Staff will not always respect a popular leader, but a respected leader will always be popular!

Holding an employee to account can require the manager to conduct a difficult conversation with the employee, and many managers are reluctant to approach this. Despite feeling apprehensive, by utilising the SIMPLE or SMART frameworks set out below to guide discussions (and documentation), the manager can approach such issues with confidence and competence. There is no easy way around this responsibility – it must be met head-on.

Although many leadership styles have been studied and documented, no one leadership style will be suitable in all situations. Traditional leadership styles include autocratic, bureaucratic, participative and laissez-faire; more contemporary styles include charismatic, connective, servant, transactional and transformational. In our view all styles of leadership have currency in various situations. In a disaster situation, an autocratic style may be necessary as there is no time for consultation and consensus; in a budget development process, a bureaucratic style may be useful; in an industrial relations conflict, a participative style may be warranted; and in a quality improvement brainstorming workshop, a laissez-faire approach may work best. Directing, supervising, coaching and delegating leadership styles are all appropriate in various situations and can all be used with the same employee concurrently, depending on the situation, even in performance management scenarios when holding a staff member to account.

Knowing that leadership is more about behaviour than personality (Kouzes & Posner, 2007) and that a leader–constituent relationship characterised by fear and mistrust will not produce positive outcomes, most leaders endeavour to develop relationships characterised by respect and confidence. Feedback delivered by a respected and credible authority holds the most value to the recipient.

Providing clear expectations

Sally is a four-year postgraduate registered nurse working in a busy medical inpatient unit. She has worked hard to develop her nursing skills since completing her graduate nurse program and is now well regarded as a senior registered nurse. In her performance appraisal and development discussion with her nurse unit manager, Sally is given the feedback that she is performing well and that her willingness to be a preceptor and mentor to new and unskilled staff has been noted and appreciated. Sally indicates she would like to work towards becoming a clinical nurse.

continued ›

continued ›

The nurse unit manager takes this opportunity to discuss with Sally the requirements for clinical nurses. Together they discuss areas for Sally to focus on developing, and Sally is provided with the clinical nurse role description and the role-specific information. Sally and her nurse unit manager document a plan for Sally to follow to facilitate her development along this pathway.

Over the next six months, Sally works to complete the development plan as laid out in the performance appraisal and development and attends a workshop designed for aspiring clinical nurses. She continues to demonstrate sound clinical judgement in the workplace and fills in as a team leader on several occasions.

At the six-month review, Sally and her nurse unit manager analyse the plan and Sally's achievements to date. Sally is then offered the opportunity to backfill in the clinical nurse role to cover a period of leave. Sally is delighted her hard work has paid off and agrees to the position.

The nurse unit manager ensures that Sally has all of the information regarding code of conduct, role description and portfolio responsibilities, and they have an in-depth discussion regarding the leadership aspects of the role. This action is recorded on the performance appraisal and development, and Sally is provided with a copy of the document. The expectations are both clear and documented.

Holding to account requires very clear communication and decisive directions so that all participants know what is expected. However, not every employee can meet every expectation all the time, and most reasonable managers will demonstrate some latitude in their expectations. When both parties share the same understanding, a failure to perform according to the manager's reasonable **expectations** may be due to one of three primary factors: skill, hill or will. Firstly, the individual may not have possessed the skills required for the tasks; for example, unforeseen barriers arose that they did not know how to approach and required further training to tackle. Or, the slope of the hill may have been too steep, meaning expectations were unrealistic: timeframes, the quality of work or the resources required may not have been clear, resulting in unachievable demands. Finally, the individual may not have had the will to complete the task: perhaps it was never explicitly determined to be a priority, or the individual involved was lazy, rude or vengeful.

Expectation
A belief that something will hap[pen]
agreed or perceived

Performance
Fulfilment of a set of obligations [or]
expectations, usually assessed a[s]
sufficient to be deemed satisfac[tory or]
complete

It is often easy to find fault in the **performance** of others and yet fail to see our own part in failures or difficulties encountered. How illuminating would it be to see our own contributions to the outcomes achieved?

Frameworks for holding to account

In management, there are many approaches to framing accountability and holding to account. Some simple frameworks are discussed below that can assist managers to approach their responsibilities and those they delegate to allow them to consistently and predictably implement accountability processes.

SMART and SIMPLE

Accountabilities and expectations should be SMART: specific, measurable, achievable, relevant and time-specific. They should be documented in clear and understandable language. The more important the accountability or expectation, the more important it is to document clearly using the SMART format. If not documented at the outset, specific expectations can be forgotten or confused, leading to argument, wasted time, renegotiation and ill-will. As a rule, committees, groups or multiple persons cannot be held accountable for making things happen. Too often, such group accountabilities result in everybody-somebody-anybody-nobody scenarios, whereby everybody is asked to achieve a goal, everybody thinks somebody will do it, anybody could do it, but in the end nobody actually does it. It is therefore important that only one person is held responsible and accountable for delivering each key assignment.

Miller (2006) articulates a SIMPLE approach to accountability whereby roles and tasks are easy to remember each time a new accountability is established. The approach helps guide managers and their teams in meeting these accountabilities:

Set expectations

Do not assume that employees know what is supposed to be done, when, and to what standard unless these are clearly explained at the outset. The clearer these expectations are, the less time is subsequently spent clarifying or arguing about them. To ensure complete understanding, expectations must be **relevant** and **realistic**.

> **nt**
> with overarching business
> es
>
> **ic**
> le within known constraints

Invite commitment

Just because employees know what to do doesn't mean they will do it. Most employees will engage if they know the goals will benefit them personally, help move the organisation forwards and be open to their input and influence (ownership). Once employees see the benefits and feel they have some control of the process, they are more likely to welcome being held to account for the results.

Measure progress

Key metrics must be quantified and communicated to inform progress and gauge whether or not the goals and expectations previously committed to have been met. Goals are measurable only when they are quantified. It is important that the measure is agreed and regularly reported so that all stakeholders can monitor ongoing performance objectively.

Provide feedback

Sharing the quantifiable measures and constructively commenting on less tangible markers (such as effort, cooperation and teamwork) can help to keep employees focused and engaged. Feedback will not solve all problems but can open up dialogue for problem-solving and follow-up actions, especially where performance is falling short of expectations.

Link to consequences

Consequences should not be confused with punishments. Punishment is something inflicted on employees that make them pay for their shortcomings. It does not usually contribute to a solution. Consequences, however, guide and focus behaviour, and encourage commitments to be taken more seriously. Consequences (positive or negative) must be certain, suitable and commensurate with goal difficulty and immediately follow the outcome or action. Both managers and employees must know that the agreed consequences will follow the action.

Evaluate effectiveness

Using preset goals, an employer can determine how successful they have been in holding employees accountable. The manager must employ self-reflection to review how processes such as communication, feedback, negotiation, compromise and consequences were managed. Reviewing their own performance and heeding supervisor and staff feedback can help a manager develop more effective ways to apply the principles of accountability. Holding oneself accountable for holding others accountable is a critical step in becoming a more effective manager and leader.

Feedback

Many employees with performance issues often have a better than average opinion of themselves, resulting in an enhanced self-worth and a disbelief in the supervisor's judgement (Brown, 2012). High-performing staff will seek feedback on performance to affirm their self-belief, while low-performing staff will resist feedback-seeking behaviour for fear it will harm their self-belief (Kuhnen & Tymula, 2012). It is critical for the supervisor to find ways to provide feedback to individuals to establish a realistic shared perspective of their performance. The most effective feedback to all staff is delivered in a supportive environment by credible and tactful supervisors (Dahling, Chau & O'Malley, 2010).

Before committing to giving feedback, it is helpful to reflect on the intent for giving the feedback, by considering these questions: What outcome is to be achieved by the feedback? What specific issue is to be addressed? Can we agree on a way forward? What impact will this have on the relationship between the parties?

Giving feedback can be a difficult and emotional undertaking. It can generate fear and other negative emotions and lead to a reluctance to deliver and a reluctance to accept. Despite this, feedback is not always delivered from a higher authority to a lower level but can be effectively delivered by employees who hold their supervisors to account despite the obvious power differential.

To be effective, feedback must come from a sincere desire to help or support the other person. It is not about fixing, but helping. Done well, feedback will be accepted as a gift; however, feedback that cannot help someone improve is simply criticism.

Real-time feedback can be delivered to a peer, subordinate or supervisor if behaviour or practice is not in line with the values, standards, expectations or performance goals of the organisation. Providing dignified, caring and honest feedback or a well-placed question immediately the concerning behaviour or practice is recognised allows for a brief pause, reflection and a teachable moment. This type of feedback may be delivered in a simple 'below the line' type of communication. Any group of people working together can, as a group, determine what is and what is not acceptable behaviour based on the organisation's standards. By simply stating that a behaviour is 'below the line' an employee provides instantaneous feedback that the concerning behaviour is not acceptable. Just in time feedback is delivered after the fact but within a timeframe that allows for meaningful action such as a correction or incorporation of change in future behaviour (Nursing Executive Center, 2011).

Whipple (2011) identifies eight 'be-attitudes' of holding others to account and providing feedback:

Be clear about expectations   People need to know what you want.

Be sure of facts   Do not accuse people of something they did not do.

Be timely   Feedback needs to follow the event closely.

Be kind   How would you like to get this input?

Be consistent   Treat everyone the same way.

Be discreet   Coach people in private, never in public.

Be gracious   Show gratitude for the things done well.

Be balanced   Holding people accountable does not always need to be negative.

Having the right attitude, being calm, managing emotions and treating others as we would like them to treat us are simple but powerful approaches. No matter how poor someone's performance may be, timely feedback can improve it (Ryvkin, Krajc & Ortmann, 2012). It is the method of delivery of such feedback that determines its effectiveness. Feedback delivered in a sensitive and supportive manner is more acceptable to the recipient and much more likely to be effective (Dahling et al., 2010).

Leaders who develop and maintain high-quality relationships with their subordinates have been found to provide feedback that is more readily received (Bezuijen, van Dam, van den Berg & Theirry, 2010). Careful, decisive, fair actions and communication are required.

Appraisal methods

Performance appraisal and development

Probably the most ubiquitous accountability tool used with staff, the performance appraisal and development is generally administered annually, with a half-yearly review. The procedure aims to guide a conversation between employee and supervisor to review the employee's performance against predetermined performance criteria, such as attendance, productivity, quality of work and error rates. The performance appraisal and development also includes important aspects that are not so easy to measure, such as attitude, teamwork and communication. The development aspect of the procedure covers not only potential deficits in knowledge, skills and abilities identified by the performance appraisal but also areas of future development for career progression.

Buddy and mentor systems

A buddy or mentor partnership can be formed to provide support to an employee who is performing to an acceptable standard. A capable and respected peer or slightly more experienced colleague acts to provide real-time and just in time feedback on behaviour that has been of concern. If the buddy or mentor process is formal, regular meetings with the supervisor may be required to discuss performance and provide feedback.

Discipline and performance improvement processes

Should feedback and guidance fail to produce the required standards of performance, a disciplinary procedure may be required. Before heading down this pathway, it is first necessary to determine that less intense options (such as buddy or mentor systems, performance appraisal and development reviews and other options) have failed or are deemed inappropriate due to the serious nature of the breach. Then, a full investigation must be conducted of the alleged poor performance, whether it is a clinical or professional, or a code of conduct breach. This can be done by the manager or an external investigator. It is vital to afford the employee the natural justice of a right of reply: they must be given an opportunity to respond to the allegations in writing before disciplinary actions are taken.

Supervisors should remain supportive in these situations, as it is not uncommon for staff who overestimate their capabilities to commence 'bullying and harassment' counterclaims towards their supervisors (Goodhew, Cammock & Hamilton, 2008). To avoid such claims it is wise to use human resources experts to inform the process to be followed. Inviting the staff member to have a support person in attendance can help all parties involved to feel safe, especially if there are feelings of distrust or animosity. The development and documentation of a formal performance improvement plan may be necessary, to address issues not resolved by this stage. It may also be necessary to vary the employee's hours of work so that greater supervision of performance and feedback is possible. For instance, bringing a nurse onto day shifts so that more frequent communication and feedback with their manager and/or buddy are possible and attendance at any education and training sessions is more achievable. Regular meetings between the supervisor and employee are important (including support persons if appropriate) to maintain momentum and adjustments as improvements are made.

Confidentiality among those participating in the discipline process is of paramount importance. Many team members will be aware of the process and will be watching to see how the manager deals with it. It can be profoundly detrimental to the team as a whole for this process to be handled poorly or, worse still, not handled at all.

Reprimands, penalties, demotions, transfers and terminations

In the healthcare sector, formal reprimands, financial penalties, demotions, transfers and terminations are severe, often last-resort responses and are generally associated with illegal or unprofessional behaviour. Such issues are beyond the scope of most supervisors to manage on their own and warrant human resources, legal, industrial and/or executive and regulatory authority involvement. The Australian Health Professional Regulatory Agency (http://www.ahpra.gov.au) is a valuable resource regarding such complex matters. They have trained managers who can provide advice and guidance on issues of professional malpractice and misconduct.

Summary

- Being accountable means being able to account for one's actions and outcomes to a higher authority. The relationship between supervisor and subordinate has explicit and implicit expectations in terms of performance, productivity and behaviour.
- Evidence suggests that supervisors and subordinates do not always have shared views or expectations of performance, and these need to be made clear and transparent.
- Performance can fall below expectations when an individual does not have the skill required, the slope of the hill is too steep, or an individual does not have the will to complete the task.
- There are many ways by which managers can hold an individual to account. By using SIMPLE and SMART frameworks as guides, managers can plan their approach despite feeling apprehensive about the process.
- A manager is like a coach who demands the best of each player for the good of the team and its supporters. Regardless of the leadership style, if clear expectations and feedback are given promptly, holding to account can be achieved effectively.

Reflective questions

1 Consider the five key accountabilities of your current role (or your next role, if you are currently a student). Rate your performance on a scale of 1 to 10 and then ask a supervisor and two peers to rate your performance on the same scale. What are the similarities and differences in the scores? Can you identify reasons for these?

2 Identify two policies in your area that make you specifically accountable for a certain behaviour or performance standard. How do you compare to your colleagues?

3 Identify two specific accountabilities of your manager that you could assist them in achieving. What could you do to help them improve current performance in each area?

4 Consider a time when you or someone you know was considered a low performer relative to peers. What was done to change the situation? How could it have been managed better?

5 Consider an event when many people were responsible for an important task but no-one did it. What was the outcome? How would you manage that situation differently next time?

Self-analysis questions

Identify your preferred management style. Imagine you are required to performance manage a staff member who has been verbally undermining your management decisions. Identify the pros and cons of using your preferred management style with this individual in the context of a multidisciplinary healthcare setting.

References

Australian Public Sector Commission. (2010). *Foundations of governance in the Australian public sector* [Employee information document]. Retrieved from http://www.apsc.gov.au/__data/assets/pdf_file/0019/5527/Foundations-2010.pdf

Bezuijen, X. M., van Dam, K., van den Berg, R. & Theirry, H. (2010). How leaders stimulate employee learning: A leader–member exchange approach. *Journal of Occupational and Organizational Psychology, 83*, 673–693. doi: 10.1348/096317909X468099

Brown, J. D. (2012). Understanding the better than average effect: Motives (still) matter. *Personality and Social Psychology Bulletin, 38*(2), 209–219. doi: 10.1177/0146167211432763

Corporations Act 2001 (Cth).

Dahling, J. J., Chau, S. L. & O'Malley, A. (2010). Correlation and consequences of feedback orientation in organisations. *Journal of Management, 38*(2), 531–546. doi: 10.1177/0149206310375467

Ehrler, M. (2005, March 7). Disregard your popularity; hold employees accountable. *Dayton Business Journal*. Retrieved from http://www.bizjournals.com

Financial Management and Accountabilities Act 1997 (Cth).

Goodhew, G. W., Cammock, P. A. & Hamilton, R. T. (2008). The management of poor performance by front-line managers. *Journal of Management, 27*(9), 951–962. doi: 10.1108/02621710810901291

Kouzes, J. M. & Posner, B. Z. (2007). *The leadership challenge* (4th ed.). San Francisco, CA: Jossey-Bass.

Kuhnen, C. M. & Tymula, A. (2012). Feedback, self-esteem, and performance in organizations. *Management Science, 58*(1), 94–113. doi: 10.1287/mnsc.1110.1379

Miller, B. C. (2006). *Keeping employees accountable for results: Quick tips for busy managers*. New York, NY: American Management Association.

National Health Act 1953 (Cth).

Nursing Executive Center. (2011). *Building peer accountability* [Study]. Available from Advisory Board Company website: http://www.advisory.com

Public Health Act 2010 (NSW).

Public Sector (Honesty and Accountability) Act 1995 (SA).

Royal Australasian College of Physicians. (n.d.). *Training site accreditation*. Retrieved from http://www.racp.edu.au/page/educational-and-professional-development/educational-overview/training-site-accreditation

Ryvkin, D., Krajc, M. & Ortmann, A. (2012). Are the unskilled doomed to remain unaware? *Journal of Economic Psychology, 33*, 1012–1031. doi: 10.1016/j.joep.2012.06.003

Smith, T. (2014). *Holding others accountable* [Video]. Retrieved from http://www.ozprinciple.com/others/holding-others-accountable

Whipple, R. (2011). *8 'be-attitudes' of holding people accountable*. Retrieved from http://thetrustambassador.com/2011/06/12/8-be-attitudes-of-holding-people-accountable

17

Critical thinking and decision-making

Richard Baldwin

Learning objectives

How do I:
- increase my understanding of the elements of critical thinking?
- counteract the barriers that might limit my critical thinking?
- improve my skills in decision-making?
- identify common decision-making errors?
- make better use of evidence in healthcare decision-making?

Introduction

It is important for managers and leaders to be able to critically analyse their own thinking and decision-making processes. Aspects of thinking and acting that managers and leaders should understand include their personal preferences, prejudices and cultural beliefs, and their personal motivations and desires. It is also important for them to understand the way these shape the biases they take to decision-making. To achieve success, leaders and managers require the ability to analyse, synthesise and establish their thoughts in a logical argument to reach a convincing conclusion.

Critical thinking

When faced with challenging management situations, the capacity to ask the right questions in order to clarify the situation helps managers to formulate appropriate responses. Critical thinking is a rational, systematic process that involves the assessment of statements and arguments, and the formulation of questions.

A statement claims that something is, or is not, the case and is not necessarily an argument. For example, three different statements that by themselves do not form an argument are: 'Smoking tobacco is bad for your health', 'Clinicians without management education make poor managers' and 'Healthcare is too expensive'. **Critical thinking** helps us decide if there is sufficient information to accept these statements.

> **thinking**
> ematic evaluation or
> ion of beliefs or statements,
> al standards' (Vaughn &
> ald, 2010, p. 119) that forms
> of problem-solving, decision-
> and emotional intelligence

To decide if the first of these statements is true requires further information, such as: 'Tobacco contains several chemicals that are known to be toxic to humans', 'Smoking tobacco releases these chemicals' and 'Epidemiological evidence indicates higher morbidity and mortality in people who regularly smoke tobacco'. Put together, these three statements form an argument. The argument is also called deductive reasoning and is distinguished from inductive reasoning, in which specific observations are used to develop broader conclusions.

The development of an argument around the other two statements above may require more than three statements and may be less well supported by evidence. Managers need the ability to assess which statements support the argument in order to analyse the arguments of others and formulate their own arguments.

Barriers to critical thinking

According to Vaughn and MacDonald (2010, p. 119), the two most common hindrances to critical thinking arise because of 'how we think' and 'what we think'. Our personal predispositions, such as preferences and appetites, influence how we think. Impediments to what we think tend to be based on beliefs about the world, our cultural heritage and upbringing. A significant influence on how and what we think can come from group pressure to conform and from our own desire to fit in.

To develop critical thinking skills, individuals need to assess the extent to which their thinking is influenced by the groups to which they belong. Group pressure can come in the form of peer pressure (the pressure to conform), appeals to popularity (a person is harder to like if they think or act differently) and appeals to common practice (doing something in the way it has always been done makes survival easier). However, group-centred thinking can degenerate into narrow-mindedness, resistance to change and stereotyping; and in this way it can limit an individual's critical thinking and problem-solving. One of the best defences against group thinking is to always evaluate a claim according to the strength of arguments – that is, to assess the statements that are being made, their underlying premises and the assumptions that these make to determine if there is a reasonable argument to support the conclusions offered. Rudinow & Barry (2007) identify the following barriers to critical thinking:

- limited frame of reference constructed because of a belief structure about the world and the source of the information – for example, placing unjustified faith in what is learned from the internet
- lack of willingness to accept different views and tendency to make hasty moral judgements
- reliance on untested assumptions, wishful thinking and self-deception – that is, being convinced that something is true because that is the easiest or least painful option or avoids difficult consequences
- ethnocentricity and cultural conditioning in thinking – that is, the inability or unwillingness to think differently from the familial, tribal or cultural group
- stereotypes or labels used to judge others – for example, holding a prejudice about someone's judgement based on their profession
- peer pressure and inappropriate reliance on authority – for example, simply believing what others say and avoiding thinking for oneself.

With regard to the final point above, critical thinking should not be confused with the need to obey a legitimate instruction, order, rule or policy. Careful judgement is needed before ignoring or disobeying legitimate authority.

Thinking is not driven by answers but by questions (Paul & Elder, 2000), and carefully constructed questions can define tasks, express problems and delineate issues. Questions are important for assessing the strengths of other people's arguments and formulating one's own arguments.

Assessing prejudice or sound decision-making

A male hospital employee who works as an administrative assistant with direct contact with patients of the mental health unit has recently informed you and his other work colleagues that he intends to commence wearing women's clothing to work. Under medical advice, he is also commencing the process of changing his sex, which will take some time. The employee has indicated to you that it is important for his own mental health that he continues to function within society as usual during his sex change process.

Two of the mental health team, claiming to represent the majority of the clinical and non-clinical staff, have come to you, as the manager, to express their concerns about the impact this sex change process will have on the patients of the mental health unit. They argue that many of the patients may find it confronting to have to deal with a man in women's clothing. They also argue that the sexual ambiguity will hamper this employee's capacity to engage with patients in a general sense. They insist that he be reassigned to work in a different part of the hospital.

As the manager, you need to consider whether the two staff members' concerns are reasonable or an exhibition of assumptions and prejudice on their part and to examine your own barriers to critical thinking that might arise as you consider your response to this situation.

Developing critical thinking skills

The Foundation of Critical Thinking lists methods that can help in the development of critical thinking (Elder & Paul, n.d.) They are discussed below.

Listen actively

Instead of hoping to passively absorb the message that someone is sending, it is useful to think about what they are saying both through the words they are using and the underlying messages. Active listening involves the listener reflecting back to the speaker what they think they heard, to confirm correct understanding. Active listening involves neither agreeing nor disagreeing; it is concerned with clarifying understanding of the speaker's meaning.

Stick to the point

When making a disciplined argument, it is important to avoid information and arguments that are irrelevant to the issue at hand and that jump from one point to another in a manner that is not logical or related. Before making an argument, the following questions should be considered: What is the main issue? What information and arguments relate directly to the main issue? What information and arguments are not relevant? How is the argument best developed to relate the relevant information to the main issue?

Be reasonable

There are two steps here: managers must be able to identify unreasonableness in others and identify their own unreasonableness. It is vital for managers to examine closely what people are saying and to form a view as to the strength of their arguments, regardless of whether they challenge the managers' own understanding, accepted position, deep-seated beliefs or cultural preferences. So, managers should be prepared to change a point of view when faced with a well-reasoned argument.

Question questions

Managers need to be skilled questioners. Successful questioners form questions that increase understanding and clarify issues. They avoid questions that come across as challenging, argumentative or loaded. One approach is to formulate a number of different questions for the same issue. Then select the one that best addresses the issue and is acceptable to the person being questioned; this is the most likely approach that will elicit the result being sought.

Decision-making

Every day we are faced with a wide variety of decisions, but not all of them relate to a problem or need deep analysis – for example, what to wear, what to eat, where to go after work. Decision-making extends to the workplace, where we need to decide if what we are facing is 'business as usual' or an issue that needs a unique decision. Unlike many personal decisions, decision-making in the workplace also has implications for others, so consideration of how to involve others in the **decision-making process** is important. The following steps guide the process of making decisions in the workplace:

> **Decision-making process**
> Steps that include identifying a [
> selecting an alternative and eva[
> the decision's effectiveness (Baz[
> & Moore, 2009; Robbins, Bergr[
> Stagg & Coulter, 2012)

- Identify the problem. Ask, 'Is there a problem?' If there is, ask, 'What is it?' Not every issue is necessarily a problem that needs a solution.
- Identify and weigh the criteria that will define the decision-making priorities. Gather and analyse information. Relatively simple analysis is often all that is necessary.
- Identify options and consult with stakeholders.
- Secure the commitment of stakeholders to the recommended option.
- Implement the solution and evaluate its effectiveness.

Biases and errors in decision-making

A number of scholars have identified possible biases and errors in decision-making, and Table 17.1 lists and summarises some of them.

Framing is concerned with how a question is shaped and defined. For example, the introduction of a ban on smoking in the workplace in the 1980s was successful because the problem was defined as an occupational health and safety issue rather than as an individual health issue for each employee. Shaping the argument against workplace smoking in this way placed legal obligations on both employers and employees to ensure a healthy workplace and removed the option of personal decisions by employees to smoke or to not smoke, even when they worked alone.

An anchoring effect occurs when a manager is faced with an unfamiliar issue but has only limited information upon which to base a decision. For example, the manager of a health service is required to negotiate the initial purchase of a new imaging machine from the only company that sells them. Although the machine is new to this country, the health service's clinicians have argued that it is essential for quality healthcare and will add to the service's prestige. No price has been mentioned, and the manager knows that the company is keen to make the first national sale. The manager's first impulse may be to ask the vendor for

Table 17.1 Possible biases and errors that occur in decision-making, according to their discussion in specific texts

Biases and errors	Description	Identified in recommended texts		
		(1)	(2)	(3)
Anchoring	Influence by others	✓	✓	✓
Availability	Bias from most recent events		✓	✓
Confirmation	Bias-based evidence	✓	✓	
Framing	Shaping the question	✓	✓	✓
Group failure	Assumption that a group of smart people can't be wrong			✓
Immediate gratification	Desire for a quick decision		✓	
Overprudence	Excessive cautiousness	✓		
Overconfidence in forecasting	Unrealistically positive views of personal decision-making	✓	✓	✓
Plunging in	Decisions made too quickly			✓
Randomness	Creation of meaning from unconnected information		✓	
Representation	Bias from other like events		✓	
Rule of thumb	Dependence on custom, practice and past experience	✓	✓	✓
Selective perception	Bias-based perception		✓	✓
Sunk costs	Protection of past mistakes	✓	✓	

Sources: Column headings are as follows: (1) J. S. Hammond, R. L. Keeney & H. Raiffa (1998). *The hidden traps in decision making. Harvard Business Review,* 76(5), 2–11; (2) S. P. Robbins, R. Bergman, I. Stagg & M. Coulter (2012). *Management* (6th ed.). Frenchs Forest: Pearson, based on D. Kahneman, P. Slovic & A. Tversky (1982). *Judgement under uncertainty: Heuristics and biases.* Cambridge, United Kingdom: Cambridge University; and S. Robbins (2004). *Decide and conquer: Make winning decisions and take control of your life.* Upper Saddle River, NJ: Financial Times Prentice Hall; (3) J. E. Russo & P. J. H. Schoemaker (1989). *Decision traps: Ten barriers to brilliant decision-making and how to overcome them.* New York, NY: Doubleday.

their price, and it comes in higher than the health service is prepared to pay. In preparing a counter offer, the manager may be influenced by the vendor's first offer; that is, the response will be anchored by the new information. Hammond, Keeney and Raiffa (1998) offer the following suggestions to avoid the possible effects of anchoring:

- Use different starting points to view the issue. (For example, ask for information on, or suggest, other imaging machines that may be available, to minimise the impression of commitment to purchasing the new machine.)
- Determine the boundaries to possible solutions. (For example, before commencing negotiations, be clear about the cost-effectiveness of the new machine to the health service and how much it is therefore worth to the health service.)

- Undertake some comparative research. (For example, seek information about the price of similar machines or the price of this machine in other countries.)
- Use anchoring proactively. (For example, as the buyer, make the first offer.)

However, strategies to avoid the impact of anchoring will vary with different situations. For example, if a manager wants new ideas from their health team about potential changes to health service design, it may be a good idea for the manager not to suggest their ideas first. Making the first suggestion may limit the team's responses. They may feel the need to respond to the suggestion, possibly negatively, rather than coming up with their own ideas. That is, going first may anchor the team's responses.

Evidence-based management decision-making

Evidence-based decision management has increased in importance in recent decades for both clinical and non-clinical managers in health organisations. One useful example of managers using evidence to guide change is clinical services redesign projects, which have been completed across a large number of health services in recent years (Ben-Tovim et al., 2008; Eagar, Masso, Robert & Bate, 2008; Ham, Kipping & Mcleod, 2003; Masso, Robert, McCarthy & Eagar, 2010; Scott et al., 2011). Typically, clinical services redesign projects are time-limited, sometimes intensive, initiatives. They involve discrete stages, and each stage is heavily based on existing data and also uses rigorously collected new data. The use of evidence in this way is crucial to the active and supportive involvement of both clinicians and managers.

In health services, research evidence may not be consistent, and opinions are often widely and strongly held. In addition, the availability of evidence does not guarantee that it will be accepted or used. Two examples are relevant to the use of evidence-based decision-making. The first concerns the discovery of the *Helicobacter pylori* bacillus by Australian scientists Barry Marshall and Robin Warren, who in 2005 were awarded the Nobel Prize for what is considered by many to be a paradigm shift in the way gastric ulcers are treated. However, 23 years after the first scientific reports emerged, Ahmed (2005, para. 3) noted that the clinical community 'met their findings, with skepticism and a lot of criticism' and that despite the existence of solid evidence it took 'quite a remarkable length of time for their discovery to become widely accepted'. The second example concerns the use of evidence in the area of public health. Botterill and Hindmoor (2012) examined this in relation to the complex issue of obesity and compared it to the simple, and often incorrect, messages articulated by policy-makers and public health officials. They concluded that advisors to decision-makers are 'boundedly rational' (p. 367); that is, complex situations are often reduced to simple messages for senior managers and policy-makers as they are bounded by their capacity to make rational decisions when faced with large volumes of conflicting information, which need to be reduced to relatively simple messages.

Summary

- Critical thinking is an essential skill for all health services managers and leaders, and techniques such as active listening, sticking to the point, being reasonable and asking thoughtful questions are elements of critical thinking.
- The barriers to critical thinking include a limited frame of reference, lack of willingness to accept different views, relying on untested assumptions, wishful thinking, self-deception, ethnocentric and cultural conditioning in thinking, peer pressure and stereotypes.
- Decision-making steps include identifying the problem, identifying and weighing the criteria that will define the decision-making priorities, and gathering and analysing information.
- There are common errors and biases that may adversely influence decisions.

Reflective questions

1 Can you recall the last time you practised the technique of active listening in your conversations with a friend or colleague? What happened?

2 Can you identify how your cultural and religious beliefs may impact on your critical thinking?

3 The director of nursing has complained to you that the previous Saturday night waiting time in the emergency department exceeded agreed targets. Is this a problem and, if yes, what is it? Reflect on whether this is a problem that needs investigation and a decision, and, if yes, what the problem is?

4 If the majority of your workforce is predominantly female and aged over 50 years, is this necessarily a problem that needs investigation? If yes, what is the problem?

5 Is a small number of complaints from patients about cancelled minor day surgery procedures (but with no serious health consequences) a problem that needs investigation and a decision? If yes, what is the problem?

Self-analysis question

Values and beliefs are often taken for granted, and we are not regularly asked to think about how they may influence our thinking. Being in touch with your own values and beliefs is important, because it enables you to be aware of the bias you may bring to your decision-making. Write down your values and personal positions concerning some everyday and some topical issues. Try to condense each value statement into a single sentence.

References

Ahmed, N. (2005). 23 years of the discovery of *Helicobacter Pylori*: Is the debate over? *Annals of Clinical Microbiology and Antimicrobials, 4*(17). doi: 10.1186/1476-0711-4-17

Bazerman, M. H. & Moore, D. A. (2009). *Judgment in managerial decision making* (7th ed.). Hoboken, NJ: Wiley.

Ben-Tovim, D. I., Bassham, J. E., Bennett, D. M., Dougherty, M. L., Martin, M. A., O'Neill, S. J. … Szwarcbord, M. G. (2008). Redesigning care at the Flinders Medical Centre: Clinical process redesign using 'lean thinking'. *Medical Journal of Australia, 188*(6 Suppl), S27. Retrieved from https://www.mja.com.au

Botterill, L. C., & Hindmoor, A. (2012). Turtles all the way down: Bounded rationality in an evidence-based age. *Policy Studies, 33*(5), 367–379. doi: 10.1080/01442872.2011.626315

Eagar, K., Masso, M., Robert, G. & Bate, P. (2008). *The NSW Clinical Services Redesign Program: Achievements and lessons.* Wollongong: University of Wollongong, Centre for Health Service Development.

Elder, L. & Paul, R. (n.d.). *Becoming a critic of your thinking.* Retrieved from http://www.criticalthinking.org/pages/becoming-a-critic-of-your-thinking/478

Ham, C., Kipping, R. & Mcleod, H. (2003). Redesigning work processes in health care: Lessons from the National Health Service. *Milbank Quarterly, 81*(3), 415–439. doi: 10.1111/1468-0009.t01-3-00062

Hammond, J. S., Keeney, R. L. & Raiffa, H. (1998). The hidden traps in decision making. *Harvard Business Review, 76*(5), 2–11.

Kahneman, D., Slovic, P. & Tversky, A. (1982). *Judgement under uncertainty: Heuristics and biases.* Cambridge, United Kingdom: Cambridge University.

Masso, M., Robert, G., McCarthy, G. & Eagar, K. (2010). The Clinical Services Redesign Program in New South Wales: Perceptions of senior health managers. *Australian Health Review, 34,* 352–359. doi: 10.1071/AH08720

Paul, R. & Elder, L. (2000). *The role of questions in teaching, thinking and learning.* [Online article taken from R. Paul & L. Elder, *Critical thinking handbook: Basic theory and instructional structures* (n.p.), Tomales, CA: Foundation for Critical Thinking]. Retrieved from http://www.criticalthinking.org/pages/the-role-of-questions-in-teaching-thinking-and-learning/524

Robbins, S. (2004). *Decide and conquer: Make winning decisions and take control of your life.* Upper Saddle River, NJ: Financial Times Prentice Hall.

Robbins, S. P., Bergman, R., Stagg, I. & Coulter, M. (2012). *Management* (6th ed.). Frenchs Forest: Pearson.

Rudinow, J. & Barry, V. E. (2007). *Invitation to critical thinking* (6th ed.). Belmont, CA: Thompson Higher Education.

Russo, J. E. & Schoemaker, P. J. H. (1989). *Decision traps: Ten barriers to brilliant decision-making and how to overcome them.* New York, NY: Doubleday.

Scott, I. A., Wills, R.-A., Coory, M., Watson, M. J., Butler, F., Waters, M. & Bowler, S. (2011). Impact of hospital-wide process redesign on clinical outcomes: A comparative study of internally versus externally led intervention. *BMJ Quality & Safety, 20*(6), 539–548. doi: 10.1136/bmjqs.2010.042150

Vaughn, L. & MacDonald, C. (2010). *The power of critical thinking* (2nd Canadian ed.). Ontario, Canada: Oxford University.

18

Managing and leading staff

David S. Briggs and Godfrey Isouard

Learning objectives

How do I:
- develop my skills in leadership of human resources as a critical component of health policy and organisational activity?
- understand the challenging role of the management of human resources in a complex, professionally dominated industry that is affected by constant change?
- determine effective strategies for retention policies and practices that are required to respond to the global maldistributions and shortages within the health profession?
- consider the requirements that human resources has for the management of four distinct generations in the substantially feminine and ageing health workforce?

Introduction

In a text on leadership and management the perspective on human resource management requires a strategic approach. Health is dominated by a large, diverse, highly professionalised workforce. Human resource management is complex and needs to properly consider three aspects of workforce development – namely, supply, demand and mobility (Narasimhan et al., 2004).

Definitions

The health workforce is globalised, with maldistributions and existing and projected shortages (Health Workforce Australia, 2012). The mobilisation and strengthening of human resources are seen as critical in sustainable health systems (Chen et al. 2004, Kabene, Orchard, Howard, Soriano & Leduc, 2006; Karimi, Cheng, Bartram, Leggat

& Sarkeshik, 2014). The health (75 per cent) and health management (61 per cent) workforce in Australia is predominantly female as compared with all industries (at 47 per cent and 36 per cent respectively) (Martins & Isouard, 2014). The health workforce is multigenerational, multicultural and substantially female. It requires collaboration across sectors on an interprofessional basis and across organisational boundaries within multidisciplinary teams and networks of service provision (Duckett, 2005).

Leadership and management

Health managers and leaders are deployed in large health systems, often distant geographically from the services and localities they manage. They are highly qualified, with the predominate field of study being health, followed by management and commerce qualifications (Martins & Isouard, 2014). Health managers are often seen to be implementing health reform but are also affected by constant reform rather than being in control (Briggs, Smyth & Anderson, 2012). Managers have been described as both victims and survivors (McKenna & Richardson, 2003) and as both heroes and villains (Greener, 2004).

Some health managers have only clinical qualifications, their management experience, both good and bad, having been learned from others. There are profession-based differences in approach to management roles (Fitzgerald & Teal, 2003) and tensions between generalist and clinically qualified managers and their peer groups where the management role is described as contested. Managers need 'to develop emotional resilience, set boundaries, develop personal support structures and understand the formal and informal sides of the organisation' (Briggs, Cruickshank & Paliadelis, 2012, p. 623). The role has moved to leadership and managing change, with emphases on sensemaking, motivating and communicating. It involves engagement, relationship-building, learning, thinking flexibly, being resilient and understanding critical thinking (Briggs, Smyth et al., 2012).

Engagement, empowerment and learning

The management of our health workforce has shifted dramatically, from a corporate function to part of all supervisors' and managers' roles (Leggat, Bartram, Casimir & Stanton, 2010). The impact of legislation and standards has ensured and made routine many practices such as industrial relations, remunerative practices, work health and safety, affirmative action and anti-discrimination. The human resources concepts of motivation and supervision are moving towards concepts of **work engagement** and empowerment, and the concept of training per se is moving towards learning, knowledge development, coaching, preceptorships and mentoring.

> **Work engagement**
> Psychological and emotional co[m]
> of an employee to their work an[d]
> workplace

Work engagement is meant to provide 'positive, fulfilling ... work related well-being ... to provide engaged, high energy work focussed staff', broadening the view about the meaning and effects of work (Bakker, Schaufeli, Leiter & Taris, 2008, p. 187). Coaching is recognised as a supportive but challenging process in developing skills in others (Isouard, Thiessen, Stanton & Hanson, 2006) and has been identified as a key competence for healthcare leadership (Henochowicz & Hetherington, 2006). Mentoring programs enhance job satisfaction of those mentored, improving knowledge, skills and career prospects (Weng et al., 2010). Mentoring is broad-based and concentrates on developing career progression, scholarly achievement and personal development, through reciprocity and accountability over time (Mills, Francis & Bonner, 2005).

Performance management

The members of the health workforce are regularly evaluated through performance reviews based on key performance indicators, competencies, organisational objectives and the perceptions of peers and consumers, a process often referred to as 360-degree reviews. Staff are also routinely measured in service and goal orientations, and in how patients and clients generally perceive the quality of teams and services.

Managers need to focus on **recruitment** and **retention** of staff, the development of the workforce, issues of workforce substitution and the achievement of a high-performance organisation that attracts and retains the right people and provides a healthy work environment. The health sector is described as 'people centred' (McConnell, 2000, p. 4) and requires an understanding of organisational behaviour, culture, power and team-based bottom-up approaches (Braithwaite, 2005).

Liang, Leggat, Howard and Lee (2013) undertook research to identify core **competencies** important in developing the capability of health managers, identifying staff development and training needs, and the implementation and conduct of performance management systems. The core competencies described are 'leadership; leading and managing change; operations, administration and resource management; evidence-informed decision making; knowledge of healthcare environment and the organisation; interpersonal, communication qualities and relationship management' (Liang et al., 2013, p. 569). Competencies reflect specific skills and attributes required of a role, and **capability** is used to describe the capacity of individuals to successfully undertake the role and utilise the competencies. Capability goes to broader concepts of 'knowledge, skills and personal attributes' (Briggs, Smyth et al., 2012, p. 73).

ment
:ess of finding and hiring the
.lified candidate

ion
ree to which an organisation is
.eep good employees satisfied
.hey want to continue to work
.organisation

tency
c skill, knowledge or attribute
of a role

lity
acity of individuals to
ully undertake the role and
e competencies

Gender

Gender is a concept based in the beliefs of society 'about what are appropriate roles and activities of men and women'. The debate is often around equality and equity and about opportunity to progress and receive promotion. Managers need to focus on how to 'improve the number, distribution and skill mix of the health workforce' (Reichenbach & Brown, 2004, pp. 792–793). Managers should also understand competing long-held beliefs and values within the workforce, including those that might be held by managers. There may also be requirements to meet institutional policies and practices on gender.

Multiple generations

The workforce now extends across four generations, described by Stanley (2010, p. 846) as 'veterans', 'baby boomers', 'generation X' and 'generation Y'. Dols, Landrum and Wieck (2010, pp. 68–69) describe the generations as 'traditionalists', 'baby boomers', 'generation X' and 'millennials'. The generational differences are described in terms of values, beliefs, expectations and behaviours. Managers need to develop strategies to engage and retain these groups.

Dols et al. (2010, pp. 70–73) suggest providing and rewarding effective mentors; managing high workloads and burnout; organising interventional staffing at difficult times; maintaining morale through acknowledgement, respect, praise and appreciation; recognising the 'extra mile'; ensuring safety as the norm; building relationships and teamwork; and being a proactive leader. Wilson, Squires, Widger, Cranley and Tourangeau (2008) focus on job satisfaction and suggest implementing shared governance, self-scheduling and job-sharing. Howell, Beckett, Nettiksimmons & Villablanca (2012, p. 720) suggest that 'enhancing and communicating career flexibility can be an effective strategy for … recruitment and retention'.

The older or ageing part of the workforce becomes more important in times of workforce shortages. In one organisation, allied health staff aged over 50 represented more than one-quarter of that occupational group, and more than half the rural health nurse workforce was over 50 (Fragar & Depczynski, 2011). Older health workers are committed productive workers affected by the impact of ageing on healthy functioning. Managing an ageing workforce requires policies and practices that are supportive and enhance their retention. Hahn's (2011) study of multiple generations drew on the ACORN mnemonic to describe imperatives:

- Accommodate employee differences.
- Create workplace choices.
- Operate from a sophisticated management style.
- Respect competence and initiative.
- Nourish retention.

Hahn (2011) encourages the use of five strategies to address generational circumstances:

- Self-assess your managerial style.
- Understand generational characteristics and core values.

- Embrace commonalities.
- Create and maintain a respectful culture.
- Bridge the generational gap.

Generational differences can be a source of frustration for managers, who need to appreciate the differences and focus on the positives and strengths in building a positive workplace (Gursoy, Maier & Chi, 2008).

Human resources

The shifted focus of human resources still sees it as a critical component of health policy and organisational activity (Dussault & Dubois, 2003) that has a more strategic planning and developmental role. The changing context of healthcare described in this chapter requires a human resource strategic approach that:

- understands the nature of the existing workforce
- focuses on maximising skills utilisation in adaptive and flexible ways
- strategically develops the workforce in sustainable ways
- emphasises retention of existing staff while also preparing for succession
- develops a responsive, adaptive and innovative workforce.

The concepts of accountability, trust and stewardship afforded to managers are important. The extent of trust is reflected in the degree of centralisation and decentralisation allowed (Rathwell & Persaud, 2002). Ideally, leaders and managers should be located close to and accessible by those delivering care. They should be capable of managing down and out to staff, clients, patients and communities as well as being capable of managing up to higher organisational levels (Briggs, 2008).

Batalden et al. (2003) suggest that leadership and quality in clinical microsystems are important and are often group activities that involve attention to processes that build knowledge, take action, review and reflect: a consistent and continuous process. The question is how best to support, develop and increase the leadership of the microsystems, where care is actually delivered. It is important that leaders possess an understanding of leadership as something more than being concerned with hierarchies and control and goes to the core of leadership at the service delivery level, within and between professions.

Skills utilisation

Dubois and Sing (2009, p. 91) suggest a move from a focus on 'staff-mix' to 'skill-mix and beyond'. These authors see the challenges as workforce shortages, societal trends towards reduced work hours, ageing and early retirement, and continued pressure on health systems over waiting times and access to services. They argue that the current focus on staff-mix is restrictive and emphasise that a focus on staff skills provides a more dynamic human resources environment that focuses effective utilisation of the available health personnel to their fullest potential.

Dubois and Singh's (2009) focus on maximising skills requires a human resources emphasis on skills assessment, training and development so that the workforce can take on new roles and functions. This occurs through role enhancement and/or role enlargement. Altering roles should be attractive to employees because it offers opportunities, new competencies and greater achievement, recognition and motivation. Evidence in support of these types of strategies is not conclusive, however, and they might cause increased tension or confusion with traditional professional roles and be seen as convenient approaches to workforce rationalisation.

Integrated care in treating chronic conditions requires multiple skills, including management, system-planning, care-planning, negotiation and teamwork, bringing clinical and management roles into alignment. These skills are also required in direct engagement, supporting patients and clients with the capacity to self-manage their disease or chronic condition. Such approaches extend the need for skill flexibility, role substitution and role delegation. Conditions need to be created that allow the organisation to maximise human resources and to utilise them flexibly (Dubois & Singh, 2009).

The health workforce is often described in terms of activity, such as hours per day of care, or in numbers or ratios, such as nurse to patient ratios. Attempts to describe the impact of these ratios in terms of quality and safety of care are inconclusive. There are also tensions between mandating ratios and allowing management to make effective decisions around staff deployment. While the evidence about what is adequate is not conclusive, increases in nursing staff levels are generally resisted, as this occupational group is the largest profession within health, and therefore a greater expense in accounting terms for those concerned with budgets. So human resource practitioners need to understand the tension when staff are seen as a resource while at the same time being accounted for as an expense (Day, Viswasam & Briggs, 2004).

Organisational behaviour and culture

Implementing human resource initiatives in the midst of what has become constant health reform requires an understanding of the impact of culture on staff and organisations. Culture is often described in contexts of transforming and empowering people to achieve a variety of objectives. There are two main theoretical perspectives on culture: that it is descriptive of what an organisation is and that it is something that organisations have. Paying attention to culture is regarded as important in implementing reform (Davies, Nutley & Mannion, 2000).

Having a consistent and coordinated approach between the organisation and its staff as to purpose or mission and the values and behaviours ascribed is an important consideration. How management value staff and how they behave towards them are also important. This requires 'shared beliefs, attitudes, values, and norms of behaviour' (Davies et al., 2000, p. 112). Often within organisations this is described as 'the way we do things around here', mostly stated in a manner that suggests opposition to change. Leonard, Graham and Bonacum (2004, p. i89) describe resistance to change and effective behaviours as communication failures and suggest that the emphasis is on 'correcting system flaws', teamwork and 'visible support from senior leadership and strong clinical leadership'. It is important to consistently practise the agreed values and behaviours so that they have real meaning within the organisation. According to Dubois and Singh (2009), an effective organisational structure for the management of human resources includes:

- relatively flat hierarchy with few supervisors
- worker autonomy
- participative management
- professional development opportunities
- relatively high organisational status for nursing
- collaboration.

Managing the challenge of the difficult worker

In most organisations there is someone perceived by management as the difficult worker, who does their job but does not engage in work activities outside the role, who is a champion of defending the status quo – 'the way we do things around here' – and is hence resistant to change, and who is admired by fellow workers for saying what they think and for standing up to management.

Is such a worker really 'the problem', or is the issue more to do with how that person is managed? From experience, I would spend informal time with this person in their work surrounds (not my office) and find out a bit more about them on a personal level. The experiences and skills that their life experience have provided may come as a surprise. I would ask them for their view or even advice about a particular problem I am confronting. I would find out if they have ever been away from work on a training course or on a visit to a similar facility or service, and if they haven't I would make sure it happens in a purposeful way. I would also tell the staff member that I appreciate that they are well liked and respected by other staff and that I see this as something positive to be built on.

This approach means practising an old but important management skill: engaging by walking and talking to staff, identifying issues and responding. If this is done skilfully, the potential of the staff member is developed, and they are empowered to want to come onside and be an effective contributor. This requires skill and effort but could be easier than performance-managing an underperformer out of the organisation.

Health teams

Increasingly, healthcare staff work in teams across sectors, in networks and in interprofessional contexts. The healthcare focus is on teamwork in safety and quality care, with one emphasis that comes from the experience of the aviation industry and its approach to crew resource management. Healthcare organisations draw on this experience to develop individual and team behaviours that alter how members communicate a problem or concern, which is viewed outside traditional approaches of apportioning blame, and how tasks are simplified and stepped. Success depends on commitment from the top and on being accepted culturally (Leonard et al., 2004). Knowledge, skills and attitudes are summarised in terms of team effectiveness as team leadership, mutual performance monitoring, backup behaviour or mutual support, communication and adaptability, shared mental models, collective orientation and mutual trust (Baker, Day & Salas, 2006; Leggat & Balding, 2013).

High-performance work systems are said to have a positive influence on employees' attitudes and behaviours (Bonias, Bartram, Leggat & Stanton, 2010). They describe human resource practices such as selective recruitment, extensive training, information-sharing, teamwork and decentralised decision-making as important influences on attitudes, behaviours and job performance (Leggat & Balding, 2013). Teamwork requires effective communication and addresses better use of resources to improve quality of care and utilises an approach where professional differences can be put aside for better outcomes. This is one of the main benefits of having a quality improvement culture embedded in the organisation (Leonard et al., 2004).

> **High-performance work sys**
> A bundle of human resource
> management practices related t
> organisational performance

Leadership of teams requires an understanding of self, often referred to as emotional intelligence. Goleman (2008) defines this in the context of self-management and relationship skills. Karimi et al. (2014) describe the importance of emotional intelligence in human resource management as a training need, linking its relevance to high-performance work systems. Briggs, Smyth et al. (2012, p. 75) suggest that a sense-making role involves the following factors:

Engagement

Communication

Interpretation and understanding

Flexible thinking

Managing competing interests

Critical thinking

Big picture visioning

Understanding and managing self

Resilience and self-confidence

Summary

- Human resource management occurs in a complex, constantly changing organisational arrangement dominated by highly skilled health professionals.
- The context is dynamic and the workforce is global.
- The supply of the workforce is maldistributed, with shortages and projected inability to meet future demands.
- Human resource leadership needs to increasingly focus on retention and on development of existing employees' skills bases.
- Critical human resource practices focus on engagement and empowerment of a flexible, adaptive workforce.

Reflective questions

1 If you were in a position to do so, how might you go about improving the number, distribution and skill-mix of the health workforce?

2 How well do you know your fellow workers or your staff? What generations are present?

3 Do you have an effective performance management review system in your organisation?

4 Do you understand the need to develop leadership at the clinical microsystem level?

5 How do you go about building knowledge by emphasising the importance of review and reflection?

Self-analysis questions

Research indicates that health service managers need a high level of self-awareness of their own abilities, sound emotional stability and personal resilience to be able to effectively lead and manage others. Develop a list of the required characteristics identified in this chapter and self-assess your current status of preparedness in these areas. Discuss with mentors and colleagues where they think you need to focus your personal development.

References

Baker, D. P., Day, R. & Salas, E. (2006). Teamwork as an essential component of high reliability organisations (Part 2). *Health Services Research*, 41(4), 1576–1598. doi: 10.1111/j.1475-6773.2006.00566.x

Bakker, A. B., Schaufeli, W. B., Leiter, M. P. & Taris, T. W. (2008). Work engagement: An emerging concept in occupational health psychology, work & stress. *International Journal of Work, Health & Organisations*, 22(3), 187–200. doi: 10.1080/02678370802393649

Batalden, P. B., Nelson, E. C., Mohr, J. M., Godfrey, M. S., Huber, M. S., Kosnik, L. & Ashling, K. (2003). Microsystems in health care: Part 5. How leaders are leading. *Joint Commission Journal on Quality and Safety*, 29(6), 297–308.

Bonias, D., Bartram, T., Leggat, S. & Stanton, P. (2010). Does psychological empowerment mediate the relationship between high performance work systems and quality of patient care in hospitals? *Asia Pacific Journal of Human Resources, 48*(3), 319–337. doi: 10.1177/1038411110381667

Braithwaite, J. (2005). Invest in people, not restructuring. *British Medical Journal, 331*(7527), 1272. doi: 10.1136/bmj.331.7527.1272-a

Briggs, D. S. (2008). SHAPE declaration on the organisation and management of health services: A call for informed public debate. *Asia Pacific Journal of Health Management, 3*(2), 10–13.

Briggs, D. S., Cruickshank, M. & Paliadelis, P. (2012). Health managers and health reform. *Journal of Management & Organisation, 18*(5), 641–658.

Briggs, D. S., Smyth, A. & Anderson, J. A. (2012). In search of capable health managers: What is distinctive about health management and why does it matter? *Asia Pacific Journal of Health Management, 7*(2), 71–78.

Chen, L., Evans, T., Anand, S., Boufford, J. I., Brown, H., Chowdhury, M. … Wibulpolprasert, S. (2004). Human resources for health: Overcoming the crisis. *Lancet, 364*(9449), 1984–1990. doi: 10.1016/S0140-6736(04)17482-5

Davies, H. T. O., Nutley, S. M. & Mannion, R. (2000). Organisational culture and quality of health care. *Quality in Health Care, 9*, 111–119.

Day, G., Viswasam, G. & Briggs, D. S. (2004). The budget and financial control. In M. Courtney & D. S. Briggs (Eds), *Health care financial management* (pp. 173–190). Sydney: Elsevier Mosby.

Dols, J., Landrum, P. & Wiek, K. L. (2010). Leading and managing an intergenerational workforce. *Creative Nursing, 16*(2), 68–74. doi: 10.1891/1078-4535.16.2.68

Dubois, C. A. & Singh, D. (2009). From staff-mix to skill-mix and beyond: Towards a systemic approach to health workforce management. *Human Resources for Health, 7*(87). doi: 10.1186/1478-4491-7-87

Duckett, S. J. (2005). Interventions to facilitate health workforce restructure. *Australia and New Zealand Health Policy, 2*(14). doi: 10.1186/1743-8462-2-14

Dussault, G. & Dubois, C. A. (2003). Human resources for health policies: A critical component in health policies. *Human Resources for Health, 1*(1). doi: 10.1186/1478-4491-1-1

Fitzgerald, A. & Teal, G. (2003). Health reform, professional identity and sub-cultures: The changing inter-professional relations between doctors. *Contemporary Nurse, 16*(1–2), 9–19.

Fragar, L. J. & Depczynski, J. C. (2011). Beyond 50: Challenges at work for older nurses and allied health workers in rural Australia; A thematic analysis of focus group discussions. *Health Services Research, 11*(42). doi: 10.1186/1472-6963-11-42

Goleman, D. (2008). *Best of HBR on emotionally intelligent leadership* (2nd ed., Harvard Business Review Article Collection). New York, NY: Harvard Business.

Greener, I. (2004). Talking to health managers about change: Heroes, villains and simplification. *Journal of Health Organisation and Management, 18*(5), 321–335.

Gursoy, D., Maier, T. A. & Chi, C. G. (2008). Generational differences: An examination of work values and generational gaps in the hospitality workforce. *International Journal of Hospitality Workforce, 27*, 448–458. doi: 10.1016/j.ijhm.2007.11.002

Hahn, J. A. (2011). Managing multiple generations: Scenarios from the workplace. *Nursing Forum, 46*(3), 119–127. doi: 10.1111/j.1744-6198.2011.00223

Health Workforce Australia. (2012). *Health workforce 2025: Doctors, nurses and midwives.* Retrieved from http://www.hwa.gov.au/our-work/health-workforce-planning/health -workforce-2025-doctors-nurses-and-midwives

Henochowicz, S. & Hetherington, D. (2006). Leadership coaching in health care. *Leadership & Organisational Development Journal, 27*(3), 183–189. doi: 10.1108/01437730610657703

Howell, L. P., Beckett, L. A., Nettiksimmons, M. A. & Villablanca, M. D. (2012). Generational and gender perspectives on career flexibility: Ensuring the faculty workforce of the future. *American Journal of Medicine, 125*(7), 719–728. doi: 10.1016/j.amjmed.2012.03. 013

Isouard, G., Thiessen, V., Stanton, P. & Hanson, S. (2006). Managing people in the health care industry. In M. G. Harris (Ed.), *Managing health services: Concepts and practices* (2nd ed., pp. 114–134). Marrickville: Mosby Elsevier.

Kabene, S. M., Orchard, C., Howard, J. M., Soriano, M. A. & Leduc, R. (2006). The importance of human resource management in health care: A global context. *Human Resources for Health, 4*(20). doi: 10.1186/1478-4491-4-20

Karimi, L., Cheng, C., Bartram, T., Leggat, S. G. & Sarkeshik, S. (2014). The effects of emotional intelligence and stress-related presenteeism on nurses' well being. *Asia Pacific Journal of Human Resources.* doi: 10.1111/1744-7941.12049

Leggat, S. C. & Balding, C. (2013). Achieving organisational competence for clinical leadership: The role of high performance work systems. *Journal of Health Organisation and Management, 27*(3), 312–329. doi: 10.1108/jhom-jul-2012-0132

Leggat, S., Bartram, T., Casimir, G. & Stanton, P. (2010). Nurse perceptions of the quality of patient care: Confirming the importance of empowerment and job satisfaction. *Healthcare Management Review, 35*(4), 355–364. doi: 10.1111/1744-7941.12049

Leonard, M., Graham, S. & Bonacum, D. (2004). The human factor: The critical importance of effective teamwork and communication in providing safe care. *Quality & Safety in Health Care, 13*(Suppl 1), i85–i90. doi: 10.1136/qshc.2004.010033

Liang, Z., Leggat, S. G., Howard, P. E. & Lee, K. (2013). What makes a hospital manager competent at the middle and senior levels? *Australian Health Review, 37,* 566–573. doi: 10.1071/AH12004

Martins, J. M. & Isouard, G. (2014). Health service managers in Australia: Progression and evolution. *Asia Pacific Journal of Health Management, 9*(2), 35–52.

McConnell, C. R. (2000). The changing face of health care management. *Health Care Manager, 18*(3), 1–17.

McKenna, S. & Richardson, J. (2003). Managing in the New Zealand health service: The interpretation of experience. *Journal of Health Organisation, 17*(2), 74–87.

Mills, J. E., Francis, K. L. & Bonner, A. (2005). Mentoring, clinical supervision and preceptoring: Clarifying the conceptual definitions for Australian rural nurses; A review of the literature. *Rural and Remote Health, 5*(410). Retrieved from http://www.rrh.org.au/publishedarticles/ article_print_410.pdf

Narasimhan, V., Brown, H., Pablos-Mendez, A., Adams, O., Dussault, G., Elzinga, G. & Chen, L. (2004). Responding to the global human resources crisis. *Lancet, 363*(9419), 1469–1472. doi: 10.1016/S0140-6736(04)16108-4

Rathwell, T. & Persaud, D. D. (2002). Running to stay still: Change and management in Canadian healthcare. *Healthcare Management Forum, 15*(3), 10–17.

Reichenbach, L. & Brown, H. (2004). Gender and academic medicine: Impacts on the health workforce. *British Medical Journal, 329*, 792–795. doi: 10.1136/bmj.329.7469.792

Stanley, D. (2010). Multigenerational workforce issues and their implications for leadership in nursing. *Journal of Nursing Management, 18*, 846–852. doi: 10.1111/j.1365 -2834.2010.01158.x

Weng, R. H., Huang, C. Y., Tsai, W. C., Chang, L. Y., Lin, S. E. & Lee, M. Y. (2010). Exploring the impact of mentoring functions on job satisfaction and organisational commitment of new staff nurses. *Health Services Research, 10*(240). doi: 10.1108/01437730610657703

Wilson, B., Squires, M., Widger, K., Cranley, L. & Tourangeau, A. (2008). Job satisfaction among a multigenerational nursing workforce. *Journal of Nursing Management, 16*, 716–723. doi: 10.1111/j.1365-2834.2008.00874.x

19

Project management

Zhanming Liang

Learning objectives

How do I:
- apply project management in health and community services?
- recognise the fundamentals and important concepts in project management?
- appreciate project-planning life cycles and major characteristics of projects?
- improve my skills in project management?
- measure project success?

Introduction

In the face of rapid change as a response to increasing health needs and financial constraints, healthcare systems and organisations are pressured to adopt innovative and effective tools to manage service delivery. Since its inception in the architectural, engineering and building sectors in the early 1900s, project management has become a systematic management tool with techniques to bring people and resources together for a single purpose (Cleland & Gareis, 2006). Its popularity in health and community services has significantly increased in the last decade. Project management has been widely used as an effective management tool to implement change, trialling new service models, developing new programs and technologies, and improving organisational structure and care processes (Dwyer, Liang, Thiessen & Martini, 2013). The inclusion of project management as one of the core competencies for health service managers, public health practitioners and those who may need to be involved in health-related projects in some way further proves its importance in health and community service provision. This chapter assists readers to develop understanding of projects and project management, how projects should be planned and implemented, ways of ensuring and measuring project success and, more importantly, how to use project management as a tool to achieve intended outcomes and generate new knowledge for future learning.

Definitions

As described by Dwyer et al. (2013, p. 20), 'a **project** is a unique set of inter-related activities designed to produce a set of deliverables and achieve a defined goal within clearly defined time, cost and quality constraints'. Dwyer and colleagues also state that the unique feature of projects can be defined as the **3D objective**, or project triangle: to deliver quality performance and meet expectations within the timeframe and budget allowed (see Figure 19.1).

Since a project is a one-off effort to achieve a specific purpose, which may not have been attempted before, project design and **project management** can be challenging. It is important that the common features of projects are well understood. There are many factors that undermine the success of a project. Some factors can be controlled by conducting proper and thorough project planning,

> **Project**
> 'A unique set of inter-related ac[...] designed to produce a set of de[...] and achieve a defined goal with[...] clearly defined time, cost and q[...] constraints' (Dwyer, Liang, Thie[...] Martini, 2013, p. 20)
>
> **3D objective**
> Meeting quality performance or[...] expectations within the timefra[...] budget allowed
>
> **Project management**
> A systematic management pro[...] with techniques to bring peop[...] resources together for a single

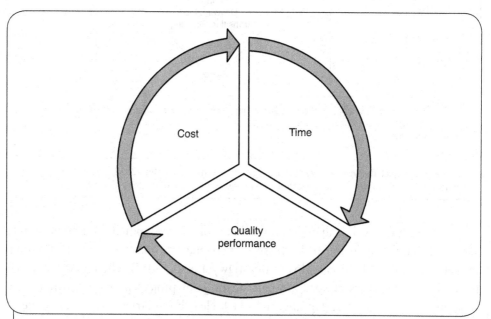

Figure 19.1 The 3D objective of a project. J. Dwyer, Z. Liang, V. Thiessen & A. Martini (2013). *Project management in health and community services: Getting good ideas to work* (p. 2). Sydney: Allen & Unwin.

building an efficient project management structure and engaging the right types of personnel, including project staff with the required project management competency and expertise.

Frameworks

Although projects are highly varied in focus, size and complexity, they move through a common basic life cycle: initiation, planning, implementation and closing. This project framework outlines the normal progression of projects from initiation to completion (Kloppenborg, 2009). Figure 19.2 shows the four-phase framework of the project life cycle.

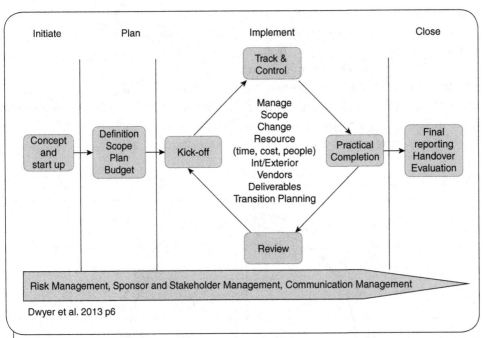

Dwyer et al. 2013 p6

Figure 19.2 Project life cycle. J. Dwyer, Z. Liang, V. Thiessen & A. Martini (2013). *Project management in health and community services: Getting good ideas to work* (p. 6). Sydney: Allen & Unwin.

However, it is worth bearing in mind that project development and management are not usually simple linear processes. There may be many cycles of planning, implementation, evaluation and variation (Dwyer et al., 2013). The phases included in the basic project framework are part of the joint project process and not truly separate. They tend to overlap and often lack clear boundaries. Moreover, projects do not generally proceed exactly as planned and can run backwards; for example, problems in the project-planning can force a rethink of the original concept. Therefore, ongoing monitoring – identifying problems or variations, modifying the plan and taking action – is a critical role for the project manager. Table 19.1 details possible steps to take during each of the four project phases.

Table 19.1 Key steps in project phases

Project phases	Key steps
Initiate	Identify a problem or opportunity. Develop and scope initial concept.
Plan	Clarify the goals and define the scope (how big is it?). Determine how, when and by whom the project will be done. Determine resource requirements. Determine evaluation measures (how project success is judged). Finalise a project plan.
Implement	Carry out all tasks as detailed in the project plan. Check work progress regularly. Keep records and collect data necessary for project monitoring and evaluation. Develop interim project reports as per funding requirements. Manage people, stakeholders and risk. Monitor budget (expenses versus income).
Close	Complete evaluation. Develop final project report. Prepare for proper handover. Maintain final communications to sponsors, funding bodies and key stakeholders. Celebrate with staff for project learning and project success.

Source: J. Dwyer, Z. Liang, V. Thiessen & A. Martini (2013). *Project management in health and community services: Getting good ideas to work* (p. 6). Sydney: Allen & Unwin.

Core components and development

A project has a clear goal to achieve, explicitly stated objectives, well-understood strategies to achieve them, well-defined benefits or changes that can be produced and measured, a specified timeline for producing all the benefits or changes, and well-defined resources to implement the strategies and produce the deliverables. Project-planning starts with defining problems to be solved, ways of solving the problems and the ultimate benefits of solving the problems. It is important that an evidence-based process should apply to the identification of problems and relevant solutions.

A rigorous **needs analysis** process plays a key role in designing a project that can ultimately address the proven problems by producing the desired outcomes via successful implementation and completion of the chosen strategies. It is also worth noting that before a project plan is completed, early consultation of key stakeholders, gaining organisational senior management support and brainstorming among the potential project team are all critical steps.

Needs analysis
A comprehensive study or evalu...
of the issues and needs of a part...
situation

Project goal

A **project goal** is a statement of what the project will achieve in response to the problems that the project will address (Dwyer et al., 2013). For example, if an identified problem is high prevalence of type 2 diabetes within the 35–44 years age group in a specific council area, a project can be planned with an overall goal of reducing the prevalence of type 2 diabetes within a certain time period among the identified target group.

Project objectives

The immediate outcomes throughout the project before achieving the overall project goal can be called **project objectives**. Like goals, objectives are statements of what the project wants to achieve at a lower level and the intermediate benefits that the project needs to produce (Dwyer et al., 2013).

Ultimately, the achievement of project objectives leads to the achievement of the overarching project goal. For example, in order to achieve a reduction in the prevalence of type 2 diabetes, a number of changes among the target population have to be brought about, such as adequate daily intake of vegetable and fruit, commitment to 30 minutes of daily physical activities, and overall body mass index reduction.

> **goal**
> ›ent of what the project will
> ›n response to the problems
> pportunities that the project
> ›ess

> **objectives**
> ›ts of what the project will
> ›t a lower level and the
> ›iate benefits that the project
> produce

Project strategies

A **project strategy** constitutes a series of related actions designed to achieve the project objectives and ultimately contribute to attaining the broader project goal (Eagar, Garrett & Lin, 2001). Once the project goal and objectives are clear, providing guidance in what to achieve, the project designer needs to decide how to realise it. Using the above example, key strategies may be the promotion of good dietary habits through a media campaign and workshops, and organisation of regular physical activities for the target group. Although projects vary in size, achieving the project goal is normally not a one-step approach. Project teams need to complete many steps, monitoring the results of these steps, before the problems can be solved and project goal achieved.

> **strategy**
> ›ion of methods to achieve
> ›oals

It is important to note that a project's goal, objectives and strategies should be closely aligned to the problems that the project is going to solve. Therefore, the development of the goal, objectives and strategies is not a linear process. A project designer needs to ensure all the intermediate changes that are important to achieving the overarching goal can be produced by implementing all the strategies. Consequently, all the intermediate changes that strategies can produce are captured in the forms of objectives.

Project plan

Once the goal, objectives and strategies for a proposed project are clear, planning the activities, timing and resources needed to achieve them is the next step. There are many tools and methods for this, such as work breakdown structures and linear responsibility charts, which can make planning easier. To complete this step, the project team needs to carry out the following tasks, identified by Dwyer et al. (2013):

- Document all the key activities and associated tasks that have to be completed; the activities and tasks of a project need to be defined and broken down into manageable chunks; a mechanism for decomposing the project goals into manageable tasks to allow estimation of project time and costs to take place (Kliem, 2007).
- Put activities and tasks in the right sequence.
- Identify the resources required to complete each of the tasks.
- Explore the relationships and dependencies between the tasks.
- Estimate how long the project will take and any deadlines (or critical points) within the project.

The above steps can be time-consuming, requiring inputs from colleagues with various levels of expertise and experience, depending on the size and complexity of the project. Project strategies cannot work unless there is a clear action plan, with the necessary staff, resources and equipment at hand. Estimation also needs to take into consideration the additional time and resources required for pretest strategies, when these are considered necessary. For example, a project team developing a training workshop for a large population group could pretest it on a small sample to discover whether the workshop is successful and the materials used are relevant and appropriate. Modifications and revisions to the workshop and relevant materials may then be required before rolling it out to the target population group. These activities should be identified in the planning stages and written into the plan.

The simplest way to make a project plan is to start with the goals, strategies and **deliverables**, breaking them down using subheadings and expanding them in a list format. In project management terms this is called creating a **work breakdown structure**, 'a tool that the project team uses progressively to divide the work of a project into smaller and smaller pieces' (Kloppenborg, 2009, p. 142) and a mechanism for decomposing the project goals into manageable tasks to allow estimation of project time and costs to take place (Kliem, 2007).

Deliverables
The products, services or outcor provided as the result of a projec

Work breakdown structure
'A tool that the project team use progressively to divide the work project into smaller and smaller (Kloppenborg, 2009, p. 142)

The concept of the work breakdown structure was initially developed by the United States Department of Defense in 1962 (Hamilton, 1964) and has been widely used in all defence services since, spreading gradually to other fields (Haugan, 2003). The process of building a good work breakdown structure forces significant issues to arise early rather than late in a project and also provides the basis for estimating the time and cost of the overall project. In fact, the work breakdown structure is a powerful tool for expressing the scope of a project in a simple graphical format.

Evaluation and learning

Project evaluation can be a powerful method of building cumulative knowledge for later projects. It provides an opportunity to reflect on outcomes, processes, organisation and methods. It also provides information to funders and community members so they can make informed decisions about whether to support the continuation or extension of a project (South Australian Community Health Research Unit, 2012).

Projects are means of trying new things, which provide unique opportunities for learning from experience and informing future practice. Project-planning is a process by which we decide the value or worth of something by observing, measuring and comparing it with an established criterion or standard (Hawe, Degeling & Hall, 1990). Therefore, evaluation, as one of the key project steps, is always of potential benefit. Regardless of whether the evaluation is simple or complex, it needs to be planned and built into the project at the planning stage (Dwyer et al., 2013). One of the reasons for compromising the benefits of evaluation is not planning it early enough to allow important data to be collected on time.

To conduct project evaluation, a range of qualitative and quantitative methods and data collection techniques can be employed. The design of project evaluation is part of the project-planning process, which guides the correct collection at the right time of the most appropriate types of information. Below are some examples suggested by Dwyer et al. (2013, p. 133) of methods that can be used to collect information for evaluation:

Analysis of records   attendance, admission and demographic details

Surveys   mail and email

Interviewing individuals   face-to-face and by telephone

Interviewing groups   focus group discussions

Documentation   journals, diaries, logs and progress reports

Triangulation   combining data from different sources and methods.

Project evaluation seeks to answer questions at different stages of the project. During project implementation, questions include: Is the project going well? Did we do what we set out to do? Is the project likely to produce the benefits as planned? Immediately after the project has been implemented, evaluation involves asking: Has the project achieved all intended objectives directly and indirectly relevant to the target population or the goal recipients? A period of time after the project has been concluded, it is important to ask: Were the benefits achieved at the end of the project sustained over time? Have the long-term benefits have been realised as anticipated? As evaluation is carried out at different phases of a project, it requires different approaches and is usually classified into four basic types: process, impact, outcome and economic evaluation.

Process evaluation

Process evaluation measures the effectiveness of the strategies and methods used in the project, and the skill of their execution. It gives people real-time feedback on what is happening, which can enhance the project's chance of success. Process evaluation also provides an indication of whether the project team has completed all the required steps essential to intended outcomes.

> **Process evaluation**
> A measure of the effectiveness strategies and methods used in project and the skill of their exe
>
> **Impact evaluation**
> A measure of the achievement of project's short-term impacts, no called project objectives
>
> **Indicator**
> Signals of the success of a proje

Impact evaluation

Impact evaluation measures the achievement of the project's short-term impacts, normally called project objectives. It should be conducted immediately after the project has been conducted or implemented, but not before all activities and strategies have been executed as planned. For large and complex projects, impact evaluation requires substantial planning, which may include choosing or designing **indicators** to make the impact of complex changes measurable.

Outcome evaluation

Outcome evaluation measures the longer term achievements of the project, which are closely related to the project goal. Both impact and outcome evaluation measure effects, benefits or intended outcomes, focusing on assessing the effects of the completed project over different time periods (Hawe et al., 1990). Since outcome evaluation takes places after the project has been completed, it is not commonly built into evaluation plans for projects, especially small projects in health and community services (Dwyer et al., 2013).

Economic evaluation

When financial constraints are present, economic considerations become paramount: resource allocation decisions should maximise efficient use of those resources. Therefore, **economic evaluation** is concerned with estimating the relative value of alternative options and is designed to help decision-makers answer the following two questions: Is this project worth doing compared with other projects we could do with the same resources? 'Are we satisfied that resources should be spent in this way rather than another way?' (Dwyer et al., 2013, p. 88)

> **Outcome evaluation**
> A measure of the longer term achievements of the project, wh closely related to the project goa
>
> **Economic evaluation**
> An estimate of the relative value alternative options using a range economic and financial techniqu

Economic evaluation of interventions or services has three main methods: cost-effectiveness analysis, cost-benefit analysis and cost-utility analysis. This type of evaluation requires specific levels of expertise and is not a common requirement for project managers. However, it is important to be aware of what it is and when it should be commissioned.

Project goal, objectives and strategies

This case study will help readers to understand the specific project-planning features and how goals, objectives and strategies are developed.

Problem statement: High prevalence of androgenic anabolic steroid misuse among Grade 10 and 11 male public school students in Wonderland City Council area

Project timeframe: One year

Project target population: Grade 8 and 9 male public school students in Wonderland High School (40 students in each grade)

Project goal: To reduce the prevalence of androgenic anabolic steroid misuse among male public school students in the Wonderland City Council area in two years

Project objectives:

- to improve the awareness of 80 per cent of Grade 8 and 9 male students in Wonderland High School of the importance of a positive attitude towards appearance and self-esteem development within 9 months
- to have 80 per cent of the Grade 8 and 9 male students at Wonderland High School demonstrate a high level of self-esteem within 12 months
- to develop among 80 per cent of Grade 8 and 9 male students in Wonderland High School a positive attitude towards appearance within 12 months.

Project strategies:

- Carry out promotional campaigns (display posters and distribute brochures) that encourage the development of positive attitudes towards appearance and self-esteem among young people at Wonderland High School for between 4 and 12 months.
- Facilitate group discussions among Grade 8 and 9 students at Wonderland High School to encourage positive and effective communications between male and female students (first round: between months 4 and 5; second round: between months 9 and 10).
- Facilitate a series of workshops for Grade 8 and 9 male students at Wonderland High School focusing on building self-confidence and self-esteem (between months 6 and 12).
- Facilitate twice-weekly after-school physical activity competitions for Grade 8 and 9 male students at Wonderland High School (between months 6 and 12).
- Provide information seminars to parents of Grade 8 and 9 male students in Wonderland High School focusing on effective communications between parents and their children (within 8 months).

Management of projects

Achieving good project outcomes depends upon good project management, which includes having the right person for the project management role. They should have the ability to get the job done and keep the project moving and be someone who understands what the project must achieve and is responsive to contingencies, open and flexible, aware of the situation and able to deal with crises. For a small project, a project manager may take on all functions that are required for the implementation of the project. However, for larger projects, many other roles may be involved that will build up a project team. These roles may include a project director, project manager, group leader, team member and technical manager.

Given the uniqueness of projects, project management requires a balance between strong content knowledge and project management ability. Therefore, as Dwyer et al. (2013 p. 63) suggest, general skills and knowledge required for project management may include some or all of the following:

- leadership ability, particularly to create and share the vision for project success and to motivate the team and stakeholders
- discipline and drive, including application to the task, taking responsibility, decisiveness and ability to work effectively at both strategic and detail levels
- excellent communication and interpersonal skills, which involves talking to the right people, influencing others, building consensus, making the project visible, negotiating, lobbying for the project and managing conflict
- initiative and organisation, including working independently, meeting deadlines and ensuring follow-through
- technical project management skills, know-how and experience
- knowledge of the working environment and ability to adapt tools and methods to suit
- analysis and reflection, which involves keeping one's eye on the ball, understanding risks, ability to read situations, flexibility and responsiveness.

Structure and stakeholders

Each project is unique in its own way; however, it does not stand alone and is part of an organisation's activities. How a project sits within the organisational structure demonstrates the line of accountability and reporting requirements and how it relates to and should interact with other parts of the organisation. Such understanding is extremely important, as it guides managers in where and how to seek help in times of doubt and when difficulties are encountered. Since a project is usually a way of trialling new ideas and is not something that has been done before, internal and external expertise and guidance can minimise mistakes in project design and implementation. Such expertise and guidance can be provided formally, by way of establishing an advisory committee.

An advisory committee consists of representatives from project sponsors, key stake-holders and key project staff usually providing advice and support, and helping the project to succeed as planned. The design of project committees, and their ways of work-ing, will depend partly on whether the project is internally or externally focused. It is important that the role of the advisory committee is clarified upon its establishment.

Project sponsors are individuals and/or organisations that provide funding or finan-cial support (including in-kind donations) to a project. Stakeholders are the individuals and/or organisations that are actively involved in the project, whose interests may be affected as a result of the project or who may exert influence over the project and its results (Project Management Institute, 2008). Stakeholders may have the power to veto or approve, delay, facilitate, derail or guide a project. Therefore, it is important that they are identified and their interests are understood in the project-planning phase. Once stakeholders are identified, it is useful to consider the impact that a particular stakeholder group may have on the project and how this will be managed.

Methods

Project management methodology is an approach that can guide the conceptualisation of project ideas, understanding of tasks required, management of a project and use of project management tools and techniques that enable projects to progress in effective, disciplined and reliable ways. However, the use of project management methods does not guarantee successful project outcomes. In fact, there is a suggestion by senior project leaders that a fixed method may not always work.

There are variations in methods according to different settings. Some government departments have adopted a specific project management method to use as a framework with or without local modifications. If the project involves a tender process or is subject to certain funding requirements, some standardised methods may be stipulated as part of the funding arrangement.

There are several methods of project management in use in the health and commu-nity services sector – for example, the Project Management Body of Knowledge (Project Management Institute, 2008), and PRINCE and PRINCE2, which stand for PRojects IN Controlled Environments (Central Computer and Telecommunications Agency, 1997). In health and community services, many organisations use their own in-house tools and methods, a hybrid of methods or occasionally no method at all. While certain principles and methods are necessary for project success, in most instances there is no one best approach (Dwyer et al., 2013).

Tools

A project team may use specific project management tools to achieve project tasks. Common tools are Gantt and PERT charts, and computerised scheduling and tracking tools such as Microsoft Project and Mac Project (Dwyer et al., 2013). Organisations may provide project teams with standard tools and templates for project proposals, plans, com-munications, risk management, and status and variation reporting. Some organisations may use specific software programs to facilitate project management processes. It is useful for project managers to check what resources are available in the workplace.

Project management is an art, not an algorithm, and it requires knowledge of when and how to use the tools and techniques available (Kliem, 2007). Project management tools may be effective in certain contexts, industries or organisations but not in others. In addition, many will be ineffective unless they are supported by strong management practices such as effective negotiation, communication, leadership, use of alliances and networks, and change management methods (Dwyer et al., 2013). In reality, organisations in health and community services generally use local adaptations of project management methods and tools to guide project design, implementation and management.

Summary

- Projects are unique, complex and vary in scope and need.
- A project is not a linear process but has a life cycle of four phases: initiation, preparation, implementation and closure.
- The rational planning approach involves the development of achievable goals, objectives and strategies in a logical order.
- Project management frameworks, models and tools can assist in understanding project management concepts and theories, but no single approach or method can guarantee project success.
- Evaluation is critical for project learning and should be included in the project-planning phase.

Reflective questions

1 What makes projects unique?
2 What are the critical factors for project success?
3 What are the key phases in a typical project life cycle?
4 Is project-planning a linear process? Explain your answer.
5 What are the purposes of work breakdown structures in project-planning?

Self-analysis question

Current understanding of projects and project management is limited among health professionals. As a manager in your organisation, how could you improve project management competence among your staff so that project management tools are properly used to implement changes and trial new ideas?

References

Central Computer and Telecommunications Agency. (1997). *PRINCE 2: An outline*. Norwich, United Kingdom: Stationery Office.

Cleland, D. & Gareis, R. (2006). *Global project management handbook*. New York, NY: McGraw-Hill Professional.

Dwyer, J., Liang, Z., Thiessen, V. & Martini, A. (2013). *Project management in health and community services: Getting good ideas to work*. Sydney: Allen & Unwin.

Eagar, K., Garrett, P. & Lin, V. (2001). *Health planning: Australian perspectives*. Sydney: Allen & Unwin.

Hamilton, R. L. (1964). *Study of methods for evaluation of the PERT/Cost Management System*. Bedford, MA: Mitre.

Haugan, G. T. (2003). *The work breakdown structure in government contracting*. Vienna, VA: Management Concepts.

Hawe, P., Degeling, D. & Hall, J. (1990). *Evaluating health promotion: A health worker's guide*. Sydney: Maclennan & Petty.

Kliem, R. L. (2007). *Effective communications for project management*. Portland, OR: Auerbach.

Kloppenborg, T. J. (2009). *Contemporary project management: Organize, plan, perform*. Mason, OH: South-Western Cengage Learning.

Project Management Institute. (2008). *A guide to the project management body of knowledge*. Newtown Square, PA: Author.

South Australian Community Health Research Unit. (2012). *Planning and evaluation wizard*. Adelaide: Flinders University.

20

Financial management

Ian Edwards

Learning objectives

How do I:
- use assets, liabilities, equity, revenues and expenses in the financial management of a service, department or organisation?
- develop an appropriate budget and cashflow?
- enhance my organisation's financial position through a casemix classification and funding system?
- use variance analysis to improve the performance of my service, department or organisation?

Introduction

The financial management of healthcare organisations is a key management responsibility for both public and private facilities. While this responsibility has always been important, it is becoming increasingly more so, with the rising costs of healthcare provision due to advances in technology, chronic disease and ageing populations. The responsible use and management of scarce healthcare resources requires knowledge and information. The accounting process provides the necessary information to develop and monitor a budget. However, it is the financial management of the budget and associated activity levels that provide the necessary framework to ensure budget integrity and financial governance.

Financial accounting is mainly concerned with the transactions of accounting, with the systematic recording of the financial events of the organisation. The main accounting groups are listed below:

Assets are items of value owned or controlled by an organisation, such as cash, inventories or land.

Liabilities are amounts owed by an organisation to external parties, such as loans or wages owing.

Equity is the funds invested in the organisation by its owner, either as capital investment or as retained earnings.

Revenues (or income) are the flows of resources into an organisation from government, grants, sales or services performed.

Expenses are outflows of resources from the organisation to purchase goods or services, or carry out its general operations.

These five basic accounting groups are the essence of how financial information that provides the means of financial management is recorded.

The basic accounting equation is represented in the relationship between the assets, liabilities and owner's equity of a business. It can be expressed as assets = liabilities + equity or equity = assets − liabilities. Perhaps the easiest way to understand this equation is to relate it to purchasing a house:

$$\text{equity (amount invested or owned)} = \text{asset (value of house)} - \text{liability (mortgage)}$$

Suppose the relationship between the asset, liability and equity in this house purchase is as follows:

$$\text{asset (\$500\,000)} = \text{liability (\$200\,000)} + \text{equity (\$300\,000)}$$

In this example, the equity (or the amount owned by the purchaser) is $300 000. The house is valued at $500 000 minus the loan or mortgage of $200 000.

Types of budgets

A budget is simply a written forecast or plan of what managers expect to happen in the future. It is quantified in terms of dollar inflows (revenue) and outflows (expenses).

There are many different types of budgets. However, each budget's use and application depend on its purpose, as well as the size and financial maturity of the organisation (King, Clarkson & Wallace, 2010). There is no one type of budget that fits all circumstances. As organisations mature, they typically move from a historical type of budget to a zero-based or activity-based budget. However, the cost of developing the information required to support construction of a more sophisticated budget needs to be taken into consideration.

Until recently, Australian public hospitals mainly used historical budgeting. Hospitals would develop budgets for the following year based upon the previous financial year's budget allocation or simply based upon the actual expenditure of the previous year. The difficulties inherent in this approach include a lack of flexibility to adjust the budget for increases in volume or activity during the course of the budget period; a lack of emphasis placed on control mechanisms to ensure that funds are being utilised in the most efficient and effective manner, and a lack of means by which to measure whether the hospital's operational plans and objectives are being met.

Budgets can be used as planning tools to allocate resources and to evaluate performance (Gapenski & Pink, 2007). There are several different approaches that can be used in constructing a budget. The major approaches include those discussed below.

Global budgets

In a global budget, funds are allocated to an organisation as a bulk amount. It is then the responsibility of the organisation to distribute the funds internally. This type of budgeting is often referred to as base budget allocation and is usually determined on an incremental basis with the previous year's final budget allocation plus a percentage increase. This method leaves little scope for any new services or initiatives other than those funded from efficiency savings.

Historical budgets

Historical budgets are also known as static, fixed or forecast budgets. They are developed on the premise that revenue and expenditure will remain relatively constant from one year to the next. Historical budgeting is designed to maintain the status quo.

Flexible budgets

This type of budget is adjusted for changes in the unit level of the cost driver. For example, a flexible budget can be based on the previous year's budget but make allowance for adjustments to the budget depending on variable factors such as ward occupancy rates and planned workload.

Zero-based budgets

Zero-based budgets take an approach that ignores (to some extent) the previous year's budget allocation and expenditure, and uses the assumption that the budget is to be developed from scratch. While zero-based budgeting encourages the supply of more detailed and strategic information into the budgetary process, it can be extremely time-consuming in its development (Dionne, Mitton, Smith & Donaldson, 2009).

Activity-based budgets

This is a method of budgeting for activities and services that incur costs in every functional area of the organisation. The budget is developed in terms of the cost of an organisation's products and services – for example, the cost of providing an occupied bed day in an orthopaedic ward. The budget is developed based on the specific activity targets that are planned for each area of the organisation. A critical part of activity-based budgeting is the development of a plan for the level of activity that is likely to be performed by the organisation (Heslop, 2012). The budget that is developed relates to the level of activity that is planned for that area of the organisation.

Budgeting for the future

Martin is the nurse manager of a busy ward in a large public hospital. He has been in this position for the previous four years. During this time he has noticed both an increase in the number of patients being cared for and the complexity of the care provided. However, there has been little change in the annual budget other than a notional increase each year that is approximately the same rate as the consumer price index. His nursing staff have also noticed the change during this period and have raised this in several team meetings, stating that nursing staff in other wards in the hospital do not have to work as hard as they do.

Martin has discussed the situation with senior management and the finance manager. However, the current historic budgeting process that is used in the facility does not enable an increase in budget without other areas receiving a lower amount. This is seen as difficult to achieve.

A new finance manager is appointed to the facility and receives executive management approval to implement a zero-based budget. Martin is sceptical that the new budgeting process will make any difference. However, on completion of the new budget, his ward receives a higher budget than expected. In discussing this with other nurse managers within the hospital, Martin discovers that several other areas were in a similar situation to his ward. Other areas had less budget than expected. In general, staff were accepting of the outcome, as the budget had been constructed in an equitable way which was transparent to all employees.

Healthcare funding

Healthcare sectors in Australia are funded differently, which can influence both the budgeting process and the ongoing management. The funding for public hospitals is provided from a range of different sources; however, the majority is provided by national and state governments. The bulk of the funding that is provided by the government is capped. This **capped funding** impacts on the development and ongoing management of the budget and on the levels of service. Both have to be managed to ensure that the budget revenue and expenses balance. In contrast, while private hospitals also receive their funding from different sources, it is not capped. This is a significant difference and enables them to provide activity-based budgets that may change during the budget period based on the levels of clinical activity that have been provided.

> **Capped funding**
> A set amount or level of funding healthcare facility to provide ser does not increase if additional se are provided above the funded activity

About two-thirds of the funding for residential aged care is provided by the Australian federal government. Subsidies are paid directly to aged care homes on behalf of their residents. The degree of funding for each resident is based on a clinical assessment which results in a set level of funding being provided for each day. Also, residents who can afford to do so contribute to the cost of their care. Aged care funding is similar in some ways to private hospitals, in that it is not capped.

Casemix

Casemix is a generic term for the method of classifying the activities that health services deliver. The origins of casemix as a classification system date back as far as the systematic diagnosis and treatment of illness. This simply means that if a patient presented with certain symptoms and a procedure was performed whose outcome was successful, the next patient presenting with the similar symptoms would be treated in the same way. The point is that casemix was founded in clinical terms, not in financial or economic terms (Heslop, 2012).

Casemix-based hospital funding was introduced in Australia in the early 1990s. It supported higher accountability. The previous standards of measuring activity, based on occupied bed days and admitted patients, evolved into a system that takes into account the **acuity** of the patient and the cost of the likely resources used.

| of clinical care required by the
ased on their condition

In order for a casemix classification system to be useful, a number of design principles must be incorporated (Madden, 2013). Firstly, classification systems in health must have clinical meaning to be useful. Patients in the same class should be similar from a clinical perspective. Episodes of care in the same class should contain similar diagnoses and treatments. Secondly, resource use homogeneity is required. The cost of the healthcare provided should be approximately the same for all patients within the same class. Finally, there should be about the right number of classes in the system – that is, not too many classes and not too few.

There are several casemix-based funding instruments being used in Australia – for example, the Aged Care Funding Instrument and the Australian National Diagnostic Related Groups (sometimes called AN-DRGs). The Diagnosis Related Groups classification was developed to classify acute admitted patient episodes in public and private hospitals, and comprises a description of body systems, separation of medical and surgical procedures, and a description of a hierarchy of procedures, medical problems and other factors that differentiate processes of care. Each episode of care is assigned to one of 24 Major Diagnostic Categories. Most of these categories are defined by body system or disease type and correspond with a particular medical or surgical specialty – for example, respiratory system. The classification of patient episodes of care to Australian National Diagnostic Related Groups allows for a more accurate method of understanding the type and level of clinical activity within a hospital. In addition, each Diagnostic Related Group is allocated a weight, which has been calculated to represent the acuity of the service provided and the average use of resources in comparison to other groups.

In Table 20.1, the various weights represent the average costs of the different types of episodes of care. The weights are relative to each other; for example, a heart transplant uses 20.53 times more resources than a carpal tunnel release (13.96 ÷ 0.68 = 20.53). The table shows that St Florence Hospital has provided 70 episodes of inpatient care. However, it is the ability to state the types of care and the total weighted separations (174.0) that is important. The average acuity for St Florence was 2.49 (174.0 ÷ 70 = 2.49). The average acuity can be used to **benchmark** with other similar facilities.

> **Benchmark**
> To measure and compare servic
> an agreed standard (Heslop, 20

Table 20.1 St Florence Hospital casemix profile

Service description	Number of cases	Casemix index[a]	Weighted separations[b]
Heart transplant	10	13.96	139.6
Carpal tunnel release	20	0.68	13.6
Renal dialysis	40	0.52	20.8
Total	**70**		174.0

Notes: (a) Relative value units per case; (b) Total relative value units per service type. The table has been constructed to clearly show the difference between simply counting the number of cases and the total weighted separations, which acknowledges the average costs for each type of case.

Reforms in funding

There has been a significant change to Australian public hospital funding arrangements, with the federal government becoming the major funder. A key feature of this reform is the national introduction of activity-based funding, which commenced in July 2012.

The Independent Hospital Pricing Authority was established as a statutory authority in December 2011 by the *National Health Reform Act 2011* (Cth). The authority is responsible for developing the national pricing framework and a consistent approach to activity-based funding of public hospitals. It is also responsible for setting the national efficient prices of the Australian National Diagnostic Related Groups that are funded to the public hospitals.

Casemix is an important tool in managing and funding healthcare systems in Australia and forms the foundation of activity-based funding for public hospitals, including funding arrangements, budgeting and performance-monitoring, at both state and federal levels (Willis, Reynolds & Keleher, 2012). It was one of the core concepts of the nation's 2010 health reform.

Management and financial performance

An organisation's financial performance must be planned and controlled with sound budgeting procedures as thoroughly as possible if acceptable results are to be achieved. This statement holds true for both public and private organisations. While public organisations do not operate for profit, they are responsible for delivering services to the public within an allocated budget. Both public and private healthcare organisations depend on the development of budgets to plan for the effective use of the available resources (Horngren, Datar & Foster, 2006). The major benefits of budgeting are listed below:

- It forces management to plan ahead and anticipate the future on a systematic basis.
- It provides management with realistic performance targets against which actual results can be compared.
- It coordinates the various segments of the organisation.
- It serves as a communication device with which the various managers can exchange information concerning goals, ideas and achievements.

Costs

The development and subsequent monitoring of a budget requires an understanding of the various types of costs and their behaviours. The total costs of an activity or service consist of three types of costs, and their relationship can be expressed as total costs = fixed costs + semi-variable costs + variable costs. Fixed costs have to be paid regardless of the level of activity or production – for example, rent, security staff and maintenance contracts. Variable costs change in direct proportion to the level of activity or production. The greater the level of activity, the greater the variable costs – for example, clinical drugs and pathology. Semi-variable costs are fixed in the short term but will vary over time or with large changes in activity or production – for example, the availability of an additional CT scanner due to patient demand.

In addition to fixed, semi-variable and variable costs, direct and indirect costs also need to be considered in developing a budget. Direct costs can be directly associated with the activity or production, and they can be either fixed or variable depending on the nature of the costs – for example, nursing services and medical supplies. Indirect costs, also called overheads, are not directly related to producing the activity or service. They can be either fixed or variable depending on the nature of the costs – for example, administrative departments and medical records department.

The budget needs to take into account the level of planned activity together with all the different types of costs. These will consist of material costs (for example, drugs and clinical supplies), direct labour and associated on-costs, and overhead costs, which are more difficult to charge directly to units of production (for example, general management salaries, power, telephone, cleaning, rent, rates and taxes).

Variance

Variance analysis is an essential financial management control function. The difference between a budgeted amount and the actual amount expended represents a variance. Managers need to investigate variances to determine their cause. Actions taken in response to variances can often dramatically improve the financial outlook of the healthcare organisation (Henderson, 2003b). There are several types of variances, which are discussed below.

Volume variance

This is caused by a change in the total numbers of services being provided. This can be both higher and lower than expected. There is a cost associated with each product, and the costs will vary according to the number produced. If a day surgery unit provides an additional 5 per cent of cases in a month, it will be reasonable to expect the variable costs of providing the service to be 5 per cent higher.

Mix variance

Mix variance is caused by a change in the proportion and types of services being provided. While the total volume of patients or services may be as planned, the complexity may increase, and this may result in an increase in nursing care.

Utilisation variance

This is caused by changes in efficiency. Efficiency variances relate to the level of resources used in producing each output and reflect a manager's performance in resource management – for example, the number of hours of nursing care per occupied bed day.

Budget development

The first stage in the development of a budget is identifying the goals and objectives. To illustrate the budget development process, we will assume that we have to develop a budget for a 30-bed ward with a planned occupancy rate of 90 per cent. As shown in Table 20.2, the level of nursing care will be 5.0 hours per occupied bed day. (An occupied bed day is a hospital inpatient bed occupied at midnight.) The number of full-time equivalents required (24.9) has been divided into fixed nursing costs, consisting of the

Table 20.2 Goals and objectives in a budget development for a hospital ward

Ward details	Required amounts
Number of beds	30
Beds per week[a]	210
Occupancy rate (%)	90
Weekly occupied bed days[b]	189
Nursing hours per occupied bed day	5.0
Nursing hours per week[c]	945
Full-time equivalent nursing staff[d]	24.9
Fixed nursing costs	
Unit managers	1.0
Assistant nursing managers	1.0
Total fixed nursing full-time equivalents	**2.0**
Variable nursing full-time equivalents	22.9
Total nursing full-time equivalents	24.9

Notes: (a) Number of beds × 7; (b) Beds per week × occupancy rate; (c) Occupied bed days × nursing hours per occupied bed day; (d) Nursing hours per week ÷ number of hours per week per full-time equivalent (1 full-time equivalent = 38 hours per week)

unit manager and the assistant; and variable nursing costs, which include the remainder of the staff.

The second task is the development of the average penalty rates for the different categories of staff. Table 20.3 calculates the average penalty rates (14.6 per cent) for the registered nurses in the ward.

Table 20.3 Calculating average penalty rates for registered nurses in a budget development for a hospital ward

Shifts	Penalty rate[a]	Frequency[b]	Total[c]
Night duty	15.0	7	105.0
Sunday and public holiday	75.0	1	75.0
Saturday	50.0	1	50.0
Evening	15.0	7	105.0
Day duty		7	0
Total		**23**	**335.0**
Average[d]			**14.6**

Notes: (a) Percentage of base pay rate; (b) Number of shifts per four-week roster; (c) Penalty rate × frequency; (d) Total ÷ frequency

The various categories of leave entitlement need to be included in the budget. This can be achieved by constructing information about the various categories. Table 20.4 calculates the leave entitlement for the variable nursing staff.

Table 20.4 Calculating leave entitlement for variable nursing staff in a budget development for a hospital ward

Types of leave	Amount of leave entitlement	Proportion of on-costs (%)
Annual	5 weeks backfill[a]	9.60
Annual loading	17.5% loading for 5 weeks[b]	1.68
Long service	1.3 weeks backfill per year[c]	2.50
Sick	1 week backfill[d]	1.90
Study	2 days (not replaced)	0
Total on-costs		**15.68**

Notes: (a) $5 \div 52 \times 100$; (b) $5 \times 17.5 = 87.5$; $87.5 \div 52 = 1.68$ (c) $1.3 \div 52 \times 100$; (d) $1 \div 52 \times 100$

Finally, all the information is used to develop an appropriate nursing budget for the ward given the initial goals and objectives. As calculated in Table 20.5, the final nursing budget requirement for the ward is $2 992 509 for the year. The fixed nursing costs are $274 314, and the variable nursing costs are $2 718 195. Understanding the various costs and how they behave assists in both the development of a budget and the ongoing management of the budget. The development of a budget requires knowledge of the staff that are to be employed and information about service delivery costs.

Few would argue that the development of an accurate budget and knowledge of how it was constructed are important. However, it is equally important that the budget is apportioned to each month (cashflowed), reflecting the planned expenses for that month (Bryans, 2007). This will support the ongoing management of the budget, as any variances between the budget and actual expenditure will be meaningful.

Therefore, to continue with the example, the annual nursing budget needs to be apportioned to each month of the year. The fixed nursing costs are not influenced by the number of patients that are in the ward. Therefore, it would be reasonable to apportion the budget to each month based on the number of days in each month. However, the variable nursing costs have a direct relationship to the number of patients in the ward. Analysis of the occupied bed days for the previous two years provides a trend over the 12-month period. As shown in Table 20.6, the annual planned occupied bed days are apportioned to each month based on the past trend. The variable nursing budget is then apportioned to each month based on the number of planned occupied bed days for each month (see Table 20.5).

The heath service delivery environment has different trends that have an impact on different types of expenditures. For example, during the winter months, medical wards in hospitals typically experience higher occupancy rates, due mainly to respiratory conditions. While all budgets need to be cashflowed, there must be a balance between the amount of the annual budget and the level of work undertaken to cashflow it. If the annual budget is small – for example, $5000 – it may be cost-effective to simply divide it by 12 months rather than understanding what the expenditure driver is for that budget and then allocating it according to anticipated monthly usage.

Table 20.5 Calculating the nursing budget in a budget development for a hospital ward

			Types of nurses			
	NM	ANM	RN	EN	AIN	Total
Number of full-time equivalents	1.00	1.00	8.00	11.9	3.00	24.90
Number of weeks employed	52	52	52	52	52	
Hourly rate of pay ($)	55.00	50.00	45.00	40.00	30.00	
Hours per week employed	38	38	38	38	38	
Annual base pay ($)	108680	98800	711360	940576	177840	2037256
Superannuation at 9.25% ($)	10053	9139	65801	87003	16450	188446
Workcover at 1.5% ($)	1630	1482	10670	14109	2668	30559
Professional development ($)	1500	1500	12000	17850	4500	37350
Uniform allowance ($)	250	250	2000	2975	750	6225
Total leave on-costs (%)	13.78	13.78	15.68	15.68	15.68	
Total cost of leave ($)	14976	13615	111541	147482	27885	315500
Shift allowance (%)	0.0	0.0	14.6	12.4	11.8	
Total cost of shift allowance ($)	0	0	103859	116631	20985	241475
Subtotal ($)	137089	124786	1017231	1326627	251078	2856811
Payroll tax at 4.75% ($)	6512	5927	48318	63015	11926	135699
Total labour costs ($)	143601	130713	1065549	1389641	263004	2992509
Fixed nursing costs ($)	143601	130713				274314
Variable nursing costs ($)			1065549	1389641	263004	2718195

Notes: NM: nurse managers; ANM: assistant nurse managers; RN: registered nurses; EN: enrolled nurses; AIN: assistants in nursing

Table 20.6 Calculating the variable nursing budget in a budget development for a hospital ward

Month	No. of days in month	% of annual days	No. of OBD	% of annual OBD	FNC ($)	VNC ($)	Total budget ($)
July	31	8.5	887	9.0	23 298	244 651	267 949
August	31	8.5	900	9.1	23 298	248 237	271 535
September	30	8.2	851	8.6	22 546	234 722	257 268
October	31	8.5	799	8.1	23 298	220 379	243 677
November	30	8.2	821	8.3	22 546	226 447	248 994
December	31	8.5	628	6.4	23 298	173 214	196 512
January	31	8.5	740	7.5	23 298	204 106	227 404
February	28	7.7	792	8.0	21 043	218 449	239 492
March	31	8.5	890	9.0	23 298	245 479	268 777
April	30	8.2	809	8.2	22 546	223 137	245 684
May	31	8.5	858	8.7	23 298	236 653	259 951
June	30	8.2	880	8.9	22 546	242 721	265 267
Total	**365**	**100.0**	**9855**	**100.0**	**274 314**	**2 718 195**	**2 992 509**

Notes: OBD: occupied bed days; FNC: fixed nursing costs; VNC: variable nursing costs

Controlling and monitoring a budget

The management of a budget should be undertaken in conjunction with other performance information. Accountable managers use strategies to ensure that processes are aligned with activity and financial goals. Monitoring and evaluation enable managers to decide when to implement changes. Short- and long-term monitoring and evaluation strategies are used to manage expenditure and activity levels to meet budget and ultimately strategic plan objectives (King et al., 2010).

Benchmarking is a quality improvement tool that allows organisations to compare their performance with others and learn from processes and systems that obtain better results, and to achieve and sustain best practice (Henderson, 2003a). A weakness of benchmarking can be that it is based on the assumption that what works in one setting can be transferred to another.

Many health services use casemix information to benchmark health services in a number of different ways, in particular to compare the average length of stay for Diagnostic Related Groups. Differences in clinical practice, the efficiency of the labour and materials utilised and the type of service delivery are other concepts that may benefit from benchmarking. The challenge in benchmarking is to balance economic outcomes with improvements in quality of care.

While undertaking budgeting activities allows a manager to forecast or plan for what may be expected to happen in the future, budget management can prove to be difficult. Where there is a lack of understanding of true costs and revenues – for example, poor understanding of cost behaviour, salaries and on-costs – a budget may be constructed upon false assumptions and therefore will not be a true indication of the costs involved in undertaking the activity or service. Also, while all care may be taken to prepare the budget based upon forecasts, if budget managers have no control over the volume of activity or resources then budget estimates may be incorrect. Finally, seasonal fluctuations may impact upon the level of the monthly budget required. In these instances, an accurate cashflow of the budget is important.

Developing an accurate budget and an appropriate cashflow for the accounting period is fundamental to the management of the budget (Gapenski & Pink, 2007). If the budget and cashflow are not prepared with accuracy, the various monthly variances will not be able to be analysed (Zelman, McCue & Glick, 2009). The variances may simply be due to the poor cashflow of the budget; if this is the case, the true position of the budget will not be known until the end of the accounting period.

With accurate budgeting and cashflow, the analysis and management of budgets becomes a manageable task. The objective of the analysis is to understand why variance has occurred. This can be achieved only with an array of performance indicators, the variance between the budget and the expenditure being only one of these. Information regarding the planned activity level and actual activity level also needs to be included, together with quality indicators.

Summary

- The five basic account groups are the essence of how financial information, which enables the development of budgets and the means of financial management and variance analysis, is recorded.
- There are many types of budgets, and their use and application depend on what they are being used for, as well as the level of maturity and the management of the organisation.
- The casemix classification system can provide significant levels of information that can be used within healthcare.
- The development of an accurate budget and cashflow based on the levels of planned outcomes is a critical part of financial governance for all types of healthcare organisations and an essential function of good financial management.
- The development of an appropriate budget and cashflow enables analysis of any variations from the planned expenses.

Reflective questions

1 Why is it important to separate fixed and variable costs in developing a budget?

2 Why do you think zero-based budgeting is considered difficult and time-consuming in its development?

3 What factors would you need to take into account in benchmarking clinical services?

4 What type of information would you require to undertake a budget variance analysis?

5 What is the role of the Independent Hospital Pricing Authority?

Self-analysis questions

Think about how budgets are developed and managed in your current or previous place of employment. What types of budgets do you think are used? How are the budgets developed? What level of transparency exists in the organisation about how budgets are developed? Do the budgets have clear objectives that need to be achieved? How are the budgets monitored? If analysis has been undertaken, did it assist with the development of strategies to maintain a balanced budget? In considering all of these questions, do you think there is an opportunity to improve financial management within the organisation? Is there an opportunity for you to do things differently?

References

Bryans, W. (2007). *Practical budget management in health and social care*. Oxford, United Kingdom: Radcliffe.

Dionne, F., Mitton, C., Smith, N. & Donaldson, C. (2009). Evaluation of the impact of program budgeting and marginal analysis in Vancouver Island Health Authority. *Journal of Health Services Research & Policy, 14*(4), 234–242. doi: 10.1258/jhsrp.2009.008182

Gapenski, L. & Pink, G. (2007). *Understanding health care financial management* (5th ed.). Chicago, IL: Health Administration.

Henderson, E. (2003a). Continuing professional development: Budgeting (Part 1). *Nursing Management, 10*(1), 33–37. doi: 10.7748/nm2003.04.10.1.33.c1919

——. (2003b). Continuing professional development: Budgeting (Part 2). *Nursing Management, 10*(2), 32–36. doi: 10.7748/nm2003.05.10.2.32.c1926

Heslop, L. (2012). Status of costing hospital nursing work within Australian casemix activity-based funding policy. *International Journal of Nursing Practice, 18*(1), 2–6. doi: 10.1111/j.1440-172X.2011.01992.x

Horngren, C., Datar, S. & Foster, G. (2006). *Cost accounting: A managerial emphasis* (12th ed.). Upper Saddle River, NJ: Pearson.

King, R., Clarkson, P. M. & Wallace, S. (2010). Budgeting practices and performance in small health care businesses. *Management Accounting Research, 21*(1), 40–55. doi: 10.1016/j.mar.2009.11.002

Madden, R. (2013). ICF and casemix models for health care funding: Use of the WHO family of classifications to improve casemix. *Disability and Rehabilitation, 35*(13), 1074–1077. doi: 10.3109/09638288.2012.720349

National Health Reform Act 2011 (Cth).

Willis, E., Reynolds, L. E. & Keleher, H. (2012). *Understanding the Australian health care system.* Chatswood: Churchill Livingstone.

Zelman, W., McCue, M. & Glick, N. (2009). *Financial management of health care organizations: An introduction to fundamental tools, concepts, and applications* (3rd ed.). San Francisco, CA: Jossey-Bass.

21

Negotiating

Sandra G. Leggat

Learning objectives

How do I:

- identify a negotiating opportunity?
- improve my skills in negotiating?
- plan a negotiation?
- decide whether I should accept the proposed solution?

Introduction

Negotiation is an important skill for a healthcare manager. According to Mealiea and Latham (1996), many managerial activities, such as budget development, performance appraisal and review, planned change, team-building, complaint-handling and resource allocation require negotiating skills. Other authors have suggested that great leaders need to be great negotiators (Nanus & Dobbs, 1999). This chapter introduces negotiating theory and tactics that can assist readers to develop their skills for use in personal and professional negotiations.

Concepts

Once two or more parties agree to enter into a negotiation, they may use either an integrative approach (win–win) or a distributive approach (win–lose). An example of an integrative approach might be the creation of a preferred health service provider relationship, in which the provider wins because they have negotiated a steady cashflow, while the organisation also wins because it has the guarantee of health services of a certain quality at an agreed price. In integrative approaches, the negotiation involves more than one factor. In the example used here, while price would be an important factor, other factors such as volume, availability, quality and mode of delivery would also be included in the negotiation. A metaphor used to describe the **integrative approach** to **negotiation** is that it increases the size of the pie to be shared.

In contrast, the **distributive approach** assumes that the factor (or pie) under negotiation cannot be increased; therefore, if one negotiator gets more, the other gets less (Bazerman & Neale, 1992). This approach to negotiation is recommended only when there is the need for a quick outcome that is more important than the longer term relationship of the negotiators. For example, there is no point in taking an integrative approach with a child who is trying to negotiate not wearing a seatbelt in the car. This is a safety issue that requires a swift resolution. However, 'most negotiations take place in the context of an ongoing relationship where it is important to carry on each negotiation in a way that will help rather than hinder future relations and future negotiations' (Fisher, Ury & Patton, 1991, p. 22).

Margin glossary boxes:

...tion
...d-forth communication
... to reach an agreement when
...the other side have some
... that are shared and some that
...sed' (Fisher, Ury & Patton,
...xxv)

...ive approach
...ation method used when the
...ors believe that both parties
...ve their goals, with neither
...or feeling like they 'lost'

...tive approach
...ation method used when
...r under negotiation cannot
...sed, and therefore if one
...or gets more, the other gets less
...an & Neale, 1992)

Frameworks for negotiating

De Janasz, Dowd & Schneider (2012) propose five stages of negotiation, each of which is discussed below.

Prepare and plan

Planning is essential to a successful negotiation, as it is important to be clear about what is wanted from the negotiation. Skilled negotiators suggest that this is the stage to identify the **BATNA,** defined as the Best Alternative To a Negotiated Agreement, which should be used as the standard against which a proposed agreement is measured. The BATNA is preferred to a set bottom line in negotiations, as it allows consideration of a wider range of solutions as more information becomes available during the negotiation process (Fisher et al., 1991).

Margin glossary box:

...rnative To a Negotiated
...ent, which should be used as
...dard against which a proposed
...nt is measured (Fisher, Ury &
...1991)

Considering a BATNA requires identification of the options available if an agreement is not reached. Once these have been outlined, the option that is considered to be the best is chosen. This becomes the BATNA, against which the terms of the proposed agreement can be evaluated. A negotiator should never accept an agreement that leaves them worse off than their BATNA.

The BATNA is influenced by the number of options available for achieving the required result from the negotiation. For example, if a person negotiating to buy a car would be happy with 10 or 12 different types of cars, their BATNA will be lower than if they want a specific car. This means it will be easier to find a negotiated solution that is better than their BATNA. If there is only one place to buy cars in the person's area, they do not have much choice. However, if there are many dealers with many different models, they can shop around for the best make, price and options. Then they can set a realistic BATNA and know when they are being offered a deal that meets their objectives.

At the preparation stage it is useful to consider the possible interests and negotiating strategies of the other party. Fisher et al. (1991) suggest that writing down both one's own interests and the possible interests of the other party helps to create a wider range of options. Consideration of the other party's BATNA might also be helpful. In the car-buying example, at the end of a slow month the dealers may be willing to reduce their profit, as one sale at a lower price is likely to be better than a BATNA of no sales at all.

Zone of possible agreement
The common ground between two or more parties to a negotiation, where possible solutions are all at least for each negotiator as their BAT

The area where negotiating parties' BATNAs overlap is known as the **zone of possible agreement**. If a car-dealer will not sell for less than $20 000 and a car-buyer has only $18 000 to spend, there is no zone of possible agreement. However, if the car-buyer has $25 000 to spend, the zone between $18 000 and $25 000 is open for possible agreement.

Calculating a BATNA

Sally works in the city, managing a health promotion service at a community health centre. Her organisation has just opened a new site in a regional town and has asked her to move there to complete the planning and development of the service.

Sally calculates her BATNA in preparation for the discussions with her manager about this new role. Her salary is currently $95 000. Not accepting the new position might mean her BATNA is $95 000. Sally will be leaving friends, family and her house in the city that she loves. She considers that a bonus of $5000 to help with the move and enable regular travel home to visit her friends and family might make her happier to move.

Sally feels that she needs to accept the move if she does not want to be disadvantaged in her current organisation. But she has the option of staying in the city and getting a new job. She looks at the jobs available for people with her education, experience and skills, and finds some with salaries of $110 000 for which she would be qualified.

Sally has therefore calculated her BATNA as a salary of $110 000 plus a $5000 incentive payment. She is ready to talk to her manager about her expectations if she were to move to the regional town for the new job.

Define ground rules

The ground rules of a negotiation may address the following factors:
- who will participate in the negotiation
- who may be present to watch or provide information and support during the negotiation
- the location of the negotiation
- the time that will be allocated to the negotiation
- the parameters for the negotiation process.

Negotiation parameters may include the requirement that all parties are polite, procedures for calling time-out, the types of issues that will be discussed and which of these may be set aside for later, and a protocol that will be followed if the negotiation process is not successful. It is more difficult to agree the ground rules to a negotiation with a negotiating partner if one has not already considered what they may entail. Documenting the ground rules that one considers important before entering the negotiation can assist in subsequent work with the other party to outline a mutually acceptable process.

Clarify and justify

During this stage of the negotiation, often referred to as principled negotiation, or separating the people from the problem, each party presents their interests and uses questions to clarify the interests of the other party. It is essential to negotiate on interests and not to get stuck on the positions of the people involved in a negotiation (Bazerman & Neale, 1992; Fisher et al., 1991). Negotiations around land claims of Indigenous people can be used to illustrate this concept. If the interests are seen to be solely about ownership of the land, the positions will be adversarial. If, however, the interests are how best to manage, preserve and develop the land, the issue becomes one of management and not property rights, and the negotiations might therefore be able to end in an agreed plan for the management of the land.

Research has shown that how issues are framed has an impact on how likely people are to accept and to be able to encourage others to accept a proposal. If people perceive that they are getting a good deal, they will be more likely to accept a proposal than if they perceive they are being taken advantage of. **Framing** issues in a positive light generally results in less risky choices, while negative framing often results in riskier choices (Tversky & Kahneman, 1981).

Negotiators often become fixated on irrelevant **anchors**, which are the initial offers made by parties to a negotiation. The anchoring effect is the common tendency to rely too heavily on anchors when making the next decision. For example, the initial price offered for the

g
choice of the language used
be an issue to make it adopt
positive or a more negative
nce

al offer made by a party to a
ion

purchase of an item sets the standard for the rest of the negotiation. This may mean that prices lower than the initial asking price seem more reasonable to a buyer, even if they are higher than the item's true worth.

There is disagreement among expert negotiators as to who should make the first offer. Some recommend that the other party should be encouraged to make the first offer, as this allows further gathering of information. Others suggest that whoever makes the first offer achieves the best outcome. If the other party makes the first offer, it may be important to follow quickly with a counter offer to avoid the first offer's becoming a strong anchor. Equally, it is suggested that if the other party rejects an offer and asks for a new, better offer, this should be declined. Instead, the other party should be asked to submit their offer. A counter offer is worth insisting upon; otherwise, one party ends up negotiating with itself.

Bargain and problem-solve

In this stage, the parties to the negotiation should be actively exploring what solutions will enable each to address their interests. Negotiators should keep an open mind and determine if there are ways to increase the size of the pie and work towards a win–win agreement.

During this stage it may be useful to check that one's style of negotiation is sensitive to the values, perceptions, norms of behaviour and mood of the other party (Fisher et al., 1991). Varying the pace and level of formality of communications, and even the location, as the negotiation progresses can be useful tactics.

If it is apparent that the parties will not be able to come to an agreement but want to continue bargaining, it may be useful to include an independent third party. De Janasz et al. (2012) suggest allowing the third party to draft a plan that considers the interests of all negotiators and then giving the negotiators the opportunity to revise the plan. This process can continue until there is agreement. A third-party **mediator** can often establish a constructive environment that requires all parties to continue to discuss issues cooperatively and objectively. Sometimes, however, unresolvable issues are sent to an **arbitrator**.

Mediator
Someone who attempts to help involved in a conflict come to ar agreement

Arbitrator
Someone who is independent fr either party in a conflict and is g the power to impose a settleme dispute

Close and implement

At this stage, either an agreement has been reached or the parties walk away from the negotiation. If an agreement has been reached it is important to summarise what has been agreed, review the key points to ensure they have been understood by all parties, confirm any areas where agreement was not reached and if necessary document the agreement for signature (de Janasz et al., 2012).

Management and negotiation

While many negotiators may use tactics to try to win a negotiation, at all times negotiators should display ethical behaviour. Spangle and Isenhart (2003, p. 172) identify the following unethical negotiating tactics:

- withholding information that has a substantial influence on the available options
- making false statements or lying to mislead the other party
- offering bribes or kickbacks
- insulting or demeaning the other party
- making promises that will not be met.

Unethical negotiation includes **negotiating in bad faith**. De Janasz et al. (2012, p. 199) advise that if the person with whom one is negotiating uses unethical means, it is 'better to end the negotiation without a resolution or contract than participate in a negotiation that compromises your values or reputation and causes you to be a victim'.

te in bad faith
ue to negotiate despite
o intention of making any
nises

Negotiation skills improvement

Researchers have spent time identifying how individuals can improve their performance in negotiating. As early as 1990 it was suggested that improving integrative abilities, through greater accuracy in judgements about the interests of the other party and high aspirations for the negotiation outcomes, is associated with better negotiation performance (Thompson, 1990). A more recent study reports a 24 per cent decrease in negotiation time when a professional negotiator is used. Also, contrary to expectation, there is no connection between the nature and duration of the relationship sustained by the negotiating parties and the time taken to reach a successful conclusion of negotiations (Malatesta, 2012). Having a great relationship does not necessarily make reaching agreement any easier.

The most important message from expert negotiators is to look for positives in all possible circumstances (Bazerman & Neale, 1992). Much of the research has explored why negotiators do not always make rational decisions, and negotiators are advised to focus on meeting their own interests as well as those of their negotiating partner (Stamato, 2004). Margaret Neale (cited in Buell, 2007, p. 1) says, 'If I can trade off issues that I care about more and you care about less, then we've been able to create value in a transaction'.

Finally, the literature suggests that females are less likely than males to engage in negotiation (Stamato, 2004); this includes negotiation regarding their salary and working conditions. Generally, women do not perceive negotiating opportunities as often as men (Babcock & Laschever, 2009). It is particularly important for female leaders and managers to develop their skills in negotiation.

Summary

- It is vital to practise, practise and practise to improve negotiating skills.
- Planning a negotiation strategy is critical and involves considering all of the information available to confirm and frame one's own interests and those of the other party.
- To achieve a win–win solution, consideration is necessary of how to increase the size of the pie.
- Negotiating tactics that could be considered unethical should never be used, as this will cause long-term damage to the relationship.
- It is important to walk away from a negotiation that does not meet the BATNA.

Reflective questions

1 Why is it important to separate the interests from the positions of people involved in a negotiation?
2 How might you calculate and use a BATNA when trying to decide whether to accept a job? What information apart from the job offer would be useful to your BATNA calculations?
3 How does the media portray negotiations between employers and unions as they aim to reach agreement on employment conditions?
4 Expert negotiators see negotiation as joint problem-solving. How is this different from the common view of negotiation being adversarial?
5 What might result from using unethical tactics in a negotiation?

Self-analysis questions

Think about times when you have attempted to negotiate an agreement with someone, either informally or formally. Identify two agreements that from your perspective were successful, and two that were unsuccessful. Write a brief description of each negotiation and look for commonalities between them. What were the conditions when you were successful? What were the conditions when you were unsuccessful? Who was involved? What preparation did you do? What can you learning from this about your negotiating style? What might you do differently in the future?

References

Babcock, L. & Laschever, S. (2009). *Women don't ask: Negotiation and the gender divide.* Princeton, NJ: Princeton University.

Bazerman, M. & Neale, M. (1992). *Negotiating rationally.* New York, NY: Free.

Buell, B. (2007). *Negotiation strategy: Seven common pitfalls to avoid.* Retrieved from http://www.gsb.stanford.edu/insights/negotiation-strategy-seven-common-pitfalls-avoid

De Janasz, S. C., Dowd, K. O. & Schneider, B. Z. (2012). *Interpersonal skills in organizations* (4th ed.). New York, NY: McGraw-Hill Irwin.

Fisher, R., Ury, W. & Patton, B. (1991). *Getting to yes.* New York, NY: Penguin.

——. (2012). *Getting to yes: Negotiating an agreement without giving in.* New York, NY: Random House Business.

Malatesta, D. (2012). The link between information and bargaining efficiency. *Journal of Public Administration and Theory, 22*(3), 527–551. doi: 10.1093/jopart/mur028

Mealiea, L. & Latham, G. P. (1996). *Skills for managerial success: Theory, experience, and practice.* Chicago, IL: Irwin.

Nanus, B. & Dobbs, S. M. (1999). *Leaders who make a difference.* San Francisco, CA: Jossey-Bass.

Spangle, M. L. & Isenhart, M. W. (2003). *Negotiation: Communication for diverse settings.* Thousand Oaks, CA: Sage.

Stamato, L. (2004). The new age of negotiation. *Ivey Business Journal,* (July–August), 1–3. Retrieved from http://iveybusinessjournal.com

Thompson, L. (1990). The influence of experience on negotiation performance. *Journal of Experimental and Social Psychology, 26*(6), 528–544.

Tversky, A. & Kahneman, D. (1981). The framing of decisions and the psychology of choice. *Science, 211*(4481), 453–458.

Part **5**

Drives Innovation

22

Creativity and visioning

Godfrey Isouard

Learning objectives

How do I:
- work with others in my organisation to develop an effective vision for the future?
- increase my ability to identify and explore creative solutions to organisational issues?
- foster creativity among the people I work with?
- assist my organisation to become a learning organisation?

Introduction

The healthcare sector is continually confronted with the issue of how to manage with less. In response, health leaders and managers must explore and use new ways to face such challenges. Such issues ultimately affect the quality and safety, and the productivity and efficiency of the health services delivered. Within each organisation, the effectiveness of the leadership and culture impact squarely on the quality of patient care delivered. In order to effectively address such challenges, leaders have started to adopt new strategies and roles focusing on visioning and creativity.

Definitions

Creativity, or creative capital, is by far an organisation's most important asset. It results from an effectively led and managed unit of creative thinkers and planners whose ideas can be transformed into valuable services and products (Florida & Goodnight, 2005). It is important to identify those factors which influence creativity within the organisation; Andriopolous (2001) identifies these as: organisational climate;

leadership style; organisational culture, resources and skills; organisational structure; and organisational systems.

Visioning is regarded as an important element that provides clear direction to an organisation. It is more than a vision statement; it is a process of assessing how fit the organisation may be to expand and function in the future. Visioning leads to strategic planning, which is the codification of strategic thinking and corporate direction into the future. The effective leader takes the essential role in building the appropriate culture through establishing the mission and

Visioning
The process of assessing how fi[t] organisation is to grow and fun[ction] the future

Vision
A clear purpose that expresses [a] sense of an organisation's futur[e]

vision, and developing plans that move beyond the certainties of today. At the organisational level, visioning exists to plan projects, enhance creativity and ensure that tasks are aligned to the vision (Foster & Akdere, 2007).

Organisations

Creativity and visioning are vital to the success of an organisation. However, it is challenging for many organisations to encourage and foster new ideas and to establish creativity and **innovation** that can benefit all concerned. Of relevance is that the need to be creative is not confined to commercial and non-health-based organisations. Innovation and creativity have an important place in **not-for-profit organisations** and in the public and government domains, where the drive has shifted to greater efficiency, effectiveness and productivity. There is increased pressure placed on these latter organisations to find new and improved means of working and innovative solutions to current and future problems.

Creativity
The act of generating new idea[s] thoughts and transforming the[m] reality

Innovation
The embodiment, combination [or] synthesis of knowledge into orig[inal] relevant, valued new products, processes or services (Luecke & 2003)

Not-for-profit organisation
An organisation that is not oper[ating] for the profit or personal gain o[f] individual members or sharehol[ders]

Systems-based approach

In Australia, strong leadership at various levels will be required to enable health reforms to succeed within healthcare organisations (Health Workforce Australia, 2012). Leading organisations use creativity and innovation to address the challenges, building cultures which foster capacity for innovation and change (Agbor, 2008). This is generally undertaken through leadership which adopts a **systems-based approach**. In such workplaces, there are common elements which characterise the culture. These are critical in ensuring that creativity and change are successfully introduced and maintained within the healthcare organisation setting. They include effective transformational

Systems-based approach
A leadership method that assum[es an] organisation is a convoluted inte[raction] of dynamic parts which work to[gether] for a common purpose

leadership, adoption of a systems-based approach and clear understanding of how to develop organisational cultures which enhance and nurture the workplace environment to embrace creativity and change. These elements are discussed and analysed in this chapter.

Learning organisations

Scott, Mannion, Davies and Marshall (2003) observe that organisational culture is a key factor in healthcare reform. They found that creativity, innovation and organisational change can be achieved only with an organisational culture that encourages adaptability to change. Once such a culture is established, the rate of innovation is dependent on how the norms, social status and hierarchy impact on employee behaviours (Rogers, 1995).

An important aspect in any organisation involves its learning capacity, by which the vision exists to ensure that all activities are aligned (Foster & Akdere, 2007).

> **g organisation**
> nisation in which employees
> achieve their target goals, new
> e enhanced, team aspiration is
> to reign, and all are inspired
> nually learn to view the whole

Learning organisations are founded on uniform engagement and collaboration by all employees, who are committed and accountable to change, each directed towards shared principles. As originally described by Peter Senge (1990) in his book *The fifth discipline*, in learning organisations employees strive to achieve their target goals, new ideas are enhanced, team aspiration is allowed to reign, and all are inspired to learn to view the whole together.

According to Senge, an emphasis on knowledge management is characteristic of learning organisations, which can change continuously, as they learn from experience in order to improve overall performance. This is achieved through continually developing, retaining and leveraging both individual and collective learning. Senge also described learning organisations as encouraging and supporting their workers towards ongoing learning while stressing information-sharing, teamwork and participation as important.

Learning organisations are readily adaptable to changes in the external environment (Costanzo & Tzoumpa, 2008). The existence of such a learning environment is fundamental to the development of creativity, and this has been shown to be achieved through a transformational approach to leadership (Gumusluoglu & Ilsev, 2009). The transformation to a learning organisation provides the necessary culture to foster innovation, creativity and change (Aragon-Correa, García-Morales & Cordón-Pozo, 2007; Sarros, Cooper & Santora, 2008).

Employees within an effective learning organisation are valued for their own contributions and are encouraged to improve and develop their individual skills and competencies. They benefit from each other's experience. Leaders in these organisation tend to respect and treat all equally within the workplace environment. In turn, employees are motivated to work towards achieving the goals set by their leaders. This ultimately provides the appropriate culture for innovative solutions, enhanced creativity and new ideas (Health Workforce Australia, 2012).

The impact on employees within such organisations has been found to be very positive (Andriopoulos, 2001). Individuals tend to acquire skills and knowledge above their position's described requirements. This allows them to accept and appreciate other roles and activities in the organisation. The use of flexible arrangements in the workplace allows employees the liberty to move freely, while removing the obstacles associated with a rigidly structured organisation. It also ensures that employees are able to cope successfully with a changing environment, as is found in healthcare today.

Management and innovation

Creating the required culture

In this context, culture is regarded as the norms and beliefs of an organisation and the ways in which it acts collectively. The culture provides the key catalyst to introducing innovation and change, and together with leadership is a main factor in providing the receptive environment for change (Gumusluoglu & Ilsev, 2009; Masood, Dani, Burns & Backhouse, 2006; Rivenburgh, 2014).

In order for a leader and manager to create a learning organisation, they must be competent in transforming and building an organisation's culture and understand how to create a culture that supports innovation and change. However, although it is widely recognised that creativity and visioning are key ingredients in a high-performing organisation (Karaman, Kok, Hasilogle & Rivera, 2008), it is often difficult to introduce, manage and sustain the required cultural change. Cummings and Worley (1995) list key activities which provide beneficial outcomes in culture change; these include motivating change, creating a vision, developing political support for change, managing the transition and sustaining momentum. Health Workforce Australia (2012) also identifies elements needed for creating the necessary culture:

- Provide a workplace environment which enables support mechanisms that allow employees to develop and trial new ideas.
- Provide flat structures with flexible teams, incorporating rewards and incentives for creative and innovative actions.
- Develop teams of managers who feel comfortable guiding flexible teams which take acceptable risks.
- Develop and provide open communication channels that build trust.
- Appoint managers to play a significant role with regard to facilitating learning and reusing effectively the knowledge received from experience.

Leading for creativity at Care Line Hospital

John is the new chief executive officer of Care Line Hospital, a tertiary referral public-funded hospital located in metropolitan Sydney. On commencing employment, John soon uncovers several serious issues in performance and service delivery, with decreased efficiency, low productivity and ineffectiveness throughout the organisation. Specifically, there are poor financial management and performance, a high level of senior management team turnover, great dissatisfaction among the employees and increased demands for services.

After wide consultation and analysis, John determines that the situation requires a new and creative model of organisation, management and service delivery. In consultation with his senior executive team, John's response is to form the following set of strategies:

- Introduce measures to change the culture so that creativity is fostered throughout the organisation through encouraging and supporting new ideas.
- Make plans to transform the culture to that of a learning organisation.
- Establish a new leadership group for the organisation, including the appointment of designated 'ideas champions', whose roles are to develop new and creative initiatives while actively targeting improvements and challenging the existing norms and processes of the organisation.
- Base the new culture on uniform engagement and collaboration by all employees, who are committed and accountable to change, each being directed towards shared principles.
- Include in the implementation plan introducing change, developing the vision, securing political agreement for change, managing the period of change and maintaining the change achieved.
- Establish a process through which all employees will be encouraged to learn from experience in an environment that encourages discussion and disagreement.
- Develop ideas on how best to negotiate change processes.

Challenges

Not all leaders and managers who seek a creative culture are successful in attaining it. Numerous challenges exist along the way which could jeopardise its development at the organisational level. These include difficulty in converting individual creativity to organisational creativity, lack of effective leadership to encourage employees to learn from experience, insufficient stimulus and motivation to generate new ideas, and barriers that impede creativity (Agbor, 2008).

Structure

The type of organisational structure in use has a clear impact on employees' ability to contribute to ideas and creativity. Vertical organisations tend to be rigid and often result in employees feeling stifled in what they can and cannot undertake. Although horizontal organisations are less efficient, there are fewer rules, and they provide employees with a sense of identification with the organisation. Employees in such work environments normally strive to achieve their target goals; through this, new ideas are fostered, and team and group aspiration flows readily (Borrill, West & Dawson, 2003).

Strategies need to be established by the leader to incorporate in the organisation smaller units with a clear direction and enabling structures that facilitate the development and trialling of new ideas. These are often referred to in the literature as innovation factories. They provide the mechanism by which to enhance innovative thinking in organisations with more traditional norms (Snowdon, Shell & Leitch, 2010).

Organisations having modern norms are generally technologically developed, rational, empathic and change-oriented, whereas those with traditional norms are the direct opposite. Those organisations embracing traditional norms have been found to diffuse creativity and innovations much more slowly within the organisation than those that have incorporated modern norms (Rogers, 1995).

Leadership

Learning organisations need a designated person to be assigned to a leadership role in developing individuals and teams to produce new and creative initiatives. These people are often called ideas champions. They aim to achieve improvements and challenge current norms and processes.

Poor leadership can result in little or no uptake of innovation or creativity within the organisation. Snowdon et al. (2010) give an account of a perceived lack of leadership in the Canadian health system and the issues that arose as a result. The authors report that innovation is an important aspect in addressing challenges in healthcare. Leadership in healthcare is critical to developing a culture that enhances and supports innovation and change for sustainability.

Converting creativity

One significant challenge for a leader is converting individual creativity into organisational creativity. As organisations aim to become more creative and innovative, the strategies employed can often lead to conditions that encourage the individual effort more than team creativity. This can result in pockets of creativity but not an overall commitment to the organisation's goals. To attain the appropriate culture, the process must be seen as long term rather than an instant solution (Andriopolous, 2001).

While it is important to commence at the individual level in order to build capacity within an organisation, creativity must then spread across all work functions and teams for the organisation to become more creative and effective. Individual effort needs to be converted across the organisation and in line with the organisation's mission and vision (Woodman, Sawyer & Griffin, 1993).

Learning from experience

Organisations need a culture in which leaders encourage their employees to learn from failings as well as successes (Hartley & Bennington, 2010). This is backed up by research which found that hospitals tend not to learn from failure, because the traditional professional approach often deters questioning, due to a tendency towards a fast fix rather than a more measured and systematic problem-solving approach (Edmondson, 2004).

Searching for new ideas

Florida and Goodnight (2005) stress that creative capital is not just the result of individual ideas but is also attained through interaction among employees and other stakeholders. The challenge for leaders is that employees need to be intellectually engaged and obstacles removed to enable organisation-wide creativity.

Leaders can sense that creativity and innovation are key components of their organisation (Klemm, 2010), and that they can be generated through extensive interaction throughout the organisation. New ideas through widespread dialogue can lead to programs which fulfil creativity targets. As such, the mission of each leader should be to create ongoing opportunities for innovation and new ideas. The leader generally promotes creativity and innovation through management strategies that create a culture which motivates employees (Sundgren & Styhre, 2007).

Leadership and innovation

Effective leadership

Healthcare leaders appreciate their responsibility in providing clear direction into the future. They need to ensure that their organisation adapts in an environment of limited resources and increased demands for services. In order to operate effectively in the long term, a visioning process should be undertaken (Kachaner & Deimler, 2008; Millett, 2006).

The quality of leadership within an organisation has been shown to affect its culture, which in turn affects creativity, innovation and performance (McGuire, 2003). It ultimately impacts on employees and their commitment and trust, on the overall effectiveness of the team, and therefore on personal and collective performance (Avolio, Walumba & Weber, 2009; Burke et al., 2006; Kouzes & Posner, 2007). In essence, effective leadership requires a vision of the future that inspires employees of the organisation. The vision must be both effective and realistic. Successful leaders are those who work towards a shared and common vision to achieve the organisation's goals (Foster & Akdere, 2007). In this context, the vision forms the unifying thread and acts as a shared goal for all employees. The leader must consider how to meet employees' needs for expression in order to encourage innovation and creativity within the workplace (Amabile, Conti, Coon, Lazenby & Herron, 1996).

Many leaders today foster lateral thinking among employees in an attempt to enhance creativity within the organisation. The optimum strategies target employees who work across various levels, including staff and line managers and the planning and strategy units. Such leaders are considered to demonstrate a vision, trustworthiness and the capability to motivate (Bass & Avolio, 1993).

Transformational leadership

The changing role of today's leaders follows contemporary leadership theories, which account for not only the leader but also the people they lead. In particular, **transformational leadership** theories focus on the role that leaders play in transforming employees in terms of their personal values and goals so that these are more consistent with those of the organisation (Bass, 1985). Transformational leadership has been found to comprise four key elements: individualised consideration, intellectual stimulation, inspirational motivation and idealised influence (Judge & Piccolo, 2004). This is widely acknowledged as the favoured framework for leadership in several current healthcare organisations (Health Workforce Australia, 2012).

Transformational leadershi
A leadership style that can inspi
positive changes in followers

There is strong empirical evidence that transformational leadership develops optimal organisational culture and positive change (Judge & Piccolo, 2004; Kouzes & Posner 2007). It has also been found to increase employee commitment and job satisfaction, and to decrease employee turnover and burnout (Borrill et al., 2003; Vandenberghe, Stordeur & D'hoore, 2002). Transformational leaders are reported to inspire their employees to higher levels of performance through transforming their attitudes, beliefs and values (Bass, 1985). Such leaders achieve change through creating shared understanding and acting as strong role models (Kinjerski & Skrypnek, 2006; Sosik & Dinger, 2007).

Vision is a key component of transformational leadership (Searle & Hamilton, 2010; Sosik & Dinger, 2007). It supports the notion that employees and others should strive to achieve goals at work (Densten, 2005). Transformational leaders leave a lasting impact on their employees, who are able to commit to the organisation's vision. Certain aspects of transformational leadership, such as intellectual stimulation and common values, have been found to result in a culture of enhanced ideas, innovation and creativity, as well as greater trust and team togetherness. This contributes to continued change due to an increased willingness by employees to accept and participate more readily in change. Such leadership transforms the organisational culture in a way that means creativity and change become the norm (Aragon-Correa et al., 2007; Sarros et al., 2008).

Summary

- Creativity and visioning are vital elements to the success of an organisation.
- Organisational visioning is used to provide clear direction to the organisation.
- Transformational leadership and a systems-based approach can help ensure that creativity and change are successfully introduced.
- Transformational leadership develops optimal organisational culture and positive change.
- Learning organisations provide the necessary culture to foster innovation, creativity and change.

Reflective questions

1 What do you understand creativity to be in an organisation? As a health leader, what measures would you take to enhance creativity in the workplace?

2 What is your understanding of organisational culture? As a health leader, what strategies would you consider to nurture a workplace environment that embraces creativity and change?

3 Do you consider it important to identify factors that influence creativity and the generation of new ideas in the workplace? Why?

4 How do you encourage existing employees to share a common vision for the organisation? Describe the approach you would take and some of the challenges you are likely to encounter.

5 In what ways can becoming a learning organisation improve the performance and effectiveness of a healthcare organisation? What impact would it have on its employees?

Self-analysis questions

List the key leadership and management characteristics identified in this chapter. Self-assess your current status and development with regard to these. Discuss with colleagues and mentors your current development in these areas and the areas that need to be focused on for future development.

References

Agbor, E. (2008). Creativity and innovation: The leadership dynamics. *Journal of Strategic Leadership*, 1(1), 39–45. Retrieved from http://www.regent.edu

Amabile, T. M., Conti, R., Coon, H., Lazenby, J. & Herron, M. (1996). Assessing the work environment for creativity. *Academy of Management Journal*, 39, 1154–1184. doi: 10.2307/256995

Andriopoulos, C. (2001). Determinants of organisational creativity: A literature review. *Management Decision*, 39(10), 834–841. doi: 10.1108/00251740110402328

Aragon-Correa, J. A., García-Morales, V. J. & Cordón-Pozo, E. (2007). Leadership and organizational learning's role on innovation and performance: Lessons from Spain. *Industrial Marketing Management*, 36(3), 349–359. doi: 10.1016/j.indmarman.2005.09.006

Avolio, B. J., Walumba, F. O. & Weber, T. J. (2009). Leadership: Current theories, research and future directions. *Annual Review of Psychology, 60*, 421–449. doi: 10.1146/annurev. psych.60.110707.163621

Bass, B. M. (1985). *Leadership and performance beyond expectation*. New York, NY: Free.

Bass, B.M. & Avolio, B. J. (1993). Transformational leadership: A response to critiques. In M. M. Chemers & R. Ayman (Eds), *Leadership theory and research: Perspectives and directions* (pp. 49–80). San Diego, CA: Academic.

Borrill, C., West, M. & Dawson, J. (2003). *The relationship between leadership, people management, staff satisfaction and intentions to leave*. Birmingham, United Kingdom: Aston Business School.

Burke, C. S., Stagl, C. S., Klein, C., Goodwin, G. F., Salas, E. & Halpin, S. M. (2006). What type of leadership behaviors are functional in teams? A meta-analysis. *Leadership Quarterly, 17*, 288–307. doi: 10.1016/j.leaqua.2006.02.007

Costanzo, L. A. & Tzoumpa, V. (2008). Enhancing organisational learning in teams: Has the middle manager got a role? *Team Performance Management, 14*(3–4), 146–164. doi: 10.1108/13527590810883424

Cummings, T. G. & Worley, C. G. (1995). *Organization development and change* (8th ed.). Mason, OH: South-Western Cengage Learning.

Densten, I. L. (2005). The relationship between visioning behaviours of leaders and follower burnout. *British Journal of Management, 16*(2), 105–118. doi: 10.1111/j.1467 -8551.2005.00428.x

Edmondson, A. C. (2004). Learning from failure in health care: Frequent opportunities, pervasive barriers. *Quality and Safety in Health Care, 13*, 3–9. doi: 10.1136/qshc.2003.009597

Florida, R. & Goodnight, J. (2005). Managing for creativity. *Harvard Business Review*, (July– August), 1–9.

Foster, R. D. & Akdere, M. (2007). Effective organizational vision: Implications for human resource development. *Journal of European Industrial Training, 31*(2), 100–111. doi: 10.1108/0309059074336

Gumusluoglu, L. & Ilsev, A. (2009). Transformational leadership, creativity, and organizational innovation. *Journal of Business Research, 62*(4), 461–473. doi: 10.1016/j.jbusres.2007.07.032

Hartley, J. & Bennington, J. (2010). *Leadership for health care*. Bristol, United Kingdom: Policy.

Health Workforce Australia. (2012). *Leadership for the sustainability of the health system: Part 1; A literature review*. Retrieved from https://www.hwa.gov.au/sites/default/files/ leadership-for-sustainability-of-health-sector-literature-review-012012.pdf

Judge, T. A. & Piccolo, R. F. (2004). Transformational and transactional leadership: A meta-analytic test of their relative validity. *Journal of Applied Psychology, 89*(5), 755–768. doi: 10.1037/0021-9010.89.5.755

Kachaner, N. & Deimler, M. S. (2008). How leading companies are stretching their strategy. *Strategy and Leadership, 36*(4), 40–43. doi: 10.1108/10878570810888768

Karaman, A., Kok, S. B., Hasilogle, S. B. & Rivera, M. (2008). Vision, creativity, strategic innovation, and transformational leadership. *Problems and Perspectives in Management, 6*(2), 104–109.

Kinjerski, V. & Skrypnek, B. J. (2006). Creating organizational conditions that foster employee spirit at work. *Leadership & Organization Development Journal, 27*(4), 280–295. doi: 10.1108/01437730610666037

Klemm, W. R. (2010). *Leadership: Creativity and innovation.* Retrieved from http://www.au.af.
mil/au/awc/awcgate/au-24/au24-401.htm

Kouzes, J. M. & Posner, B. Z. (2007). *The leadership challenge.* San Francisco, CA: Jossey-Barry.

Luecke, R. & Katz, R. (2003). *Managing creativity and innovation.* Boston, MA: Harvard
Business.

Masood, S. A., Dani, S. S., Burns, N. D. & Backhouse, C. J. (2006). Transformational leadership
and organizational culture: The situational strength perspective. *Proceedings of the
Institution of Mechanical Engineers, Part B: Journal of Engineering Manufacture, 220*(6),
941–949. doi: 10.1243/09544054JEM499

McGuire, J. B. (2003). *Leadership strategies for culture change: Developing change leadership
as an organizational core capability* [White paper]. Retrieved from Center for Creative
Leadership website: http://www.ccl.org/leadership/pdf/community/connectedleadership.pdf

Millett, S. M. (2006). Futuring and visioning: Complementary approaches to strategic decision
making. *Strategy and Leadership, 34*(3), 43–50. doi: 10.1108/10878570610660591

Rivenburgh, D. (2014). Creating a vibrant, thriving, responsible culture. *Journal for Quality and
Participation, 37*(1), 4–9.

Rogers, E. (1995). *Diffusion of innovations.* New York: Free.

Sarros, J. C., Cooper, B. K. & Santora, J. C. (2008). Building a climate for innovation
through transformational leadership and organizational culture. *Journal of Leadership &
Organizational Studies, 15*(2), 145–158. doi: 10.1177/1548051808324100

Scott, T., Mannion, R., Davies, H. T. O. & Marshall, M. N. (2003). Implementing culture change
in health care: Theory and practice. *International Journal for Quality in Health Care, 15*(2),
111–118. doi: 10.1093/intqhc/mzg021

Searle, G. D. & Hamilton, S. J. (2010). Leading to inspire others: Charismatic influence
or hard work? *Leadership & Organization Development Journal, 32*(7), 736–754.
doi: 10.1108/01437731111170021

Senge, P. (1990). *The fifth discipline: The art and practice of the learning organization.* London,
United Kingdom: Century Business.

Snowdon, A., Shell, J. & Leitch, K. (2010). *Innovation takes leadership* [Report by Ivey Centre
for Health Innovation and Leadership]. Retrieved from Ivey website: http://sites.ivey.ca/
healthinnovation/files/2010/09/White-Paper.pdf

Sosik, J. J. & Dinger, S. L. (2007). Relationships between leadership style and vision content:
The moderating role of need for social approval, self-monitoring, and need for social power.
Leadership Quarterly, 18(2), 134–153. doi: 10.1016/j.leaqua.2007.01.004

Sundgren, M. & Styhre, A. (2007). Creativity and the fallacy of misplaced concreteness in
new drug development: A Whiteheadian perspective. *European Journal of Innovation
Management, 10*(2), 215–235. doi: 10.1108/14601060710745260

Vandenberghe, C., Stordeur, S. & D'hoore, W. (2002). Transactional and transformational
leadership in nursing: Structural validity and substantive relationships. *European Journal of
Psychological Assessment, 18*(1), 16–29. doi: 10.1027//1015-5759.18.1.16

Woodman, R. W., Sawyer, J. E. & Griffin, R. W. (1993). Toward a theory of organizational
creativity. *Academy of Management Review, 18*(2), 293–321. doi: 10.5465/
AMR.1993.3997517

23

Evidence-based practice

Sandra G. Leggat and Denise M. Jepsen

Learning objectives

How do I:

- determine when to look for evidence to assist in decision-making?
- source relevant evidence for my management practice and decision-making?
- critically appraise evidence for its strengths, weaknesses and relevance to a particular health services management question?
- apply relevant evidence to my management practice and decision-making?
- find out more about evidence-based management?

Introduction

Building on the concepts of evidence-based medicine and evidence-based policy, the concept of evidence-based leadership and management suggests that leaders and managers find, evaluate and use the best available scientific evidence to inform their practice. An early definition of evidence-based management was 'translating principles based on best evidence into organisational practices' (Rousseau, 2006, p. 256). This chapter discusses when and how to look for evidence and outlines how to apply it to the leadership or management decision or situation at hand.

Use of evidence

While there are studies linking doctors who practise evidence-based medicine with better clinical outcomes (Pfeffer & Sutton, 2006), and despite the inherent logic of basing decisions on evidence, we could find no studies linking **evidence-based management** with better organisational outcomes. In fact, there is a large body of research that suggests that managers have difficulty finding and applying evidence to their management practice generally (Hemsley-Brown & Sharp, 2003), and to health-care leadership and management specifically (Finkler & Ward, 2003).

Studies have found that health service managers believe using evidence will improve management effectiveness (Adily & Ward, 2005; Liang, Howard, Leggat & Murphy, 2012), and most health service managers report a desire to use and apply evidence (Mitton & Patten, 2004). However, they make little regular use of evidence in their decision-making, especially neglecting scientific or research evidence (Liang et al., 2012; Lomas, Culyer, McCutcheon, McAuley & Law, 2005).

:e-based management
ng principles based on best
into organisational practices'
u, 2006, p. 256)

It is recognised that management research has had a much shorter timeframe than other areas of research (Axelsson, 1998), which has led to the dearth of robust evidence. In addition, there have been many articles written that outline the divide between those who use the evidence and those who produce the evidence, with suggestions that researchers need to better understand context and decision-making processes (Black, 2001). With an evidence-based approach there should be more demand for systematic research reviews and meta-analyses (Axelsson, 1998) that clearly describe what is known and what is still to be learned. A framework for improving the use of evidence in managerial decision-making is proposed by Liang et al. (2012). As outlined in Figure 23.1, the writers suggest roles for a range of players in the healthcare system.

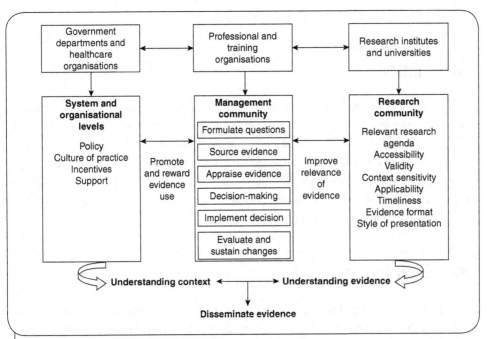

Figure 23.1 Framework for improving the use of evidence in managerial decision-making. Z. Liang, P. F. Howard, S. G. Leggat & G. Murphy (2012). A framework to improve evidence-informed decision-making in health service management. *Australian Health Review, 36*(3), 287. doi: 10.1071/ah11051.

Managers and leaders should encourage an evidence-based organisational culture by asking for evidence and its potential application to their organisation. Recognising there is a long way to go to bridge the research–practice gap (Walshe & Rundall, 2001), managers should also participate in scholarly or scientific management research if invited to do so. Further, managers can capitalise on the supports offered by educational institutions to learn the skills and techniques to find, evaluate and apply their own relevant evidence.

It is clear that organisations must have a coherent approach if evidence-based management is to be embraced. This will encourage a significant power shift in organisations, replacing formal authority and opinion with facts and data (Pfeffer & Sutton, 2006). Organisational factors critical to the success of evidence-informed decision-making in health service management are supportive systems for access to evidence and information-sharing (Lavis et al., 2005), and provision of incentives to promote the use of evidence (Nutley & Davies, 2000). Shortell (2006) highlights the important role of health service boards in driving the necessary cultural change to implement such supportive organisational systems.

Frameworks for evidence-based management and leadership

In evidence-based management and leadership, managers and leaders need to formulate questions and then source and appraise the available evidence. This is then interpreted and used for decision-making, with implementation and evaluation following. This method is consistent with a report published by Barends, Rousseau & Briner (2014, p. 2), which suggests six steps to evidence-based management, to be taken

> through the conscientious, explicit and judicious use of the best available evidence from multiple sources by
> 1 Asking: translating a practical issue or problem into an answerable question
> 2 Acquiring: systematically searching for and retrieving the evidence
> 3 Appraising: critically judging the trustworthiness and relevance of the evidence
> 4 Aggregating: weighing and pulling together the evidence
> 5 Applying: incorporating the evidence into the decision-making process
> 6 Assessing: evaluating the outcome of the decision taken.

Pfeffer and Sutton (2006) suggest that everyone in an organisation needs to take responsibility for the implementation of evidence-based management. They propose that managers ask for evidence of efficacy every time someone outlines a change. Managers should also ensure that decision-makers have all of the available supporting (and non-supporting) data.

Source the evidence

Managers should consider all sources of evidence, ranging from scientific to opinion or stakeholder evidence (Barends et al., 2014). It is important to acquire the *best* available evidence to address the issue at hand, while recognising that in most instances issues such as time and access mean that not *all* available evidence will be included in a review. Four specific sources of evidence, and questions to ask when considering them, are given below.

Scientific, scholarly or academic research findings

What has been studied, researched and established in peer-reviewed studies on this topic? Which databases should we search? What might a librarian be able to do to help us find out about this topic?

Stakeholders' values and concerns

Who may be affected by this decision? Whose views are important when coming to this decision? Who should we involve in interviews or discussions about this topic?

Organisational data, facts and figures

What do we know about this issue within our organisation? What information and metrics are available to inform and support our decision-making? Which reports could we use or ask for that would help our deliberations about this topic?

Professional experience and judgement

Who has experience or expertise in this area, either within or outside this organisation? Who has experience or expertise in a similar area and therefore could usefully inform this decision? Who else might we discuss this topic with?

Performance review system change enhanced by evidence

As a result of policy change at government level, annual performance reviews have become compulsory in a large metropolitan public healthcare organisation. Forms, tools, communications and other activities associated with the performance review system need to be updated. The policy directive includes a reading list to justify the policy, but no resources have been supplied on how to implement the performance review system.

The education and implementation team have many questions as they begin to revise and update their system. They want to know, for example: Which are the critical parts of the performance review system that need particular attention? What needs to be emphasised in the training, both to managers conducting reviews and to staff being reviewed? Is an overall or summary numerical rating system always required? Should managers or employees have the 'last word' on the performance review? Should staff be able to leapfrog their supervisor's rating and seek a second opinion?

The managers implementing the new system are all former clinicians now working in management roles, well used to routinely checking evidence-based sources for clinical treatments and treatment options. However, these managers have not been trained in

continued ›

continued ›

how to design, implement or conduct training on a performance review system. Their typical way of implementing a management intervention is to discuss similar interventions with other healthcare services, ask about their successes and learnings, and adapt those experiences to their own situation. Sometimes, they may ask to see what books on the topic are available in their institutional library.

After reflecting on the lack of solid evidence regarding how to implement a revised performance review system, the responsible manager recommends that the department join the Center for Evidence-Based Management (www.cebma.org) to gain access to peer-reviewed journals that are specifically in the management field. They can then find out what is already known about effective performance review system implementation. By adding peer-reviewed journals to their evidence base, they introduce a scientific rigour to the department that has previously been absent.

Appraise the evidence

All types of evidence can be useful for decision-making, but managers and leaders must be aware of how the evidence applies to their situation and the strengths and weaknesses presented. When appraising the evidence, it is important to take into account how and where the evidence was gathered, and under what conditions. Who conducted the research or spoke of the experience, and what biases or other limits might have applied in that instance? What else was occurring at the time that may provide an alternative explanation for the results?

Evidence can be of variable quality, even within the scientific literature, and difficulties sometimes arise when comparing studies using different methodologies. There is fierce debate between researchers who see the randomised controlled trial, systematic review or meta-analysis as the gold standard for research evidence, and those who privilege other forms of evidence (see, for example, O'Halloran, Porter & Blackwood, 2010). On the other hand, many research organisations acknowledge that a large number of questions are best answered by qualitative and cross-sectional studies (National Institute for Health and Clinical Excellence, 2009). Figure 23.2 outlines a hierarchy of evidence in which the higher volume stakeholder evidence, such as background information, organisational information and expert opinion, at the bottom of the pyramid and the empirically based lower volume information at the top.

Apply the evidence to decision-making

Some decisions are novel and apply at one time to perhaps unknown or uncertain circumstances or environments. Consider, for example, the one-off change in the performance review system discussed above, which needs a series of decisions at the implementation stage. Other decisions are applied routinely as a matter of normal

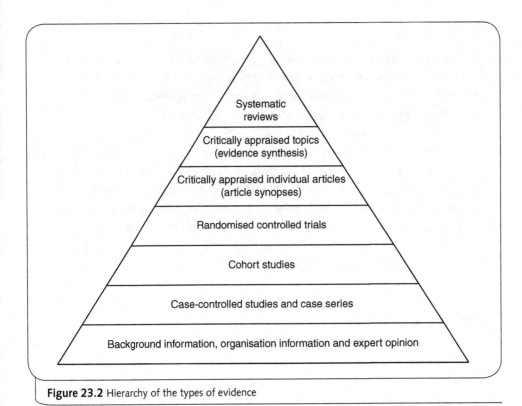

Figure 23.2 Hierarchy of the types of evidence

business practice, such as recruiting, hiring or other selection decision-making. In all these circumstances, it is preferable to consider the best available evidence, critically appraised, that can be applied to the particular circumstances.

A range of biases may impact on decision-making processes. While it is beyond the scope of this chapter to provide detailed discussion of decision-making biases, there are two to which managers should pay attention. The first is **group think**, which occurs when an individual feels pressure (real or imagined) to agree with the group. Group think is dangerous because the group can be lulled into believing that because many think this way, it is the best way. The second is **sunk-cost bias**, which means that a wrong decision was made based on what had previously been invested, be it financial resources or time. It is sunk-cost because resources have already been expended which are unlikely to be recovered, so it becomes irrelevant for the next decision.

think
at occurs when an individual
ssure (real or imagined) to
th the group

st bias
at occurs when an individual
makes a decision based on
ey have previously invested

Summary

- Managers need to look for evidence when they or others plan a significant change in the workplace.
- Evidence is acquired from four areas: scientific research findings; stakeholders' values and concerns; organisational data, facts and figures; and professional experience and judgement.
- The quality of the different forms of evidence must be taken into account by examining aspects such as the source, method, context and analyses used.
- The relevant evidence should be used appropriately in decision-making strategies.

Reflective questions

1 Why do you think there is debate in the field about the importance of randomised controlled trials as compared to expert opinion as evidence?

2 Even scientifically rigorous studies can often be contradictory, leading to apparently opposite results. How might you deal with conflicting evidence?

3 How might you justify your selection of experts when you call on people in your personal network to give you advice?

4 To what extent does your own experience with an issue or topic form part of the evidence base?

5 Many scholarly studies include sophisticated statistical analyses to reach their conclusions. How might you deal with this evidence when you do not understand the statistics used?

Self-analysis question

Lynn McVey (2013, para. 10), chief executive officer and president of Meadowlands Hospital Medical Center, in New Jersey, claims, 'When a [doctor] tells me, "The nurses on the 3rd floor suck." Immediately I know he hasn't yet been baptized by evidence-based management. After I drill down his statement several layers, I ultimately discover he could not find nurse Janie Friday morning when he needed her. I then explain I can actually help him when he uses evidence-based statements, but nobody can do anything with, "The nurses on the 3rd floor suck"'. How does this relate to your understanding of evidence-based management in healthcare?

References

Adily, A. & Ward, J. E. (2005). Enhancing evidence-based practice in population health: Staff views, barriers and strategies for change. *Australian Health Review, 29*(4), 469–477. doi: 10.1071/AH050469

Axelsson, R. (1998). Towards an evidence based health care management. *International Journal of Health Planning and Management, 13*(4), 307–317. doi: 10.1002/(SICI)1099 -1751(199810/12)13:4<307::AID-HPM525>3.0.CO;2-V

Barends, E., Rousseau, D. M. & Briner, R. B. (2014). *Evidence-based management: The basic principles.* Amsterdam, Netherlands: Center for Evidence-Based Management.

Black, N. (2001). Evidence based policy: Proceed with care. *British Medical Journal, 323*(7307), 275. doi: 10.1136/bmj.323.7307.275

Finkler, S. A. & Ward, D. M. (2003). The case for the use of evidence-based management research for the control of hospital costs. *Health Care Management Review, 28*(4), 348–365. doi: 10.1097/00004010-200310000-00007

Hemsley-Brown, J. V. & Sharp, C. (2003). The use of research to improve professional practice: A systematic review of the literature. *Oxford Review of Education, 29*(4), 449–470. doi: 10.1080/0305498032000153025

Lavis, J. N., Davies, H., Oxman, A., Denis, J., Golden-Biddle, K. & Ferlie, E. (2005). Towards systematic reviews that inform health care management and policy-making. *Journal of Health Services Research & Policy, 10*(1), 35–48. doi: 10.1258/1355819054308549

Liang, Z., Howard, P. F., Leggat, S. G. & Murphy, G. (2012). A framework to improve evidence-informed decision-making in health service management. *Australian Health Review, 36*(3), 284–289. doi: 10.1071/AH11051

Lomas, J., Culyer, T., McCutcheon, C., McAuley, L. & Law, S. (2005). *Conceptualizing and combining evidence for health system guidance*. Ottawa, Canada: Canadian Health Services Research Foundation.

McVey, L. (2013). *Lessons from Beyonce: Hospitals need evidence-based management*. Retrieved from http://www.hospitalimpact.org/index.php/2013/08/19/beyonce_hospitals_need_evidence_based_ma

Mitton, C. & Patten, S. (2004). Evidence-based priority-setting: What do the decision-makers think? *Journal of Health Services Research & Policy, 9*(3), 146–152. doi: 10.1258/1355819041403240

National Institute for Health and Clinical Excellence. (2009). *The guidelines manual*. London, United Kingdom: Author.

Nutley, S. & Davies, H. T. O. (2000). Making a reality of evidence-based practice: Some lessons from the diffusion of innovation. *Public Money and Management*, (October–December), 35–42. doi: 10.1111/1467-9302.00234

O'Halloran, P., Porter, S. & Blackwood, B. (2010). Evidence based practice and its critics: What is a nurse manager to do? *Journal of Nursing Management, 18*(1), 90–95. doi: 10.1111/j.1365-2834.2009.01068.x

Pfeffer, J. & Sutton, R. I. (2006). Evidence-based management. *Harvard Business Review, 84*(1), 62–74.

Rousseau, D. M. (2006). Is there such a thing as 'evidence-based management'? *Academy of Management Review, 31*(2), 256–269. doi: 10.5465/AMR.2006.20208679

Shortell, S. M. (2006). Promoting evidence-based management. *Frontiers of Health Services Management, 22*(3), 23–29.

Walshe, K. & Rundall, T. G. (2001). Evidence-based management: From theory to practice in health care. *Milbank Quarterly, 79*(3): 429–457. doi: 10.1111/1468-0009.00214

24

Successfully managing conflict

Gary E. Day

Learning objectives

How do I:

- recognise the types and origins of conflict in my workplace?
- determine which is the best approach to managing conflict?
- develop my skills to be more successful in managing conflict within my workplace?
- analyse conflict situations and design an appropriate conflict management strategy?

Introduction

Dana (2001) claims that over 50 per cent of voluntary resignations from organisations can be directly attributed to unresolved conflict. Managers need to understand that conflict does not resolve itself; rather, it tends to gather intensity and energy. Gupta, Boyd and Kuzmits (2011, p. 395) have found that 'employees spend as much as 42 percent of their time engaging in or attempting to resolve conflict and 20 percent of managers' time is taken up by conflict-related issues'. Managing conflict is one of the prime responsibilities of managing staff and teams. It is critical, then, that managers are able to detect initial symptoms of conflict and adopt the most effective behaviours to resolve it (Vivar, 2006). In this chapter, different types and origins of conflict are discussed, as well as approaches to managing and resolving conflict.

Types and origins of conflict

Conflict is best defined as unresolved, protracted disagreements between individuals or groups that negatively impact on staff, organisations and working relationships. Conflict between team members and workgroups can be highly disruptive, leading to poor team outcomes and lack of team cohesion and trust. At its worst, conflict can lead to staff turnover (Dana, 2001); absenteeism (Vivar, 2006); negative patient outcomes, organisational loyalty and work commitment (Jehn, 1995; Jehn & Chatman, 1999); low staff morale (Iglesias & Vallejo, 2012); and a negative workplace culture.

There are numerous ways of defining the types, levels and origins of **conflict**. Gupta et al. (2011, p. 396) divide conflict into four areas: 'this recognises that entities (people, parties, groups) might become involved at different points in time in conflict, and that conflict can be between organizations (inter-organizational), groups (inter-group), individuals (inter-personal) and also with oneself (intra-personal)'. Malloch and Porter-O'Grady (2005) offer a different perspective on the origins of conflict by highlighting five primary causes, which are discussed below. Healthcare managers should be cognisant that any given conflict may originate in a combination of two or more of these causes.

ed, protracted disagreements
individuals or groups that
y impact on staff, organisations
king relationships

Relationship-based conflict

Relationship-based conflict involves a fundamental and intractable difference between two individuals and is probably most commonly seen between staff members within a department. The conflict might be quite heated or quietly insidious, and outwardly manifested through harassing, bullying, gossiping or denigrating behaviours.

Values-based conflict

This is seen in a clash of values between the organisation and the staff. Commonly, the organisation's 'lived' values will be at odds with its 'espoused' values, which causes friction with staff. Conflict concerning values can occur when staff feels the organisation is not true to its stated values or deviates from the reason they decided to join the organisation in the first place.

Interest-based conflict

Interest-based conflict may be seen when different professional groups in an organisation have conflict over a common issue. While there may be mutual commitment to the overall aims of the organisation, there remains conflict based on a shared interest. This might be seen, for example, if nursing and medical staff identify a different solution or approach to the same problem. The conflict arises when each professional group is unwilling to move from their stated or professional position.

Structure-driven conflict

Structure-driven conflict happens when inequities in the system cause discordance between groups. It may be a result of inadequate or unfair polices, rules, practices or protocols, or of contextual or organisational factors that inhibit cooperative professional relationships (Malloch & Porter-O'Grady, 2005). This may be seen in the unequal treatment of different groups within a health system or hospital, when one group receives favourable treatment in terms of services, pay increases or privileges over other clinical groups that are working under the same conditions in the same organisation.

Data-based conflict

Differences of opinion can be based on the use of data to support a given argument or point of view. Data may be used or manipulated to support a position, and this may be the source of conflict between groups. Alternatively, one group may be given more access to data than another group, or one group may not be given the same information to assist in a decision-making process.

Is all conflict bad?

While it is often thought that all conflict is inherently bad and that organisations should always be peaceful and harmonious, conflict can in fact be functional, as well as dysfunctional. Parkin (2009) claims that functional conflict focuses on disagreements about content and issues of tasks, with their surrounding decisions, opinions, ideas and points of view. In the right surroundings and with the correct management, functional conflict can actually energise groups and improve team performance. According to Parkin, functional conflict can increase understandings of alternative and multiple views, stimulate questioning and effective use of information, improve the evaluation of alternatives and enhance critical thinking.

Functional conflict can be achieved only when there is mutual respect for all parties involved, maturity among the team members and open and honest communication throughout – not when teams are in turmoil or are harbouring dysfunctional, unresolved conflict. Heifetz, Grashow and Linsky (2009) go further, by suggesting that managers can orchestrate functional conflict to achieve real, not superficial, harmony within teams.

Management of conflict

Most people dislike dealing with conflict or actively avoid it, because it is often heated, takes considerable emotional capital and is confronting. Human nature, through the 'fight or flight' mechanism, either encourages people to run away from conflict or, when cornered, compels them to fight.

Managers often avoid dealing with conflict, hoping that it will self-rectify, disappear or calm down. Unfortunately, failure to adequately address and actively manage conflict can lead to its escalation. Health managers need the correct tools and approaches to adequately address and manage conflict. Just as one type of fire extinguisher will not extinguish every type of fire, so one single approach to conflict resolution will not manage every type of conflict, and health managers need to develop a suite of methods to deal with the range of conflicts they will face. Lencioni (2005) claims that avoiding conflict is one of the main types of team dysfunctions, and that a fundamental requirement of managers is to address and deal with conflict.

Katz and Flynn (2013) suggest that leaders and employees give different definitions of conflict and have varying opinions on the effectiveness of the systems in place. There is also little awareness of the tools and strategies available to mitigate conflict in the workplace. It is therefore critical that health managers have open conversations with staff to discuss conflicts that detract from the team's performance and how to adequately address them.

Health managers need to be in a position to actively deal with or 'call' conflict when they see it. By making it explicit within the team that the manager will address conflict, the team effectively gives permission for conflict management and resolution to occur. Openly discussing conflict also demonstrates to the team that dealing with conflict is another management function, like staffing and budgeting. This active approach can take the mystique and stress out of managing conflict at a local level.

While it is important to consider the health manager's role in managing and dealing with conflict, there is also an important leadership function in conflict resolution, in preventing and dealing with conflict situations as they arise. Demonstrating strong leadership is as important as developing sound management strategies to deal with conflict. Healthcare workers at any level can demonstrate leadership and effect positive strategies to prevent conflict from occurring or escalating.

Showing leadership to prevent conflict

One afternoon, Susan, a second-year registered nurse, is sent from her usual ward to assist an understaffed medical unit. On arrival, she does a quick scan of her patients and notices that the family of one patient, Mrs Smith, is distressed and angry, beginning to use abusive language and to become verbally intimidating. Susan asks the family to sit down and tell her their concerns.

She discovers that Mrs Smith has been in pain and discomfort for several hours. The family has tried to alert the staff numerous times without success. The family's frustration has developed into anger at what they perceive to be a lack of care and attention.

Susan outlines a plan to Mrs Smith and her family, and then carries it out. She immediately organises the necessary pain relief, repositions her in bed and makes sure she is comfortable. After that, Susan ensures that she goes to Mrs Smith's bed and checks on her condition every hour.

Susan could have made the excuse that she was only relieving on the ward, or she could have referred the complaints to the nurse manager or had the family removed from the hospital for inappropriate conduct. However, by listening to the family, she has de-escalated what could have been a conflict situation between the patient's family and the ward staff and has re-established a rapport with the family and patient.

Approaches to conflict resolution

The seminal works of Kenneth Thomas and Ralph Kilmann and of M. Afzalur Rahim categorise approaches to conflict resolution based on a dynamic interaction between co-operation and assertiveness. Before being discussed in detail, Thomas and Kilmann's (1974) categorisations are listed below followed in brackets by the corresponding categorisations by Rahim (1983):

- avoiding (avoiding)
- compromising (compromising)
- collaborating (integrating)
- accommodating (obliging)
- competing (dominating).

When all parties in a conflict feel they have achieved a win–win result and that each party was treated with respect, and when none of the parties feels they have had to compromise their own position, the conflict has been adequately addressed. But when one group feels they have lost out in the negotiations, there is a high probability that the conflict will recur.

Unfortunately, managers often choose the wrong approach when attempting to manage conflict. Iglesias and Vallejo (2012) report that the most common style used by nurses is compromising, followed by competing, avoiding, accommodating and finally collaborating.

Avoiding

Unfortunately, avoidance is a common approach to conflict resolution. It should be noted that avoidance may be used as a deliberate stalling or delaying tactic; however, it usually ends in a lose–lose situation for the conflicted parties. Avoiding behaviours can be seen to reduce the importance of the issues causing the conflict, and they exhibit a low concern for others. Avoidance is failure to address the issues and look for suitable solutions.

Compromising

Conflict resolution strategies that rely on compromise result in an outcome where there is moderate concern for each party (Rahim, 2011). This approach relies on moderate levels of cooperation and assertiveness, focusing primarily on a mutually agreeable outcome that only partly satisfies the parties involved. While compromise appears to lead to conflict resolution, neither party gets exactly what it needs, and each has to give ground from its initial position. While relationships are left largely intact, parties may feel emotionally or professionally deflated. It could be argued that a compromised solution produces a lose–lose outcome for the parties.

Collaborating (integrating)

Collaborating strategies are used when parties have a high level of concern for each other. An outcome is reached that satisfies the needs of all parties, meaning a win–win result. Gupta et al. (2011, p. 397) say that the collaborative approach to conflict resolution is superior, as it 'promotes creative problem solving and fosters mutual respect and rapport'.

Accommodating (obliging)

Rahim (2011) says that obliging strategies demonstrate a low concern for oneself and a high concern for the other party. Obliging is often associated with self-effacing or timid behaviour by one party and results in unilateral possessions and unconditional promises. Accommodating produces lose–win outcomes in which one party has to give up ground or their position at the expense of the other. In some cases, accommodating resolution strategies are used to maintain harmony. Managers may adopt an accommodating (or avoiding) approach to reduce the immediate heat in the issue until a more appropriate long-term strategy is developed.

Competing (dominating)

Competing is characterised by one party imposing their will on others in an aggressive, threatening and power-driven approach (Rahim, 2011), which results in a win–lose outcome. It is worth noting that both competing and accommodating strategies may be heavily influenced by power dynamics in the workplace and used to either keep the peace or demonstrate superiority. Neither strategy achieves lasting resolution, as they divide rather than unite the parties.

Conflict resolution strategies

When considering an approach to conflict resolution, it is important to understand the influence of culture on the different parties. Leung (2008) claims that Asian cultures typically view conflict or disputes from a harmony perspective that is associated with collectivism, placing emphasis on the avoiding and accommodating approaches, whereas Western cultures often view conflict from the perspective of individualism, relying more heavily on the dominating approach.

A contemporary conflict resolution tool is called the evaporating cloud approach (Gupta et al., 2011; see Figure 24.1). It involves three key steps: identifying and displaying all elements of a conflict situation, identifying all underlying assumptions that cause the conflict to exist and developing solutions that invalidate one or more of the assumptions.

The Evaporating Cloud Framework, as described by Gupta et al. (2011), provides structure to a formal discussion to work through conflict situations. One of the issues with unresolved conflict is that the parties often do not want to or know how to go about resolving the matter. By using the framework to guide the discussion, a structured solution can be arrived at. The framework leads the parties through the following process: 'D and D¹ represent two opposing wants or actions … B and C represent the basic needs to be satisfied, and … A represents the common objective for which B and C are needed' (p. 399).

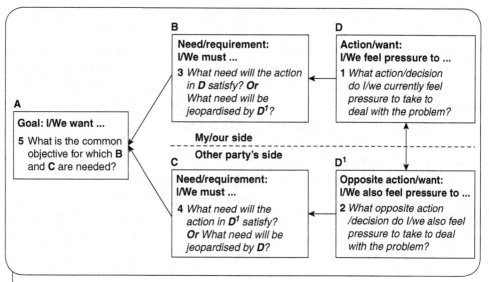

Figure 24.1 Evaporating Cloud Framework. Adapted from M. Gupta, L. Boyd & F. Kuzmits (2011). The evaporating cloud: A tool for resolving workplace conflict. *International Journal of Conflict Management*, 22(4), 394–412 (399, fig. 3). doi: 10.1108/10444061111171387.

In using the evaporating cloud approach, the manager must take an active role in bringing the conflicted parties together. The process requires each party to verbalise what they need or require and at the end of the process to identify common objectives. The process enables the manager to depersonalise the conflict by separating the issue from the personalities involved and by concentrating on the shared interests rather than the individual positions of each party. It also focuses the parties on possibilities, options and solutions. This approach is useful for interest-driven, structure-driven and data-based conflicts and stops the issue from becoming relationship-based.

Considerations when managing conflict

Managers must be able to step outside the conflict they are managing. If the manager is central to the conflict and a party in it, they should consider asking someone else to mediate and negotiate an outcome.

It is essential to collect all of the data and clarify all of the concerns and questions before developing a strategy to resolve the conflict. In relationship-based conflicts, it may be necessary to remove one or more of the parties for a time to bring the team back into equilibrium. The manager should also set out the ground rules and process by which the negotiation will take place. Each group must be heard by the other, and there should be mutual respect and honesty between the parties.

During negotiations it is important to concentrate on the similarities shared by the parties rather than on the differences between them; in many situations there will be more of the former than of the latter. Establishing the similarities between the parties changes the management of conflict into a more positive exercise, from which it is easier to work through the points of misalignment. This approach is particularly successful with interest-based and structure-driven conflict situations.

Managers need to look for small wins and then build on them. Having 'wins' in conflict negotiations enables all parties to see that progress is being made. Wins also develop trust between the parties and the manager.

Finally, after the conflict has been resolved, the manager can play an important role in refocusing the team and rebuilding trust within it. This is essential to re-establish robust, professional working relationships and team norms and to ensure the team is focused on its core business. The manager also needs to continually monitor the team's progress, so it does not slip back into the conflict situation.

Summary

- Conflict can be intrapersonal, interpersonal, intergroup and interorganisational.
- Conflict is a major cause of team dysfunction and the basis of negative team, organisational and patient outcomes. Managers need to take a leadership role in identifying conflict and constructively dealing with it.
- Preventing and de-escalating conflict is both a management and leadership function.
- Managers need to be able to draw from a range of approaches when dealing with conflict, including avoiding, compromising, collaborating, accommodating and competing, and must choose the correct approach for each conflict situation.
- Conflicts can be relationship-based, values-based, interest-based, structure-driven, data-based or a combination of these. Management of a conflict may therefore mean addressing more than one root cause.

Reflective questions

1 In what way is preventing or de-escalating conflict a leadership and a management function?

2 Why is it important to understand the different types of conflicts that occur in the workplace?

3 Based on your experience (both professionally and personally), what is your predominant style in dealing with conflict, and why?

4 Which among the types of conflicts discussed in this chapter would you find most difficult to manage, and why?

5 Can all conflict in the workplace be categorised as bad? Justify your answer.

Self-analysis questions

Consider the last time you were involved in a conflict situation (at home or at work). What sort of conflict was it, and how would you categorise it? What role did you play? What did the situation tell you about your leadership and management style? What did you learn from the situation?

References

Dana, D. (2001). *Conflict resolution: Mediation tools for everyday worklife*. New York, NY: McGraw-Hill.

Gupta, M., Boyd, L. & Kuzmits, F. (2011). The evaporating cloud: A tool for resolving workplace conflict. *International Journal of Conflict Management, 22*(4), 394–412. doi: 10.1108/10444061111171387

Heifetz, R., Grashow, A. & Linsky, M. (2009). *The practice of adaptive leadership: Tools and tactics for changing your organization and the world*. Boston, MA: Harvard Business.

Iglesias, M. E. L. & Vallejo, R. B. (2012). Conflict resolution styles in the nursing profession. *Contemporary Nurse, 43*(1), 73–80. doi: 10.5172/conu.2012.43.1.73

Jehn, K. (1995). A multimethod examination of the benefits and detriments of intragroup conflict. *Administrative Science Quarterly, 40*(2), 256–282.

Jehn, K. & Chatman, J. (1999). The influence of proportional and perceptual conflict composition on team performance. *International Journal of Conflict Management, 11,* 56–73. doi: 10.1108/eb022835

Katz, N. H. & Flynn, L. T. (2013). Understanding conflict management systems and strategies in the workplace: A pilot study. *Conflict Resolution Quarterly, 30*(4), 393–410. doi: 10.1002/crq.21070

Lencioni, P. (2005). *Overcoming the five dysfunctions of a team: A field guide for leaders, managers and facilitators.* San Francisco, CA: Jossey-Bass.

Leung, A. S. M. (2008). Interpersonal conflict and resolution strategies: An examination of Hong Kong employees. *Team Performance Management, 14*(3–4), 165–178. doi: 10.1108/13527590810883433

Malloch, K. & Porter-O'Grady, T. (2005). *The quantum leader: Applications for the new world of work.* Boston, MA: Jones & Bartlett.

Parkin, P. (2009). *Managing change in healthcare: Using action research.* London, United Kingdom: Sage.

Rahim, M. (1983). A measure of styles of handling interpersonal conflict. *Academy of Management Journal, 26,* 368–376. doi: 10.2307/255985

——. (2011). *Managing conflict in organizations* (4th ed.). Westport, CT: Transaction.

Thomas, K. W. & Kilmann, R. H. (1974). *Thomas-Kilmann conflict mode instrument.* Mountain View, CA: Xicom.

Vivar, C. G. (2006). Putting conflict management into practice: A nursing case study. *Journal of Nursing Management, 14,* 201–206. doi: 10.1111/j.1365-2934.2006.00554.x

25

Building positive workplace cultures

Gary E. Day and Kirsty Marles

Learning objectives

How do I:

- understand the key concepts associated with workplace cultures?
- identify the impacts of positive and negative workplace cultures on the functioning of an organisation, particularly in the area of patient safety and quality?
- identify different types of workplace cultures?
- understand the impact a health manager or leader can make on the culture of an organisation or department?
- build positive workplace cultures?

Introduction

Understanding, managing and building culture within a workplace are key responsibilities of leadership and management. This chapter outlines what workplace culture is, the impact of poor culture on an organisation and what managers can do to improve workplace culture.

Peter Drucker (as cited in Fernández-Aráoz, 2014, para. 2) once famously said, 'Culture eats strategy over breakfast'. This might seem implausible, because there is an expectation on healthcare managers to plan, set out, implement and then evaluate strategy. Drucker's point is that unless there is a positive culture in a workplace, seeing a strategy move to successful implementation and adoption is very difficult, sometimes impossible.

Definitions

Workplace culture (also called organisational or corporate culture) has been well defined in the literature. Culture has often been described as the particular beliefs or values of an organisation that distinguish it from other similar organisations. Local definitions include 'the way we do things around here' and 'our corporate DNA'. These descriptions of workplace culture hold true and describe the unique and often hard-to-define 'feel' of an organisation. Scott, Mannion, Davies and Marshall (2003, p. 925) describe workplace culture as 'a wide range of social phenomena, including an organization's customary dress, language, behaviour, beliefs, values, assumptions, symbols of status and authority, myths, ceremonies, and modes of deference and subversion; all of which help to define an organization's character and norms'.

> **ace culture**
> icular beliefs, norms or values
> ganisation that distinguish it
> er similar organisations

While we may talk about a single defining culture, the truth is that in larger organisations there may be several cultures or subcultures. Manley, Sanders, Cardiff and Webster (2011, p. 4) state that 'organisational culture in the past has been assumed to be singular and pervasive, monolithic and integrative, but all organisations have multiple cultures usually associated with different functional groupings or geographical locations'. Subcultures can be routinely seen in large hospitals, where individual departments may have cultures that are slightly different from but aligned with that of the organisation overall. Subcultures are commonplace and contribute to the overall feel, function and direction of an organisation.

On the other hand, countercultures – a form of organisational incivility – work at odds with the organisation and can be quite disruptive or destructive to its overall functioning. Andersson and Pearson (1999, p. 457) describe organisational incivility as 'low intensity deviant behaviour with ambiguous intent to harm the target, in violation of workplace norms for mutual respect'. One of the key responsibilities of a healthcare manager and leader is the cultivation of positive, productive workplace cultures. Schein (1992, as cited in Graber and Fitzpatrick, 2008, p. 194) says that one of the prime responsibilities of leaders is the management and creation of culture.

Typology of workplace cultures

While setting the culture of an organisation is the prime responsibility of the chief executive officer and the executive team, managers are expected to support and promote the desired culture. In order to understand what sort of culture prevails in an organisation, it is necessary to be able to categorise culture types. Categorisation allows the health manager to determine whether there is a need to redefine and change the culture in which they work. Self-aware health managers also need to ask themselves the following questions: How am I contributing to the culture in this organisation? If I don't like the present culture in the organisation, what am I going to do to change it?

The literature categorises culture in many ways, ranging from three-culture models (Westrum, 2004) to quadrant models (Quinn and Rohrbaugh, 1983; Wolniak, 2013) to cultures depicted as animal types (Line, 1999). A cultural framework that has been used widely in a number of industries, including health, is the **Competing Values Framework** (Cameron & Quinn, 2011; see Figure 25.1). It categorises four main cultural types and describes how each of these predominantly functions.

Competing Values Framew
A research-informed framework
describes four key culture types
hierarchy, adhocracy and marke
(Cameron & Quinn, 2011)

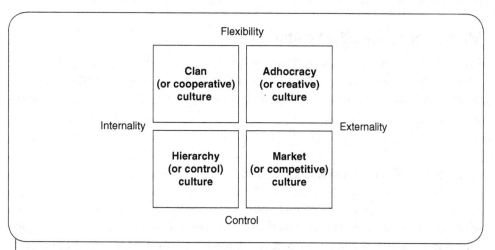

Figure 25.1 Competing Values Framework. Adapted from K. S. Cameron & R. E. Quinn (2011). *Diagnosing and changing organizational culture: Based on the Competing Values Framework* (3rd ed.). San Francisco, CA: Jossey-Bass.

The Competing Values Framework runs along two axes forming a cross. The vertical axis focuses on organisations that have flexibility and discretion through to those with high levels of stability and control. The horizontal axis highlights organisations with a strong internal focus and integration through to those that are externally focused and differentiated. Using these axes, Cameron and Quinn (2011) have categorised four predominant cultures, which are discussed below. Healthcare organisations may identify any one of these types. Each has its benefits and limitations depending on the type of organisation and the direction in which a healthcare facility is heading. Healthcare managers need to be aware of how they impact the culture and how they should support staff in their specific cultural type.

Clan (or cooperative) culture

This culture is characterised by a strong internal focus and flexibility. Organisations with a clan culture exhibit strong family-like, nurturing, cohesive and collaborative traits. Teams within such organisations work with a level of autonomy and self-direction.

Hierarchy (or control) culture

The hierarchy culture is characterised by an internal focus with strong control processes. Organisations with a hierarchy culture have defined hierarchies or bureaucracies, and command and control structures with a focus on policies, procedures, processes and protocols. They aim to be stable, consistent and dependable.

Adhocracy (or creative) culture

This culture is characterised by flexibility and an external focus. Organisations with an adhocracy culture promote rapid change, creativity and innovation, and they can be high-pressured, as they search for the next new product and aim to be 'ahead of the game'.

Market (or competitive) culture

The market culture has strong internal control and is externally focused. Organisations with a market culture focus on the external customer rather than the internal staff and can be very competitive, as they seek new customers and have an emphasis on customer service.

Measuring workplace culture

There are several ways in which to measure culture within organisations, from the subjective (having a general sense of what the organisation is like) to the objective (validated survey instruments and other qualitative approaches). Researchers have recently tried to understand the scope and range of quantitative instruments to measure workplace culture in healthcare organisations, and Scott et al. (2003) have identified 13 such instruments. However, while all of these examined employee views, perceptions and opinions of their working environments, only two considered the values and beliefs that might inform those views. The authors conclude that 'it is unlikely that any single instrument will ever provide a valid, reliable, and trustworthy assessment of an organisation's culture, and so a multi-method approach will always be desirable (p. 942)'. Organisations tend to use a range of approaches to measure their culture, including measurements focusing on staff and patients.

Organisational implications of different workplace cultures

The healthcare manager's role in proactively managing culture is critical to the overall functioning and success of the organisation. The culture of an organisation can impact positively on its operation, profitability and ability to work through challenging circumstances. While the culture of an organisation may seem a soft, non-core issue to some, the positive and negative impacts of culture can have substantial financial and operational implications.

Workplace culture can lead to positive outcomes in many areas of a health organisation. Along with improved teamwork, cohesion and employee involvement, and patient satisfaction (Gregory, Harris, Armenakis & Shook, 2009), lower patient mortality and improved nurses' health, job satisfaction, organisational commitment, emotional exhaustion and intention to stay have been recorded (Laschinger, Cummings, Wong & Grau, 2014). Positive culture also leads to more optimism among staff about the organisation's ability to meet future challenges, improved working relationships, greater accountability and efficiency, better cost management, more devolvement of management to clinicians, and facilities that are more strategically placed and patient-focused (Braithwaite et al., 2005). A reduction in medical errors has also been reported as a result of positive workplace culture (Stock, McFadden & Gowen, 2007), as have improved quality of care (Siourouni, Kastanioti, Tziallas & Niakas, 2012) and positive clinician attitudes in adopting new technology (Callen, Braithwaite & Westbrook, 2007).

However, negative workplace culture, the consequences of which are regularly discussed in healthcare reports and reviews, can manifest itself through unethical and possibly illegal activity (Casali & Day, 2010), higher staff turnover and lower staff morale and productivity (Siourouni et al., 2012). It can also result in a lower quality of care (Mid Staffordshire NHS Foundation Trust Public Inquiry, 2010) and higher levels of workplace bullying (O'Farrell & Nordstrom, 2013).

The effect of culture on the provision of care

A number of commissions of inquiry in Australia have shed light on the link between organisational culture and patient care. The Garling (2008, p. 3) Report closely examined the provision of acute care services in New South Wales public hospitals. The report recommended that 'a new culture needs to take root which sees the patient's needs as the paramount central concern of the system and not the convenience of the clinicians and administrators'.

These issues are not unique to Australian healthcare facilities, and similar culture and patient care issues have been raised in the United Kingdom. The Francis Inquiry, which began in 2010, highlighted poor clinical outcomes attributed to inappropriate culture within the Mid Staffordshire NHS Trust. Examples of poor culture leading to substandard and dangerous care can be seen in these excerpts from one of the inquiry's reports:

> [The chief executive of the trust] described the Trust's culture as being inwardly focused and complacent, resistant to change and accepting of poor standards. (Mid Staffordshire NHS Foundation Trust Public Inquiry, 2010, p. 22)

continued ›

continued ›

When [a patient's daughter] was asked to describe the nursing culture on Ward 11, she said, 'They were bullies. They bullied … the other staff and they bullied the patients. There was no word for it. … particularly during the two weeks that Mum was dying, effectively, they were calling out for the toilet and they would just walk by them.' (p. 45)

Management imperatives in building positive workplace cultures

The contemporary literature highlights several critical success factors for creating and maintaining positive workplace cultures, of which four are mentioned regularly: positive and supportive leadership, workplace learning, collaboration, and a focus on the patient or client.

Tyler and Parker (2011) claim that role-modelling of positive attitudes by managers and leaders promotes high levels of teamwork. Working collaboratively, rather than as a group of individuals, is essential for improved workplace culture. Laschinger et al. (2014) found that positive and supportive leadership empowers staff, lowers patient mortality, improves nurses' health and job satisfaction and reduces absenteeism, staff turnover and incivility. Additionally, managers who build emotional resilience in their workforce and team members create a healthier workplace culture, reducing absenteeism, improving teamwork and raising morale (Sergeant & Laws-Chapman, 2012). To ensure that staff feel engaged, managers need to be highly visible, provide feedback and coaching to employees and make sure that doctors are included as part of developing the culture (Hegland, Tarcon & Krueger, 2010).

The literature also emphasises the development of staff as a key component in developing positive workplace cultures. Tomlinson (2010), when reviewing an organisation that had a culture of high employee engagement, identified emphases on leadership, employee and organisational development, employee recognition and internal communication. Similarly, Goh, Chan and Kuziemsky (2013) suggest that to develop positive workplace cultures, managers need to foster collaborative learning among staff, to rid their organisation of a blame culture and to prioritise patient safety.

Finally, in an examination of the establishment of sustainable, healthy work environments through the standards set by the American Association of Critical-Care Nurses, Hickey (2010) claims that central to establishing and sustaining positive work environments are skilled communication from managers, true collaboration with staff, effective decision-making, appropriate staffing levels, meaningful staff recognition and authentic leadership.

Changing an organisation's culture

Changing organisational culture is not easy; it takes time and effort. There are often long-held, deeply taken-for-granted behaviours, attitudes and values that form the cultural reality of the organisation (Schedlitzki & Edwards, 2014). Any attempt to effect a change in culture requires relationships and leadership that through the use of systems embed shared values, beliefs and purpose in everyday practice.

Changing to a more desired culture takes concerted and persistent effort by all levels of management over an extended period. It probably took years for the culture to reach its current state, so any attempt to change it is likely to take as long. Building trust with the organisation's staff, creating new norms, rewarding new behaviours, establishing new customs and rituals: these all take time, effort and consistent messages from the executive.

When embarking on major cultural change, continued and continual communication from the executive to the staff should be implemented. The executive team needs to be adept at 'selling the vision', creating a level of excitement and anticipation about where the organisation is heading and making sure staff buy into this. Both formal and informal approaches may be used to ensure staff are aware of what is being proposed. Also, the espoused vision of the organisation must match the lived vision: the leadership and management should make sure that what they are actually doing is in line with what they say they are doing. For example, new staff should be selected and recruited in line with the organisation's values and beliefs. Failure in this area leads to staff confusion and lack of trust.

Managers should maintain or create rituals and customs that are unique to the organisation. This might be as simple as celebrating birthdays or anniversaries, and celebrating 'wins' in the organisation. The leadership need to be specific about the kinds of behaviours that are in line with the new culture and to be proactive about addressing behaviours that are not in line with the organisation's vision and values.

Leadership imperatives in building positive workplace cultures

Leadership and culture are often discussed within the organisational development literature as being mutually dependent. Many researchers believe that the most important role of a formal leader is to create and manage culture (Schedlitzki & Edwards, 2014). To understand workplace culture, to know what is a positive culture and to know how to develop a positive culture are essential for formal leaders in healthcare settings.

Leaders must be clear about the type of culture they want for their organisation. They must strategise and plan to create the conditions required to support a positive workplace culture. It is essential to deliver consistent messages through all the workplace mechanisms to contribute to building positive organisational culture.

Edgar Schein is recognised for his notable research into organisational development. In his text *Organizational culture and leadership* he describes primary and secondary embedding mechanisms (Schein, 2010). These are drawn on below to describe the role of the formal leader in building and embedding positive workplace cultures.

'What leaders pay attention to, measure, and control on a regular basis has a critical impact on organisational culture' (Schein, 2010, p. 237). This is a particularly powerful mechanism in highly regulated industries such as health and aged care, which have tight measures and controls set by regulators outside the organisation. In creating a positive workplace culture within these industries, the leader must be conscious of how compliance measures, such as legal, ethical, clinical and quality measures, impact on the culture within the organisation.

'How leaders allocate resources' influences workplace culture (Schein, 2010, p. 245). However, this needs to be considered within the context of the quantity of resources that are available and the financial risks involved. Carney (2011, p. 523) states that health leaders need to be able to 'place excellence at the forefront of care delivery, whilst at the same time being capable of managing the tensions that exist between cost effectiveness and the quality of care'. Decisions about how to allocate scarce resources are not value- or risk-free. It is the act of deciding how they are allocated that will reveal important aspects of an organisation's culture and attitude to risk.

'Deliberate role modeling, teaching, and coaching' contribute to dispersing a positive workplace culture (Schein, 2010, p. 246). Leaders must themselves be conscious of the behaviour they are modelling. Similarly, those who are promoted to supervisory positions or who are responsible for training or coaching others must be champions of the positive workplace culture. This is particularly important when inducting or orientating new staff.

'How leaders allocate rewards and status' can also influence workplace culture (Schein, 2010, p. 247). Both Tomlinson (2010) and Hickey (2010) say that there needs to be meaningful employee recognition that exemplifies and rewards the sorts of behaviours and outcomes the organisation is promoting. For example, if internal customer service is a priority within a values-based culture, then the reward and recognition program must reflect this.

The use of the performance appraisal process by managers and leaders acts as an important means for linking rewards and behavioural change to the type of culture and organisational values that they wish to promote. Schein (2004, p. 259) states that 'if the founders or leaders are trying to ensure that their values and assumptions will be learned, they must create a reward, promotion and status system that is consistent with those assumptions'. The system and process that are established in effect provide the means for evaluating the effectiveness of change on an ongoing basis.

'How leaders recruit, select, promote and excommunicate' has a significant impact on changing, reinforcing and promoting an organisation's culture (Schein, 2010, p. 249). In the first instance, managers and organisations need to look at recruiting practices. 'Creating cultures starts with hiring the right people and then helping them develop critical relationships' (Hegland et al., 2010, p. 57). Ideally, leaders should use their selection and recruitment process to recruit and advance those they perceive as having the values they want and to remove those they consider not to share these values. Schein (2004, p. 11) describes secondary embedding mechanisms that leaders must be conscious of in creating the desired organisational culture to include the following:

- Organizational design and structure
- Organizational systems and procedures
- Rites and rituals of the organization
- Design of physical space, facades, and buildings
- Stories about important events and people
- Formal statements of organizational philosophy, creeds, and charters.

Summary

- Workplace culture is formed by an organisation's unique behaviours, beliefs, values, ceremonies, experiences and history.
- A widely used approach to categorising workplace cultures is the Competing Values Framework, which identifies four main cultures: clan, hierarchy, adhocracy and market.
- A health manager's actions (or inactions) – their approach to organisational systems, policies and procedures, and customs and rituals – have a direct impact on the culture of a department or organisation.
- A health service manager can build a positive workplace culture through role-modelling, teaching and coaching, by ensuring new staff are recruited, selected and promoted according to the organisation's stated values, and through clear, transparent, regular and purposeful communication with staff.

Reflective questions

1 What is your role and function in developing the culture of your organisation or department?

2 What are some of the rituals, beliefs, values and assumptions in your organisation that differentiate it from others?

3 Look at the mission, vision and values statements of your organisation. How is the culture reflected in them?

4 Are the actions of your organisation in line with its stated vision, values and mission? What is the impact of the lived and the espoused values on the culture of your organisation?

5 Using the Competing Values Framework as a guide, identify the type of culture in your department or organisation.

Self-analysis questions

Consider the culture in your organisation or in an organisation you have worked in. What role do you or the healthcare manager play in contributing to that culture? What would you do personally to change or improve the culture you are in? What leadership and management traits would you have to call on to make this change or improvement?

References

Andersson, L. M. & Pearson, C. M. (1999). Tit for tat? The spiraling effect of incivility in the workplace. *Academy of Management Review, 24,* 452–471. doi: 10.2307/259136

Braithwaite, J., Westbrook, M. T., Iedema, R., Mallock, N. A., Forsyth, R. & Zhang, K. (2005). A tale of two hospitals: Assessing cultural landscapes and compositions. *Social Science and Medicine, 60,* 1149–1162. doi: 10.1016/j.socscimed.2004.06.046

Callen, J. L., Braithwaite, J. & Westbrook, J. I. (2007). Cultures in hospitals and their influence on attitudes to, and satisfaction with, the use of clinical information systems. *Social Science and Medicine, 65,* 635–639. doi: 10.1016/j.socscimed.2007.03.053

Cameron, K. S. & Quinn, R. E. (2011). *Diagnosing and changing organizational culture: Based on the Competing Values Framework* (3rd ed.). San Francisco, CA: Jossey-Bass.

Carney, M. (2011). Influence of organizational culture on quality healthcare delivery. *International Journal of Health Care Quality Assurance, 24*(7), 523–539. doi: 10.1108/09526861111160562

Casali, G. L. & Day, G. E. (2010). Treating an unhealthy organisational culture: The implications of the Bundaberg Hospital Inquiry for managerial ethical decision making. *Australian Health Review, 34*(1), 73–79. doi: 10.1071/AH09543

Fernández-Aráoz, C. (2014). Creating a culture of unconditional love. *Harvard Business Review,* (January 8). Available from https://hbr.org

Garling, P. (2008). *Final report of the Special Commission of Inquiry: Acute Care Services in NSW Public Hospitals; Overview.* Retrieved from New South Wales Department of Premier and Cabinet website: http://www.dpc.nsw.gov.au/__data/assets/pdf_file/0003/34194/Overview_-_Special_Commission_Of_Inquiry_Into_Acute_Care_Services_In_New_South_Wales_Public_Hospitals.pdf

Goh, S. C., Chan, C. & Kuziemsky, C. (2013). Teamwork, organizational learning, patient safety and job outcomes. *International Journal of Health Care Quality Assurance, 26*(5), 420–432. doi: 10.1108/IJHCQA-05-2011-0032

Graber, D. & Fitzpatrick, A. (2008). Establishing values-based leadership and values systems in health care organisations. *Journal of Health and Human Services Administration, 31*(2), 179–197.

Gregory, B. T., Harris, S. G., Armenakis, A. A. & Shook, C. L. (2009). Organizational culture and effectiveness: A study of values, attitudes, and organizational outcomes. *Journal of Business Research, 62*, 673–679. doi: 10.1016/j.jbusres.2008.05.021

Hegland, L. T., Tarcon, K. A. & Krueger, M. (2010). Building culture from the ground up in a new hospital. *Physician Executive, 36*(1), 56–60.

Hickey, P. A. (2010). Building a culture of excellence in Boston and beyond. *World Journal for Pediatric and Congental Heart Surgery, 1*(3), 314–320. doi: 10.1177/2150135110380240

Laschinger, H. K. S., Cummings, G. G., Wong, C. A. & Grau, A. L. (2014). Resonant leadership and workplace empowerment: The value of positive organizational cultures in reducing workplace incivility. *Nursing Economic$, 32*(1), 5–15.

Line, M. B. (1999). Types of organisational culture. *Library Management, 20*(2), 73–75. doi: 10.1108/01435129910251520

Manley, K., Sanders, K., Cardiff, S. & Webster, J. (2011). Effective workplace culture: The attributes, enabling factors and consequences of a new concept. *International Practice Development Journal, 1*(2), Article 1.

Mid Staffordshire NHS Foundation Trust Public Inquiry. (2010). *Independent inquiry into care provided by Mid Staffordshire NHS Foundation Trust, January 2005 – March 2009: Volume 1* (Chaired by R. Francis QC). Retrieved from National Archives website: http://webarchive.nationalarchives.gov.uk/20130107105354/http://www.dh.gov.uk/prod_consum_dh/groups/dh_digitalassets/@dh/@en/@ps/documents/digitalasset/dh_113447.pdf

O'Farrell, C. & Nordstrom, C. R. (2013). Workplace bullying: Examining self-monitoring and organizational culture. *Journal of Psychological Issues in Organizational Culture, 3*(4), 6–17. doi: 10.1002/jpoc.21079

Quinn, R. E. & Rohrbaugh, J. (1983). The spatial model of effectiveness criteria: Towards a competing values approach to organizational analysis. *Management Science, 29*(3), 363–377. doi: 10.1287/mnsc.29.3.363

Schedlitzki, D. & Edwards, G. (2014). *Studying leadership: Traditional and critical approaches.* London, United Kingdom: Sage.

Schein, E. (1992). *Organizational culture and leadership* (2nd ed.). San Francisco, CA: Jossey-Bass.

——. (2004). *Organizational culture and leadership.* (3rd ed.). San Francisco, CA: Jossey-Bass.

——. (2010). *Organizational culture and leadership* (4th ed.). Hoboken, NJ: Wiley.

Scott, T., Mannion, R., Davies, H. & Marshall, M. (2003). The quantitative measurement of organizational culture in health care: A review of available instruments. *Health Services Research, 38*(3), 923–945. doi: 10.1111/1475-6773.00154

Sergeant, J. & Laws-Chapman, C. (2012). Creating a positive workplace culture. *Nursing Management, 18*(9), 14–19. doi: 10.7748/nm2012.02.18.9.14.c8889

Siourouni, E., Kastanioti, C. K., Tziallas, D. & Niakas, D. (2012). Health care provider's organizational culture profile: A literature review. *Health Science Journal, 6*(2), 212–233. Available from http://hsj.gr

Stock, G. N., McFadden, K. L. & Gowen III, C. R. (2007). Organizational culture, critical success factors, and the reduction of hospital errors. *International Journal of Production Economics, 106*, 368–392. doi: 10.1016/j.ijpe.2006.07.005

Tomlinson, G. (2010). Building a culture of high employee engagement. *Strategic HR Review, 9*(3), 25–31. doi: 10.1108/14754391011040046

Tyler, D. A. & Parker, V. A. (2011). Nursing home culture, teamwork, and culture change. *Journal of Research in Nursing, 16*(1), 37–49. doi: 10.1177/1744987110366187

Westrum, R. (2004). A typology of organisational cultures. *Quality and Safety in Health Care, 13*(Suppl 2), ii22–ii27. doi: 10.1136/qshc.2003.009522

Wolniak, R. (2013). A typology of organizational cultures in terms of improvement of the quality management. *Manager, 17*, 7–21.

26

Leading and managing change

Gary E. Day and Elizabeth Shannon

Learning objectives

How do I:

- plan and lead change within a workplace?
- choose a relevant change management framework?
- plan the change process and the human management component of the change?
- develop my skills in leading organisational change?

Introduction

This chapter provides an introduction to the world of change management. Firstly, it sets out the case for change – why change management matters – then looks at the theories concerning individual and organisational change. Finally, the role of the professional change manager is discussed.

Definitions

For the purposes of this chapter, change is viewed from an organisational perspective. Organisational change is a systematic approach to reshaping organisations in line with their future goals, aims, vision and philosophy. By its very nature, organisational change needs to be actively managed to ensure the desired outcomes. Organisational change management requires the manager to take account of the range of internal and external forces that can augment, shape, hinder or derail organisational change. The internal forces can include organisational objectives, work standards, personnel, staff expertise and profit, while the external forces can include economic, technical, political, governmental and sociocultural factors, as well as the operating environment (Pathak, 2010).

The manager should realise that any number of these internal and external forces may need to be actively managed simultaneously to ensure a successful outcome.

Management of change

The Change Management Institute identifies 13 knowledge areas that change managers need to understand (Change Management Institute, 2013, p. 16); these are listed below:

1   A Change Management Perspective – The overarching theories behind change
2   Defining Change – What is the change?
3   Managing Benefits – Ensuring change delivers value
4   Stakeholder Strategy – How to identify and engage stakeholders
5   Communication and Engagement – Communicating change effectively
6   Change Impact – Assessing change impact and progress
7   Change Readiness, Planning and Measurement – Preparing for change
8   Project Management – Change initiatives, projects and programmes
9   Education and Learning Support – Training and supporting change
10 Facilitation – Facilitating group events through a change process
11 Sustaining Systems – Ensuring that change is sustained
12 Personal and Professional Management – Developing personal effectiveness
13 Organizational Considerations – Critical elements of awareness for professional Change Managers

As part of the accreditation of professional change managers, the Change Management Institute (2012) also identifies 11 competencies that managers of **organisational change** need to display. These are described as change management skills, but change managers *lead* change, so the skills have clear links to those outlined in the Health LEADS Framework (Health Workforce Australia, 2013), as described below.

The **change management** competency that relates to the 'Leads Self' element of LEADS is *self-management*. Change managers must be self-managers. Self-management requires resilience, flexibility and emotional intelligence; it means taking on personal responsibility for the change management effort.

sational change
atic approach to reshaping
tions in line with their future
ms, vision and philosophy

management
ured and intentional approach
ge that may involve a detailed
broader but deliberately
approach

The competencies that relate to 'Engages Others' are *influencing others and communicating effectively*. Change managers influence others through relationship-building, networking and writing *communications*. They also *facilitate meetings* to reach agreement between key stakeholders to the change.

Change managers 'Achieve Outcomes' through skilfully applying *project management* knowledge, tools and techniques. They structure and *facilitate change* to provide the required outcomes. They undertake *impact assessments* to gather evidence that these outcomes have been achieved.

Change managers 'Drive Innovation' as part of their job and in themselves, through continuous *professional development*. They acquire *specialist expertise in communications*, and in *training*, learning and development. They coach others to share their skill set and promote change management as a profession. Strategic thinking, analytical thinking and a holistic perspective are key intellectual skills for change managers.

In order to facilitate change, change managers must understand the environment in which the change will occur and 'Shape Systems': what kind of organisational culture exists, and how ready is the organisation for change? Change managers need to apply their *thinking and judgement* to the principles of change within their environment (Change Management Institute, 2012).

Kotter (2012) suggests that individuals and organisations will continue to see increasing rates of change into the 21st century. An environment of constant change will make an adaptive organisational culture and 'teamwork at the top' essential requirements. People who can communicate vision will be required to lead flatter hierarchies of semi-autonomous teams. Greater and more skilful use of change management methodologies is essential in order to achieve personal and organisational benefit.

People and change

Actively managing the change process requires a focus on the human element of change. The negative consequences of poor change management can be seen in time and cost blowouts, false starts and failure to complete projects, as well as adverse health outcomes in staff. The literature is clear that failing to manage change effectively can have serious psychological and physiological impacts on staff, and human resource implications such as increased staff turnover and absenteeism. For example, the human impact of a poorly managed change process can lead to deterioration in employee health and wellbeing, resulting in an early exit from the labour market (Vahtera & Virtanen, 2013). Some studies have reported employees experiencing disrupted sleep, depression, weight gain and high blood pressure (Ferrie, Shipley, Marmot, Stansfeld & Smith, 1998). Other negative impacts reported include an increased number of sick days (Hansson, Vingard, Arnetz & Anderzen, 2008) and a significant increase in staff receiving stress-related medication (Dahl, 2011). In the context of health services, poorly managed change can also have negative patient outcomes, including increased length of stay and mortality rates (Timmers, Hulstaert & Leenen, 2014).

To ensure that change is truly successful, change and **transition** are required (Bridges & Mitchell, 2000). Therefore, the manager needs to be cognisant of the two elements: change is the external process that impacts on the individual staff member (most organisational change could be considered external, such as policy, practice and structure), while transition is internal – the personal, emotional and mental process the staff member goes through to accept and adapt

Transition
The personal, emotional and me[ntal]
process a person goes through t[o accept]
and adapt to a change

to the change. Through transition, the staff member accepts the change as personally 'safe' and perceives a personal and organisational benefit to modifying their practice or behaviour. Managers must fully engage their staff and assist them to transition from one process to another, working through all their employees' issues and concerns with them so they embrace the proposed change.

When staff experience a series of change cycles and go through the psychological stages of change repeatedly, it can lead to **change fatigue** (Bernerth, Walker & Harris, 2011). Upcoming change can also lead to **anticipatory grief** (Kubler-Ross & Kessler, 2005), associated with the future stress of change, particularly if previous change has been distressing to the individual. The prospect of a new round of change will stimulate grieving for the loss of the current situation, even before the change has occurred. The sense of loss can be due to perceived or actual loss, of status, influence, power, work history or emotional investment in a project, and to changes in the team and the prevailing culture. A clear change management plan provides a structured approach that may give some comfort to staff damaged by poorly managed processes in the past.

fatigue
, apathy or passive resignation
duals or teams as a result
and continual organisational

atory grief
g that occurs before an
g or known loss

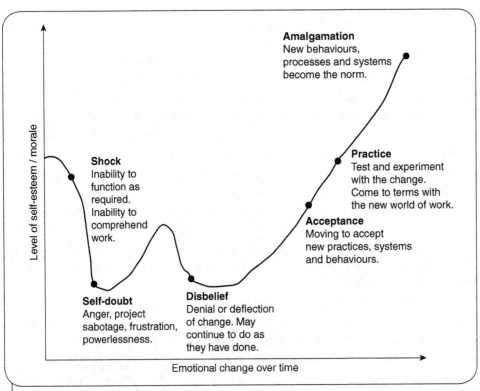

Figure 26.1 The stages of grief / change model

In many ways, particularly during large-scale change, managers need to take staff through a process similar to the grief process described by Kubler-Ross and Kessler (2005). The stages of grief model has been adopted over the years to be used in the change process, as many staff feel similar levels of loss, grief and distress during organisational change. Managers should expect staff to go through a range of psychological stages until the change is fully integrated, including shock, disbelief, doubt in their own abilities, acceptance that the change is happening and finally practice and amalgamation. During this process, the individual and the team will experience self-esteem and morale highs and lows as they realign themselves to the new world of work (see Figure 26.1).

Frameworks for change management

Lewin's field theory and force field analysis

The earliest popular framework of change, developed by Kurt Lewin (1947), is the simplest. It is because of its simplicity that it is a useful starting point. Lewin introduces the idea of the change process taking three steps: 'unfreezing' the original situation, 'moving', or introducing the change, and 'refreezing' the new situation in order to make the new standard permanent. He describes change as occurring through the interaction of social forces, some of which support change while others oppose it, within a 'field of action'.

However, while Lewin does describe the opposing forces as a kind of force field, he does not recommend that change managers undertake the kind of force field analysis that commonly bears his name today. Force field analysis lists the forces for change on one side of a page and the forces against change on the other side. It simply and graphically illustrates where arguments and stakeholders sit in relation to the change. A popular tool for change managers, it is sometimes criticised as being too simplistic to be effective (Burnes & Cooke, 2013).

Kotter's theory of organisational change

Fifty years later, John Kotter (2012) took Lewin's (1947) three steps and expanded them into eight steps for successful change, as outlined below. Kotter's work has been used extensively in a range of fields, including the health industry, to frame a structured approach to change management.

'Establishing a sense of urgency'

In Kotter's first step, the health manager must get enough staff to see there are challenges or opportunities that need to be addressed in the short term. Without an adequate sense of urgency, the manager will find it nearly impossible to achieve the necessary traction to start staff moving and taking the problem seriously. The manager may need to work through a range of staff emotions, such as complacency, anger, self-protection, pessimism, change fatigue, self-interest or reluctance. Each of these negative staff attitudes will need to be worked through to find the issues that unite the team to move forwards to address the problem in a coordinated fashion (Kotter, 2012, pp. 37–52).

'Creating the guiding coalition'
Creating the guiding coalition relies on the manager developing a cohesive team to help drive and guide the change. Central to this stage of the process is to bring together the right people with the right skills to do the right job. The manager's roles at this stage are to ensure good two-way communication, motivate staff and create a sense of excitement, share important information to developing trust, and establish team norms and protocols (Kotter, 2012, pp. 53–68).

'Developing a vision and strategy'
The manager's role in this crucial step is to help staff, and the guiding coalition, to see possibilities, what the future might be. The manager also needs to develop a solid strategy (plans and budgets) to underpin the future possibilities. They should ensure that they build on the sense of urgency and the reason staff accepted the change in the first place (Kotter, 2012, pp. 69–86).

'Communicating the change vision'
At this stage the manager needs to communicate a clear and unambiguous vision. Staff are likely to have a lot of questions by this point, and the manager should be proactively answering questions and communicating to maintain momentum. It is important to keep on message and ensure that the message is communicated in clear language that staff can understand. It may be necessary for the manager to repackage the same message in different forms for all staff to be clear about why the change is important (Kotter, 2012, pp. 87–104).

'Empowering employees for broad-based action'
The manager needs to remove barriers and allow staff to make the necessary changes. Barriers may be restrictive policies and protocols, outdated management practices, insecure managers and negative language regarding the change (Kotter, 2012, pp. 105–120). Kotter and Cohen (2002) suggest that at this stage, the manager should not try to do everything at once, instead breaking the solution down into smaller projects and allowing staff to act on these smaller, bite-sized objectives.

'Generating short-term wins'
At this stage, the manager should try to achieve a number of small wins. This will bolster the guiding coalition and demonstrate that the overall process can be successful.

Wins creates confidence in the change process and help build momentum. Each win must be appropriately celebrated and communicated. The manager needs to provide constructive feedback to staff. Each win stage also provides a perfect opportunity to evaluate how the project is proceeding and what learnings can be used in other elements of the process (Kotter, 2012, pp. 121–136).

'Consolidating gains and producing more change'

There is a danger of celebrating wins too early and stopping there. In this step, the manager needs to keep up the urgency and ensure that there is continued enthusiasm for the project. It is a good time to remind staff about how far they have come to date and how close the finished project is. Continuing to sell the vision is a positive way of encouraging staff to consider why they signed on in the first place and what is at stake if they finish the change prematurely (Kotter, 2012, pp. 137–152).

'Anchoring new approaches in the culture'

At this final stage, the manager is responsible for ensuring the project doesn't slip or the staff return to old habits, processes and approaches. New approaches and behaviours should be highlighted, recognised and rewarded. The manager needs to build the change into everyday work practices, including orientation of new staff and revised protocols and documentation. The completed change process must be communicated to staff and the improvements that have arisen from the new change emphasised (Kotter, 2012, pp. 153–166).

Involving staff in change

As the newly arrived director of clinical services in an organisation that had been through a significant number of senior staff changes over the preceding years, I identified a gap in the clinical capability that could have a negative impact on patient clinical outcomes. I tried to create a sense of urgency based on adverse patient outcomes, but I had trouble convincing the nursing staff to adopt a new clinical service to close this service gap.

After nearly six months of resistance to change I identified a group of nurses who were the opinion-makers and informal leaders in the organisation. All of them had been in the organisation a long time, and despite their not having any formal management role in the hospital, staff turned to them for guidance on organisational decisions. I decided to send the group on a study tour to several organisations running similar clinical services to those I hoped to introduce in our facility. When the nurses came back from the tour they owned the idea, and rather than resist change they became the change champions. I had found my guiding coalition and had a core of staff to communicate the vision to the other staff. The new service was up and running in four months. I wished I had recognised this group earlier.

ADKAR model

Hiatt (2006, p. 2) proposes a stepped model of change management which integrates individual change and organisational change: by changing individuals within an organisation, he claims, it is possible to change the organisation as a whole. Individual change requires the following qualities, from which the ADKAR mnemonic is taken:

- Awareness of the need to change
- Desire to support and participate in the change
- Knowledge of how to change
- Ability to implement required skills and behaviors
- Reinforcement to sustain the change

Awareness and desire take the individual away from the current way of doing things. Knowledge and ability guide them through the transition. Reinforcement takes the change securely into the future (Hiatt, 2006).

The amount of change management required in any circumstance is a function of the extent or scope of change required and the time in which the process must occur (Hiatt & Creasey, 2012). In other words, small-scale, incremental change requires less management than large-scale, radical change.

The amount of change management required will also depend on an organisation's past history. How has change been managed before? What outcomes have resulted from earlier change processes? If change has been managed poorly, it may be more difficult to engage people in the current change (Hiatt & Creasey, 2012).

Hiatt and Creasey (2012) describe change management as supported when certain individual roles and organisational conditions are fulfilled. In the first instance, communication about the change must be delivered by the appropriate individual. Corporate messages – the big picture – should be communicated by senior managers. Immediate supervisors should be available to discuss the personal impacts on individual staff. While senior managers have the authority to mandate and sponsor the change, immediate supervisors can help staff become more comfortable and less resistant to the change.

The change management process described by Hiatt and Creasey (2012) has clear links to project management methodology (Project Management Institute, 2008), and the ADKAR model has been recognised as the preferred change management model for project managers by the industry's international professional organisation, the Project Management Institute, as well as by the Australian Institute of Project Management. The model has also been criticised for this close alignment with project management by some change management proponents (Lawler & Sillitoe, 2010).

Summary

- Change management is an important emerging discipline.
- Managers must consider both the external process of change and the internal process of transition for change to be successful.
- Several change models can be applied to organisational change.
- Change managers must possess skills in areas such as education and training, communication and engagement, and facilitation, as well as a detailed understanding of change and change processes.

Reflective questions

1 What is the most recent change process you have experienced? Was it successful in achieving its goals? What kind of impact did it have on you and your team?

2 Can you describe what is meant by 'organisational change'?

3 What do you think is the relationship between individual and organisational change?

4 Have you ever experienced the six psychological stages of grief in relation to a change? How long did it take from start to finish?

5 Can you apply Lewin's (1947) three-step model of change to a recent change experience?

Self-analysis questions

Think about a time when you were intensely involved in a significant change – either leading or being affected by it. How effective was the change? Did it achieve what it set out to do? How did you feel about it? Which one of the change management frameworks presented in this chapter best describes that change process? If you knew then what you know now about change and change management, might you have acted any differently?

References

Bernerth, J. B., Walker, H. J. & Harris, S. G. (2011). Change fatigue: Development and initial validation of a new measure. *Work and Stress*, *25*(4), 321–337. doi: 10.1080/ 02678373.2011.634280

Bridges, W. & Mitchell, S. (2000). Leading transition: A new model for change. *Leader to Leader*, *16*(Spring), 30–36.

Burnes, B. & Cooke, B. (2013). Kurt Lewin's field theory: A review and re-evaluation. *International Journal of Management Reviews*, *15*, 408–425. doi: 10.1111/j.1468 -2370.2012.00348.x

Change Management Institute. (2012). *Change manager master level: Competency model.* Freemantle: Author.

——. (2013). *The effective change manager: The change management body of knowledge.* Freemantle: Vivid.

Dahl, M. S. (2011). Organizational change and employee stress. *Management Science*, 57(2), 240–256. doi: 10.1287/mnsc.1100.1273

Ferrie, J. E., Shipley, M. J., Marmot, M. G., Stansfeld, S. & Smith, G. D. (1998). The health effects of major organisational change and job insecurity. *Social Science and Medicine*, 46(2), 243–254. doi: 10.1016/S0277-9536(97)00158-5

Hansson, A.-S., Vingard, E., Arnetz, B. B. & Anderzen, I. (2008). Organizational change, health and sick leave among health care employees: A longitudinal study measuring stress markers, individuals and work site factors. *Work and Stress*, 22(1), 69–80. doi: 10.1080/02678370801996236

Health Workforce Australia. (2013). *Health LEADS Australia: The Australian health leadership framework*. Adelaide: Author.

Hiatt, J. M. (2006). *ADKAR: A model of change in business, government and our community*. Loveland, CO: Prosci Learning Center.

Hiatt, J. M. & Creasey, T. J. (2012). *Change management: The people side of change* (2nd ed.). Loveland, CO: Prosci Learning Center.

Kotter, J. P. (2012). *Leading change* (2nd ed.). Boston, MA: Harvard Business.

Kotter, J. P. & Cohen, D. S. (2002). *The heart of change*. Boston, MA: Harvard Business.

Kubler-Ross, E. & Kessler, D. (2005). *On grief and grieving: Finding the meaning of grief through the five stages of loss*. New York, NY: Scribner.

Lawler, A. & Sillitoe, J. (2010). Perspectives on instituting change management in large organisations. *Australian Universities Review*, 52(2), 43–48.

Lewin, K. (1947). Frontiers in group dynamics: Concept, method and reality in social science; Social equilibria and social change. *Human Relations*, 1(5), 5–41. doi: 10.1177/001872674700100103

Pathak, H. (2010). *Organisational change*. Delhi, India: Pearson Education.

Project Management Institute. (2008). *A guide to the project management body of knowledge* (4th ed.). Newtown Square, PA: Author.

Timmers, T. K., Hulstaert, P. F. & Leenen, L. P. H. (2014). Patient outcomes can be associated with organizational changes: A quality improvement case study. *Critical Care Nursing Quarterly*, 37(1), 125–134. doi: 10.1097/CNQ.0000000000000011

Vahtera, J. & Virtanen, M. (2013). The health effects of major organisational changes. *Occupational Environmental Medicine*, 70, 677–678. doi: 10.1136/oemed-2013-101635

27

Quality and service improvement

Martin Connor

Learning objectives

How do I:
- apply the principles of quality improvement in a healthcare setting?
- describe the key differences between a traditional hierarchical management approach and the quality improvement approach?
- use the eight main characteristics of the quality improvement approach to facilitate change in my organisation?
- ensure I structure my quality improvement change processes to engage the clinicians?
- determine the data needed to embark on a quality improvement process?

Introduction

Quality improvement has a specific history and tradition, a particular approach and a repertoire of techniques that have been repeatedly shown to be effective in delivering sustainable improvements in healthcare delivery (Chassin & O'Kane, 2010; Kurth, 2013; Shewhart, 1980; Warrier & McGillen, 2011). Along with a description of each of these characteristics, this chapter provides readers with a series of techniques associated with them, establishing a quality improvement framework within which problems can be best addressed.

Definitions

Despite the fact that it is in widespread use, there is no definitive account of what constitutes quality improvement. The language of quality improvement, however, is used widely in healthcare settings around the world. Many people use the term as a vague generalisation for 'trying to make things better', but this chapter argues that it is a specific term of art and science. **Quality improvement** offers a profoundly different approach to management in healthcare from that of the traditional hierarchical system. The traditional approach is based on the idea that managers know best and that organisations will best fulfil their missions if workers do what they are told. Managers who believe this respond to problems by seeking ever closer mechanisms of 'control' and 'accountability' to try to make people comply with management wishes. In the alternative view offered by quality improvement, the most important knowledge in the organisation is that held by the people who do the work. In healthcare, this is the clinicians themselves, and the clinical teams they work in on a daily basis.

In the hierarchical approach, it is management's job to distil strategy, issue instructions and create a system of compliance. In the quality improvement approach, it is management's job to enter a deep and authentic listening relationship with the clinicians and teams within the organisation, to remove the barriers to achieving high-quality outcomes and to ensure that the systems that support the work are efficient and effective enough for financial balance and the delivery of strategic goals.

Whereas traditional hierarchical management focuses on control and as a consequence tends to centralise power (State Services Authority, 2013), the quality improvement approach focuses on alignment and tends to decentralise power – ultimately to clinical teams. In many healthcare organisations, the traditional model of management is still dominant, and managers who adopt a quality improvement approach have to display considerable courage and resilience to achieve results in this quite different way of seeing the world.

History of quality improvement

Walter Shewhart and W. Edward Deming

In 1924, Walter Shewhart was working in the inspection engineering department of the Western Electric Company in the United States when he produced a single-page memorandum for his boss that contained two revolutionary ideas that remain at the heart of quality improvement thinking to this day. The first was that to improve the quality of a finished product, the organisation should stop taking an 'inspection' approach, which examined products that had already been made, and instead focus on the processes that went into production and ensure these were working properly to deliver the required outcomes. The second idea was that the organisation should apply statistical methods to look at data over time, studying variations in processes to identify where changes needed to be made to improve outcomes (Berwick, 1991; Best & Neuhauser, 2006).

These ideas come together to form one of the basic building blocks of quality improvement: that of **statistical process control**, which is defined as a philosophy, a strategy and a set of methods for ongoing improvement of systems, processes and outcomes. It is based on learning through data and founded on the theory of variation (Carey, 2003). In its simplest form, this idea states that there are two basic types of variations in processes. Common cause variation arises inevitably, because of the nature of the process under consideration, and needs to be accepted as a natural part of the management system. Special cause variation arises because of unusual factors bearing on the process (Kolesar, 1993; Mohammed, Cheng, Rouse & Marshall, 2001).

> **Statistical process control**
> A philosophy, a strategy and a s[...]
> methods for ongoing improvem[...]
> systems, processes and outcom[...]

Shewhart's work came to be known to the young physicist and mathematician W. Edward Deming in the 1920s, and Shewhart became a mentor to Deming in the 1920s and 1930s. Deming both internalised Shewhart's work and extended and developed it in the course of his career (see https://www.deming.org). He had a more philosophical outlook than Shewhart and developed the ideas of process management by providing a more comprehensive conceptual framework, with four main principles (Anderson, Rungtusanatham & Schroeder, 1994). Taken together, these create a particular way of seeing the world. The four principles are discussed below.

Work happens in systems

This is important in thinking about improving healthcare for two main reasons. Firstly, it warns against falling into the trap of blaming individuals when things go wrong – it is important to look first at the system they are operating within for causes of quality or safety problems. When thinking about changing systems, it is also crucial to continually remember the importance of teams rather than individuals. Secondly, the principle gives power to thinking about what is happening in the wider care system when trying to address a particular improvement.

Understanding variation is fundamental

One of Shewhart's basic principles of quality management is that there are two types of variations in a system, which have been introduced already: common cause variation and special cause variation (Berwick, 1991). The basic idea behind the principle is that the process with the smallest possible range of variation will be the most efficient.

It is essential to appreciate psychology

In healthcare improvement, appreciating psychology is of particular importance in developing leadership relationships necessary to gain commitment and permissions to design and sustain positive changes. To lead change effectively in a clinical environment, it is essential to acknowledge that almost all health professionals feel a vocational commitment to their work, have the interests of patients at heart and come to work wanting to do a good job. It is more often poor systems rather than bad people that cause problems with quality.

To act as a change agent, we must develop a theory of knowledge

In both individual change projects and leadership as a whole, it is important for leaders to continually reflect on how they are interpreting information and developing their view of the world, as individuals and within teams. Over time, one of the challenges of creating sustainable change is to grow the capability of teams to better grasp their situation and to have the confidence to experiment to improve it. This can be done only when people feel they understand their system, and to lead teams to this understanding requires the development of a theory of knowledge.

Brent James

After attending one of Deming's seminars in the late 1980s, Dr Brent James went on to lead the development of the quality improvement movement at Intermountain Healthcare in Utah. The Intermountain system was cited by President Barack Obama (2009, June 15) in 2009 as a place 'where high quality care is being provided at a cost well below average … excellence that we need to make the standard in our healthcare system', and James was named fourth among *Modern Healthcare*'s '50 most influential physician executives' (n.d.) in 2013. These results have been achieved through the systematic implementation of a quality improvement philosophy.

The seminal text that brought quality improvement into the mainstream of healthcare leadership was *Crossing the quality chasm*, published in 2001 (Institute of Medicine, 2001). It should be required reading for all practising and aspiring healthcare leaders.

Work happens in systems

An outpatients service has a chronic problem with access, and there is pressure from funders and the local hospital board to reduce waiting times for patients referred by local general practitioners. Without taking a systems view, managers might be tempted to simply increase capacity by putting on extra clinics for a time. This will give short-term benefits, but the problem is likely to recur and may get worse. With a quality improvement perspective, a deeper reform approach will look at what happens before and after the outpatients clinic, and it will include general practitioners and surgeons at the start of the process of designing the solution, so that the reasons for referral can be addressed, as well as the potential need for more operations after patients have been seen in outpatients.

Characteristics of quality and service improvement

There are eight characteristics of a quality improvement approach (Buttell, Hendler & Daley, 2008; Health Foundation, 2010). In healthcare, the method is patient-centred, professionally respectful, team-based, disciplined in project management, information-rich, evidence-based, process-focused and sustainable. From the literature and the author's experience, each of these is essential to delivering sustainable improvements at the level of the clinical team, organisation, region or nation.

Patient-centred

The term patient-centred in healthcare settings refers to the respect of and response to patient and consumer values, needs and preferences. The Australian Commission on Safety and Quality in Healthcare (2010, p. 7) lists the dimensions of patient-centred care as: 'respect, emotional support, physical comfort, information and communication, continuity and transition, care coordination, involvement of family and carers, and access to care'.

Many clinicians will quickly and rightly claim that their work is automatically patient-centred; after all, what do we think is going on in each clinic, ward or operating theatre? And on the one hand, this is certainly true. The sort of patient-centredness defined here, though, goes beyond the duty of the clinician to give the best care possible to the patient in front of them. It extends to whether patients feel valued, whether they have been involved in decisions about their care, whether they have had their preferences respected and whether the overall services (including all the steps that lead into the clinic room as well as those that continue beyond it) have been thought about from a patient's point of view.

Also of great importance in public health systems is the leadership role to organise care so that it is not only the patients who get seen whose interests are looked after, but also those patients who are not seen. In other words, while a doctor may have a paramount duty to the patient in the room, healthcare leaders also have to think about the populations that may need diagnoses or interventions and how best to organise services based on the disease in populations rather than just on those who are accessing services today. The technique associated with this characteristic involves leaders truly internalising in their own thinking a radically patient-centred outlook as one of the cornerstones for their quality improvement approach (Berwick, 2009).

Professionally respectful

There are many managers who behave as if they do not understand the value of clinical professionals, or allied health professionals; or, even if they do understand it, they do not behave appropriately. Almost all senior doctors, nurses and allied health professionals will have completed more than 15 years of education, training and experience to achieve their standing and will have a vocational commitment to their work (Elston, 1991).

Unless healthcare managers and leaders begin their work (before the first conversation has been held) from a position of essential respect for the authority and status of clinicians, they are both unlikely to succeed in working with individuals and teams in a healthcare environment and – worse – likely to do harm to either morale or patient outcomes. Paradoxically, professional respect is also the only approach through which an effective challenge can be made to clinical practice. This is because it is only when a healthcare leader is in a relationship of mutual respect and trust with senior clinicians that a challenge from 'outside' the professional circle will be accepted and given attention (Harrison & Ahmad, 2000). Without this relationship, any changes beyond the superficial level will be ignored, rejected or subverted.

The technique associated with this characteristic involves leaders understanding that professional respect should not be an attitude, but a discipline – and one that should be practised daily. Out of this discipline comes the ability to discern whether concerns being raised should lead to abandoning a plan or finding a different way forwards, or whether the time is simply wrong to make a change. Professional respect is essential to remaining open to the possibility that some unsuspected safety risk has been highlighted.

Team-based

Because of Deming's insistence on focusing on the system as a whole, quality improvement changes can be properly designed only on the basis of respectful engagement with the interprofessional care team. The simple reason for this is that even the simplest interactions between patients and the care system will involve at the very least managers plus doctor, or managers plus nurse or allied health professional. The more complex interventions, of course, involve multiple teams and particular sequences of care. It is simply not possible to get the information needed to design and implement a change without having reasonable representation in the process, and any changes made without this rounded perspective are highly likely to fail, or indeed be unsafe.

The technique associated with this characteristic involves leaders identifying at the beginning of a change process the key people who need to be involved in leading the change (McGrath et al., 2008). This may not always be the people in the most senior positions (though they will need to give their permissions), but it must include key representatives from each of the main professional groups, and administrators.

Disciplined in project management

There are several standard methodologies for project management internationally, perhaps the most widespread for major projects being PRINCE, which stands for PRojects IN Controlled Environments (United Kingdom Department of Finance and Personnel, 2014). While these can have a tendency to be overelaborate, it is essential to initiate quality improvement work within a formalised framework of project management discipline.

The techniques associated with this characteristic involve the following elements. Firstly, an unambiguous top-management sponsorship must be secured that includes an emotional commitment to the goals of the project. This is essential, since it is rare that a sustainable improvement can be delivered without some changes to resource allocation (in terms of money or time), investment, policy, procedures, leadership or structures. Solutions will often have all or many of these ingredients – it is the recipe that is unknown at the outset of the work. Top-management sponsorship is crucial because of the risk clinicians and clinical teams take in agreeing to embark on a change process, and healthcare leaders should be able to give a true and authentic agreement that the organisation shares the goals of the team and will do what is necessary to support the change.

Secondly, every change process should commence with a project initiation document containing a clear statement of who will be involved in the process (refer to the discussion above about whole-team involvement), what the goals of the project are and who the top-management sponsors are.

Finally, at the outset of the change, a clear statement of the criteria of success for the change should be clarified and agreed with the team concerned, expressed as **SMART** or **SMARTT** targets. These criteria can be changed or added to in the course of the project, but only by reference back to, and with the agreement of, the team concerned.

> **SMART**
> Targets that are Specific, Measu
> Achievable, Reasonable and Tim
> bound
>
> **SMARTT**
> Targets that are Specific, Measu
> Achievable, Realistic, Timely and
> Tangible

Information-rich

All information should be considered in terms of whether it is actionable: whether the data have the potential to change decisions made about how things are done. If they do not, the data should be disregarded – literally, not paid any attention. With this approach, all data becomes either 'so what?' data, which can ultimately elicit only a shrug, or 'aha!' data, which elicit a conversation about what should be done in response. 'Aha!' data promises changes in behaviour, resources or policies that could make a difference. These sorts of data are the basis for quality improvement, but healthcare organisations are often replete with 'so what?' data and have precious little 'aha!' data.

Therefore, recognising, defining and generating 'aha!' data are key technical challenges associated with quality improvement. Often, organisations and managers invest considerable time and capital in snapshot analyses – that is, analysis of a situation taken at a specific point in time and not repeatable. While this is better than having no information at all, it is categorically not the right sort of approach to deliver sustainable quality improvement. Instead, a key property of the information needed for quality improvement is that it is **time series data**, information built on a run chart whose x axis is a time period and whose y axis is the number associated with the process being improved. An example of a run chart is shown in Figure 27.1.

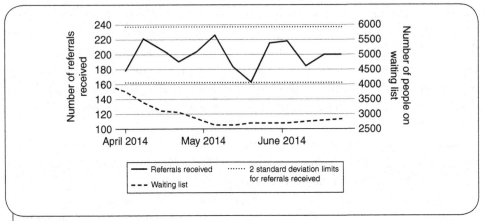

Figure 27.1 Run chart showing referrals received by an orthopaedic department. Gold Coast Hospital and Health Service, Management Information System.

Figure 27.1 is an example of the type of analysis that is powerful when planning to tackle outpatient waiting lists. In this chart, each data point along the x axis is a week. The left-hand y axis (plotted by the solid line) shows the number of orthopaedic referrals received into a district hospital service. The right-hand y axis (plotted by the dashed line) shows the overall number of patients who are waiting for a first outpatient appointment. The process demonstrated is that of a general practitioner deciding which patients out of a population of about 550 000 need to see a specialist orthopaedic surgeon or related service. The information retrieved from the time series demonstrates the power of the process: in order to provide the right capacity to meet the demand, there will need to be an average of 200 new clinic slots per week (referrals received), with a maximum of 230 and a minimum of 160 (2 standard deviation limits for referrals received).

The dotted lines on the chart represent two standard deviations from the mean, and because none of the weeks go above or below the lines, the process can be assumed to have had stable, normal variation, with no special cause variation in the time period. Information about the waiting list for the service does not reveal what capacity variation the department needs to plan for in order to manage without queues; only the weekly data on referrals reveals this.

The techniques associated with this characteristic involve leaders assessing the information to be used for quality improvement in terms of its frequency, quality, aggregation and time lag. Each of these aspects is discussed briefly below.

Frequency

The frequency of data-sampling should be directly related to the types of decisions that might be made, based on the process being managed. For example, monitoring vital signs of patients in an intensive care unit may require sampling many times an hour, and some of the processes associated with emergency departments may need to be sampled daily, or three times a day. On the other hand, most scheduled care processes can be sampled weekly, because the decisions associated with managing waiting lists are not made more frequently than weekly, and many safety and quality, coded activity and financial data items are available only monthly. For a quality improvement project, the frequency of the data required will depend on the nature of the process to be improved, and the frequency with which decisions can realistically be made related to the process.

Quality

Data quality is always an important issue and relates to the accuracy with which the data item represents the process to which it relates. For example, if 20 per cent of the referrals shown in Figure 27.1 were clinically inappropriate or duplicated, then the capacity requirement would be lower than if every single referral needed a clinic slot. People often think that there is no point in looking at such data frequently because they are of poor quality, but there is an important paradox about data quality which should be borne in mind: unless data are being used to make decisions, there will be no drive to improve their quality. The answer to this is to establish processes as if decisions will be made on the basis of the data (assemble the right group of people, agree the measures, get the data flowing, discuss the data at the right level of frequency) but also to focus effort in the early period on resolving the data quality issues. The answer from a quality improvement perspective to the assertion that data quality is poor is that now is the time to fix it.

Aggregation

Aggregation, which is defined as the 'combination of related categories, usually within a common branch of a hierarchy, to provide information at a broader level' (Organisation for Economic Co-operation and Development, 2013), is another key factor in quality information. Data to drive quality improvement should be as disaggregated as possible. Patient- and physician-level data should be sought where possible and de-identified as appropriate. Aggregated data mask variation and hide the real causes of problems.

Time lag

Finally, time lag is a major factor in how effective information is to drive change. This relates to the time between the period of data collection and the point at which the team analyses the data. Long time lags and high levels of aggregation can combine to create a great deal of 'so what?' data. A solid approach is to have the time lag being no longer than the frequency. Therefore, daily data should be viewable the next day, weekly data within a week, and so on.

Evidence-based

There are many thoughtful researchers and policy-makers troubled by the fact that real-world healthcare problems capable of being solved by reference to well-attested and high-quality evidence in the scientific literature form a very small percentage of the problems faced by the health system. There is a major problem in health policy (and in many other policy areas) of 'translation'. The problem has two components: firstly, the work that researchers do is often not relevant to practising leaders, so it doesn't get used (Bartunek, 2007); and secondly, the leaders who are effective at leading change and making improvements are too busy doing that work to write and publish.

The technique associated with this characteristic involves leaders making reasonable efforts to research solutions and explore the evidence available while acknowledging it will often disappoint. It has been estimated that 50 per cent of clinical practice has no high-quality evidence to support it; 30 per cent has some evidence, suggesting it might be more beneficial than doing nothing; and only about 20 per cent is supported by high-quality evidence.

Process-focused

The focus on process allows the quality improvement approach to avoid excessive emotion and focus on the practical workings of the system as it is, with a view to asking how it might be improved. Processes, their variations and their capacity to be standardised are the currency of all quality improvement initiatives (Mohammed, 2004; Shewhart, 1980).

The concept of becoming process-focused is utterly foundational to quality improvement, and all other considerations must ultimately find their expression in leaders' understanding of the processes involved and the variations expressed by them. Some people describe problems in terms of insufficient resources, but a quality improvement perspective reduces this to what process problem can be seen as a result of the claim of insufficient resources. Others look at behaviours as problems, but the quality improvement perspective reduces this to what process problem can be seen as a result of the claim that behaviours are not all they should be. The technique associated with this characteristic involves leaders constantly asking which clinical process is driving the outcome.

Sustainable

Sustainable change is different from a quick-fix change. The processes are distinct, and the change process for sustainability takes longer to establish, because the right levels of top-management support and local team commitment are prerequisites for success. This is true to the extent that wise quality improvement leaders will walk away from a problem unless the right conditions for change are in place.

Also, the work needed to identify and establish (often novel) information flows can take more time than the alternative, which is 'best efforts' based on existing data. This can include creating automated information environments in which data can flow on specific algorithms with programmed frequency to support and monitor higher levels of performance.

A direct positive corollary, however, is that sustainable high performance has a transformational impact on organisations or systems. It shows that 'it can be done', it undermines scepticism, it creates a world of learning that can transfer to other situations, and it engenders a spirit of confidence that better outcomes are possible.

The technique associated with this characteristic involves leaders sustaining focus on the agreed goals within the quality improvement project. It also involves their acting as buffers between any unrealistic expectations of results from the organisation that may distract from the improvement team doing the right thing when this runs counter to the alternative option, which may produce a quick return but be unsustainable.

Summary

- Quality improvement is the only management philosophy that combines the ethics of patient-centredness with the values of professional respect, the rigour of statistical process control and the discipline of project management.
- Quality improvement in a healthcare setting is a particular approach with a repertoire of techniques that have been repeatedly shown to be effective in delivering sustainable, positive change in healthcare delivery.
- The four process management principles are that work happens in systems, understanding variation is fundamental, it is essential to appreciate psychology, and to act as a change agent, we must develop a theory of knowledge
- Quality improvement has eight main characteristics; it is patient-centred, professionally respectful, team-based, disciplined in project management, information-rich, evidence-based, process-focused and sustainable.

Reflective questions

1 What does quality improvement mean in healthcare settings?
2 What were the two revolutionary ideas around quality improvement?
3 What is meant by statistical process control?
4 How does the traditional hierarchical management approach differ from Deming's and James's alternative quality improvement approach?
5 What does patient-centredness mean within a quality improvement framework?

Self-analysis questions

Which of the main elements of the quality improvement approach described in this chapter is most evident within your workplace? Thinking about yourself as a leader, which one of the principles would you implement to create sustainable improvements in your workplace or education setting?

References

50 most influential physician executives – 2013. (n.d.). *Modern Healthcare*. Retrieved from http://www.modernhealthcare.com

Anderson, J. C., Rungtusanatham, M. & Schroeder, R. G. (1994). A theory of quality management underlying the Deming management method. *Academy of Management Review, 19*(3), 472–509.

Australian Commission on Safety and Quality in Healthcare. (2010). *Patient-centred care: Improving quality and safety by focusing care on patients and consumers; Discussion paper*. Retrieved from http://www.safetyandquality.gov.au/wp-content/uploads/2012/01/PCCC -DiscussPaper.pdf

Bartunek, J. M. (2007). Academic-practitioner collaboration need not require joint or relevant research: Towards a relational scholarship of integration. *Academy of Management Journal, 50*(6), 1323–1333.

Berwick, D. M. (1991). Controlling variation in health care: A consultation from Walter Shewhart. *Medical Care, 29*(12), 1212–1225. doi: 10.1097/00005650-199112000-00004

———. (2009). What 'patient-centered' should mean: Confessions of an extremist. *Health Affairs, 28*(4), w555–w565. doi: 10.1377/hlthaff.28.4.w555

Best, M. & Neuhauser, D. (2006). Walter A Shewhart, 1924, and the Hawthorne factory. *Quality and Safety in Health Care, 15*(2), 142–143. doi: 10.1136/qshc.2006.018093

Buttell, P., Hendler, R. & Daley, J. (2008). Quality in healthcare: Concepts and practice. In K. H. Cohn & D. E. Hough (Eds), *The business of healthcare: Vol. 3. Improving systems of care* (pp. 61–95). Westport, CT: Praeger.

Carey, R. G. (2003). *Improving healthcare with control charts: Basic and advanced SPC methods and case studies.* Milwaukee, WI: ASQ Quality.

Chassin, M. R. & O'Kane, M. E. (2010). History of the quality improvement movement. In March of Dimes, *Toward improving the outcome of pregnancy III* (pp. 1–8). Retrieved from http://www.npic.org/MOD/MOD_TIOPIII_FinalManuscript.pdf

Elston, M. A. (1991). The politics of professional power: Medicine in a changing health service. In J. Gabe, M. Calnan & M. Bury (Eds), *The sociology of the health service* (pp. 58–88). London, United Kingdom: Routledge.

Harrison, S. & Ahmad, W. I. U. (2000). Medical autonomy and the UK state 1975–2025. *Sociology, 34*(1), 119–146. doi: 10.1177/S0038038500000092

Health Foundation. (2010). *Quality improvement made simple: What every board should know about healthcare quality improvement* [Information document]. Retrieved from http://www.health.org.uk/public/cms/75/76/313/594/Quality_improvement_made_simple.pdf?realName=uDCzzh.pdf

Institute of Medicine. (2001). *Crossing the quality chasm: A new health system for the 21st century.* Washington, DC: National Academies Press.

Kolesar, P. J. (1993). The relevance of research on statistical process control to the total quality movement. *Journal of Engineering and Technology Management, 10,* 317–338. doi: 10.1016/0923-4748(93)90027-G

Kurth, D. (2013). Introducing quality improvement. *Pediatric Anasthesia, 23,* 569–570. doi: 10.1111/pan.12167

McGrath, K. M., Bennett, D. M., Ben-Tovim, D. I., Boyages, S. C., Lyons, N. J. & O'Connell, T. J. (2008). Implementing and sustaining transformational change in health care: Lessons learnt about clinical process redesign. *Medical Journal Australia, 188*(6), 32–35.

Mohammed, M. A. (2004). Using statistical process control to improve the quality of health care. *Quality and Safety in Health Care, 13*(4), 243–245. doi: 10.1136/qshc.2004.011650

Mohammed, M. A., Cheng, K. K., Rouse, A. & Marshall, T. (2001). Bristol, Shipman, and clinical governance: Shewhart's forgotten lessons. *Lancet, 357*(9254), 463–467. doi: 10.1016/S0140-6736(00)04019-8

Obama, B. (2009, June 15). *Remarks by the president at the annual conference of the American Medical Association* [Press release]. Retrieved from http://www.whitehouse.gov/the-press-office/remarks-president-annual-conference-american-medical-association

Organisation for Economic Co-operation and Development. (2013). *Glossary of statistical terms: Aggregation.* Retrieved from http://stats.oecd.org/glossary/detail.asp?ID=68

Shewhart, W. A. (1980). *Economic control of quality manufactured product.* Milwaukee, WI: American Society for Quality.

State Services Authority. (2013). *Organisational design* [Information document]. Retrieved from
    http://www.ssa.vic.gov.au/images/stories/product_files/109_lpo_organisational_design.pdf
United Kingdom Department of Finance and Personnel. (2014). PRINCE: Management of
    projects in general. In *Northern Ireland guide to expenditure appraisal and evaluation* (10.4).
    Retrieved from http://www.dfpni.gov.uk/eag_prince_management_of_projects_in_general
Warrier, S. & McGillen, B. (2011). The evolution of quality improvement. *Medicine and Health
    Rhode Island*, 94(7), 211–212.

Part **6**

Shapes Systems

28

Workforce-planning

Ged Williams and Ben Archdall

Learning objectives

How do I:
- improve my skills in workforce-planning?
- understand the principles of workforce-planning?
- consider the Australian health workforce in relation to the structures, processes and trends in global health workforce-planning?
- take into account workforce issues in the Australian healthcare sector in workforce-planning?

Introduction

Workforce-planning in the healthcare system is becoming a politically charged issue in many countries due to a looming shortage of various health professional groups and the subsequent costs and liabilities to governments hoping to generate improvements and efficiencies. In 2010 the World Health Organization (2010) released *Models and tools for health workforce planning and projections* in an attempt to optimise the sharing of countries' experiences and best practices worldwide. Subsequently, both developing and developed nations are attempting to establish more sophisticated approaches to workforce-planning at national and regional levels (DalPoz, Gupta, Quain & Soucat, 2009; Dussault, Buchan, Sermeus & Padaiga, 2010; Lacerda, Caul Liraux, Spiegel & Neto, 2013).

The policy direction on health workforce sustainability set out in the World Health Organization's (2008) code on international recruitment of health workers recommends countries aim for workforce self-sufficiency with regard to workforce-planning. This requires a defined population base, such as a region or country, to facilitate the ongoing production of health workers at a volume sufficient to meet its own healthcare needs.

Australia has made policy statements about the desirability of health workforce self-sufficiency (Productivity Commission, 2005), but the evidence shows that it falls far short of this measure and continues to actively recruit health professionals from developing nations (Australian Institute of Health and Welfare, 2014c). There is need for wider discussion, involving not just health professionals but the entire community, about what is required of a health system, its workforce capacity and its budget (Buchan, Naccarella & Brooks, 2011). This chapter discusses the principles, practices and pitfalls of workforce-planning in the healthcare sector, giving particular emphasis to the Australian perspective.

Definitions

Workforce-planning is an ongoing business process aimed at ensuring the right people with the right skills are in the right place at the right time and at the right cost. A continuous cycle of workforce-planning ensures a timely and effective response to changes in an organisation's business objectives (Chief Information Office, 2013).

> **Workforce-planning**
> An ongoing business process air
> ensuring the right people with t
> skills are in the right place at the
> time and at the right cost

Workforce-planning is not a rigid linear process. Many considerations are needed to inform the plan, and yet the future is never static, so the plan must remain dynamic if it is to serve the purpose for which it has been designed. To this end the World Health Organization (2010, p. 3) notes, 'It is therefore critical that [workforce] plans include mechanisms for adjustment according to changing ongoing circumstances. Making projections is a policy-making necessity, but is also one that must be accompanied by regular re-evaluation and adjustment'.

Furthermore, health services are forever being asked to curtail costs, forcing workforce plans to find innovation and reform that can reduce ever-growing workforce costs. In 2005 the Australian Productivity Commission (2005, p. 9) noted that 'productivity enhanced improvements in health workforce arrangements are critical to ensuring a sustainable health care system, particularly given the constraints on government funding for health care'. The expectations on healthcare executives to provide efficient and effective workforce plans now and into the future are clear.

Australia's healthcare workforce

In the 2006 Australian census, it was estimated that 550 000 people worked in healthcare occupations and a further 300 000 worked in community care services such as aged care, social welfare and child protective services. Since 2001, healthcare occupations such as those listed in Table 28.1 had grown by an average of 22 per cent, while the national growth in jobs was around 6 per cent, making healthcare the fastest growing occupational group in the country. Furthermore, healthcare expenditure had grown from $89 billion in 2001–02 (8.4 per cent of gross domestic product) to $140 billion in 2011–12 (9.5 per cent of gross domestic product), with the highest cost burden being that of labour, at about 70 per cent of the total budget (Australian Institute of Health and Welfare, 2014b).

The many anomalies identified in the Australian health workforce profile possibly represent the consequences of poor workforce-planning. For instance, the number of overseas-born doctors and nurses in Australia has increased in recent years. In 2011, more than half of general practitioners (56 per cent) and just under half of specialists (47 per cent) were born overseas, up from 46 per cent and 37 per cent respectively in 2001. In comparison, less than a third (28 per cent) of the total employed population in 2011 were born overseas. In 2011, it was identified that one-third (33 per cent) of nurses in Australia were born overseas, compared with one-quarter (25 per cent) in 2001 (Australian Bureau of Statistics, 2013). Australia is a signatory to a number of global and regional codes of practice relating to the recruitment of internationally trained health professionals. Under the codes, Australia must refrain from actively recruiting health professionals from those countries that are experiencing a lack of trained health professionals (World Health Assembly, 2010).

Conversely, the globalisation of the nursing profession has facilitated more Australian nurses to move overseas to work (Australian Institute of Health and Welfare, 2013b). This may assist in balancing the impact of migration flows, although the current and historical data informing this analysis need to be reviewed for anomalies.

Some aspects of the allied health workforce also have idiosyncrasies that may contribute to adverse workforce outcomes for Australia. Mak, Clark, March and Gilbert (2013) performed a number of studies on the pharmacist workforce in Victoria and South Australia, finding a significant proportion of pharmacists were not in clinical roles. There was also a level of dissatisfaction related to various factors within the profession, which could affect future attrition, something that professional leaders and policy-makers need to address to avoid future adverse outcomes.

Significant efforts have been made to increase the number of graduating healthcare professionals in Australia in recent years. For instance, the number of student enrolments leading to provisional registration as a medical practitioner more than doubled from 7900 in 2001 to 16 900 in 2011, with more women enrolled than men. The proportion of medical student enrolments completed by international students increased from 15 per cent in 2001 to 18 per cent in 2011. There were 45 400 students enrolled in a general nursing course required for initial registration in 2011; this is twice the number of enrolments in 2001 (22 600). During this time, the proportion of

Table 28.1 Healthcare occupation totals in Australia, 2012

Occupation	Status/type breakdown	No. of status/type	% of all healthcare workers	Total no. in occupation	Changes as % of 2008 figures
Medical practitioners	Practising	81 910	89.5	91 504	+ 16.4
	Non-practising	9 594	10.5		
Nurses and midwives	Practising	290 144	86.8	334 078	+ 6.8
	Non-practising	43 934	13.2		
Allied health professionals	Psychologists	29 414	23.2	126 788	n/a
	Pharmacists	27 005	21.3		
	Physiotherapists	23 962	18.9		
	Occupational therapists	14 327	11.3		
	Medical radiation practitioners	13 312	10.5		
	Other	18 768	14.8		
Registered dental practitioners	Dentists	14 596	75.0	19 462	+ 26.0
	Therapists/hygienists	4 865	25.0		

Source: Australian Institute of Health and Welfare. (2013a). *Allied health workforce 2012* (National Health Workforce Series no. 5, Cat. no. HWL 51) [Report]. Retrieved from http://www.aihw.gov.au/WorkArea/DownloadAsset.aspx?id=60129544590; (2013b). *Nursing and midwifery workforce 2012* (National Health Workforce Series no. 6, Cat. no. HWL 52) [Report]. Retrieved from http://www.aihw.gov.au/WorkArea/DownloadAsset.aspx?id=60129545314; (2014a). *Dental workforce 2012* (National Health Workforce Series no.7, Cat. no. HWL 53) [Report]. Retrieved from http://www.aihw.gov.au/WorkArea/DownloadAsset.aspx?id=60129545958; (2014c). *Medical workforce 2012* (National Health Workforce Series no. 8, Cat. no. HWL 54) [Report]. Retrieved from http://www.aihw.gov.au/WorkArea/DownloadAsset.aspx?id=60129546076.

nursing students who were international students also increased, from 3 per cent in 2001 to 15 per cent in 2011 (Australian Bureau of Statistics, 2013).

Notwithstanding some improvement in health workforce data and statistics, the Australian government identified the need for a unifying, whole-of-country approach to health workforce-planning and advice and so commissioned the formation of Health Workforce Australia in 2009 to improve national-level health workforce-planning and -training arrangements. The first reports on **health workforce projections**, covering all medical practitioners and nurses, were released in April 2012 (Health Workforce Australia, 2012a), followed by a report focusing on medical specialty projections in November 2012 (Health Workforce Australia, 2012b).

> **workforce projection**
> st or estimate of what the
> e delivering health services may
> in the future

In the baseline (comparison) scenario, Australia is expected to have a shortage of 2701 physicians and 109 490 nurses by 2025. These Health Workforce Australia (2012a) projection models were based on scenario methods (see below). Despite these gloomy predictions, between 2011 and 2014 Australia experienced a relative oversupply of nurses. In South Australia, newly graduating nurses (37 per cent) and graduating midwives (15 per cent) were not able to gain entry positions to the Transition to Professional Practice Program, while in Tasmania it was reported that many graduates of nursing found themselves moving interstate or leaving the profession altogether, as there were simply not enough jobs for them all (Australian Nursing Federation, 2013).

The irony of this bizarre situation is not lost on Australian health system policy-advisors, who on the one hand state that the country cannot afford to support the current numbers of healthcare graduates from the nation's universities, and on the other must concede that all of them (and more) are needed if Australia is to achieve **health workforce sustainability** by 2025. The need for careful and considered workforce-planning has never been as important to the survival of Australia's healthcare system as we currently know it (Mason, 2013).

> **workforce sustainability**
> ance of the specific staff
> , nurses, allied health
> ›nals, specialist support staff)
> to meet the health needs of the
> ›a or population

Framework for workforce-planning

Organisations that do not follow a structured cyclical model of workforce-planning expose themselves to reactive workforce-planning activities such as international recruitment campaigns, which may become necessary as a response to acute increases in service demand or shortages in workforce supply. Many conceptual models have been developed to provide a framework through which workforce-planning can be understood and followed, and several are easy to find online (for example, see Advisory Group on Reform of Australian Government Administration, 2010; Chief Information Office, 2013; Department of Human Services, 2012).

The World Health Organization (2010) and several partners developed the HRH (Human Resources for Health) Action Framework (see Figure 28.1), which includes

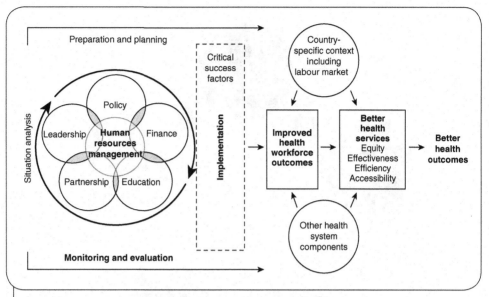

Figure 28.1 HRH Action Framework. World Health Organization. (2010). *Models and tools for health workforce planning and projections* (Human Resources for Health Observer, Issue no. 3, p. 4, fig. 1). Retrieved (29 January 2015) from http://whqlibdoc.who.int/ publications/2010/9789241599016_eng.pdf?ua=1. Reproduced with the permission of the publisher.

six action fields (human resources management systems, leadership, partnership, finance, education and policy) and an action cycle, which illustrates the phases to follow in applying the framework (situational analysis, planning, implementation, and monitoring and evaluation). To ensure a comprehensive approach to a given challenge, users of the framework are advised to address all action fields and phases of the action cycle, paying particular attention to the set of critical success factors. (For more detailed analysis and background information, see the HRH Action Framework website: http://www.capacityproject.org/framework.)

By adapting the four HRH Action Framework action cycle phases to create five cycle phases with minor modifications to language and emphasis, we have developed a simple action-planning or change management cycle involving an ongoing, sequenced process to facilitate the stakeholder engagement critical to successful planning outcomes (see Figure 28.2). Before being discussed in detail, the five action cycle phases are listed below followed in brackets by the corresponding HRH Action Framework phases:

- environmental scanning (situational analysis)
- scenario-based projections (planning)
- demand and supply gap analysis (planning)
- strategy development and implementation (implementation)
- monitoring and evaluation (monitoring and evaluation).

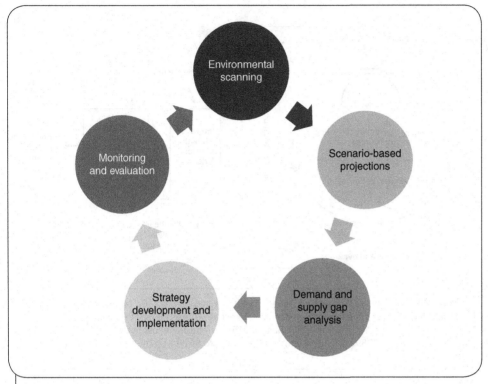

Figure 28.2 Action-planning cycle involving an ongoing, sequenced process

Environmental scanning

Also known as situational analysis, environmental scanning requires planners to understand the existing workforce and the factors (internal and external) that will affect the
organisation and its workforce needs in the future. Analysis of the existing workforce
should consider the following elements:

Demographics age, sex, length of tenure and location

Health context service, hospital, district, province and country

Human capital key people, core positions and job satisfaction

Critical role types new or emerging roles

Capability education and training, qualifications and general wellbeing

Capacity productivity, skill mix, role or service redesign.

Environmental scanning can be used in the development of assumptions used in future
workforce attrition and can inform staff development, recruitment or retention strategies.
A review of factors that will affect the workforce in the future should also consider those
listed below:

- organisational priorities
- service demands
- capital infrastructure
- technology

- fiscal constraints
- industrial awards, policy and legislative reform
- other strengths, weaknesses, opportunities and threats (a SWOT analysis).

These factors, associated assumptions and validated existing workforce data can form the metric drivers used in future scenario-based projections.

Scenario-based projections

This phase involves linking the results of environmental scanning to realistic scenario-based workforce projections for both the existing workforce and the supply chain. When deciding which factors to include as drivers in workforce projections, both their likelihood of occurring and their impact should be considered.

In their simplest form, workforce projections can be produced by linking the existing workforce profiles, head count and/or full-time equivalents with future service demands in a linear algorithm; for example, if demand increases by 50 per cent, so will the workforce. This demand-driven model is then adjusted based on further assumptions and scenarios identified in the environmental scanning process. Attrition and supply calculations are based on similar principles but use different drivers; for example, attrition can be driven by a number of workforce demographics, while supply can come from several different sources.

Health Workforce Australia (2012a) uses a projection model exploring three different categories of scenarios based on different policy options. These are innovation and reform, immigration, and other impact scenarios. In each scenario, Health Workforce Australia calculated the number of graduates from Australian medical and nursing education programs that would be required to achieve a balance between projected supply and demand. By using this model, Health Workforce Australia was able to conclude that among the many strategies that could be deployed, the best strategy to improve the gap between supply and demand was retention (Crettenden et al., 2014).

Demand and supply gap analysis

The objective of this phase is to provide a set of findings around which strategies and implementation plans can be based. Considering both head count and full-time equivalent variations, some critical gaps to explore and report may include the following:

- workforce versus budget
- attrition versus new graduates and external recruitment (including overseas)
- education pathways versus critical roles or specialties
- minimum number of staff required to operate a service (critical mass) versus service demand volume and ability to respond to peaks and troughs in demand.

Furthermore, the profile of the workforce projection requires articulation and refinement, especially in terms of occupation types, broad skill sets and specialist skill sets. This analysis can inform which education sector to target or partner with to fill the identified gap – for example, schools, universities or TAFEs.

Strategy development and implementation

Strategic workforce-planning outcomes should link with and support the organisation's objectives. Strategies may need to address the factors listed below:

- workforce development
- workforce re-engineering and substitution
- recruitment and retention
- service redesign, research and innovation
- industrial or policy reform.

All strategies will require consultation and must be documented, understandable, specific, measurable, affordable, accountable and timely (DUSMAAT). Documented and in an accessible place, preferably online, the strategy must be understandable, meaning that employees and all other stakeholders can read it and understand the intent. It should identify specific tasks and actions that are clear and linked directly to the goal; measures must also link to the goal and be easy to obtain, update and review to inform progress and performance. As with any business strategy, the plan must be affordable, or at the very least cost-neutral, and each action must have an accountable officer – that is, a specific person or position named as responsible for the completion of the task within a certain timeframe. Essentially, this is good change management theory applied to workforce-planning, and it relies on good leadership for execution.

Monitoring and evaluation

Once clear measures and accountabilities are documented, staff, unions, managers and other stakeholders can monitor and review progress. A shared level of ownership and transparency will allow dialogue on performance metrics as required. It is during this phase that adjustments can be made to respond to changing dynamics, needs and projections. This will contribute to improvements in future workforce-planning iterations and provide a basis to evaluate the return on investment.

Gold Coast University Hospital workforce-planning

Background

The Gold Coast University Hospital is a $1.75 billion, 750-bed tertiary level public healthcare facility collocated with Griffith University. It opened in 2013 to service a population of over 600 000 people located within the greater Gold Coast region. The hospital was built on a green-field site and replaced the 450-bed Gold Coast Hospital, which was decommissioned immediately following the transfer of beds and services to the new site. In 2009 the executive management team for the Gold Coast Health Service established a six-month workforce-planning project to assess the impact on the workforce of the Gold Coast University Hospital and associated services.

continued >

continued ›

Workforce-planning framework

The framework applied by the workforce-planning project involved environmental scanning of 270 services, workforce projections over a five-year commissioning period, workforce demand and supply gap analysis by clinical professionals and provision of strategic recommendations.

Findings

The execution of the workforce-planning activities was generally constrained by the scale and volume of services involved. New systems and processes were developed to improve service-planning coordination across clinical professions and identify erroneous baseline data.

The workforce-planning framework resulted in a projected workforce growth of 83 per cent during the proposed five-year commissioning period for the Gold Coast University Hospital. The demand drivers for this growth identified by the environmental scanning included a projected increase in clinical activity, associated with expanded and new services; the impact of new capital infrastructure, including the design and scale of the new facility; and an increase in patient acuity, resulting from new and expanded tertiary level services being offered.

The gap analysis between workforce demand and supply found that the existing supply chains within the regional education network would be inadequate to meet the projected growth for some clinical professions, such as nursing. This supply shortage could be compounded by retention issues related to an ageing workforce.

A number of recommendations were made and strategies implemented, including the development of partnerships with the local education sector to 'grow our own' workforce to meet the projected workforce demand.

Management and workforce-planning

Automation

An automated electronic tool able to receive data from numerous sources that inform assumptions and algorithms is critical in the workforce-planning process. Queensland Health, for example, developed the WorkMAPP system, which is used to manage and forecast workforce-planning data for the entire public health workforce across the state of Queensland – almost 80 000 people. Through this tool Queensland Health is able to constantly review various scenario projections and speculate on the possible outcomes from an almost infinite series of scenarios – provided the raw data sources are reliable and accurate.

Retention and satisfaction

As identified by the Health Workforce Australia (2012a) workforce modelling projections, retention is the most profitable investment to minimise workforce shortage.

In addressing retention and staff satisfaction needs, it is critical to identify strategies that have been proven to make a difference (Buykx, Humphreys, Wakerman & Pashen, 2010; Shacklock & Brunetto, 2012), as well as those that are most affordable, and then use a knowledgeable stakeholder group to decide how and when to implement such strategies.

Retention strategies may be organisation-wide, such as the establishment of employer of choice programs to improve reputation, or targeted, such as the Medical Rural Bonded Scholarship Schemes funded by the Australian government, which per student per year of study provide around $25 000, which is tax free and indexed annually, in exchange for a commitment to work six consecutive years in a rural or remote area of Australia (Department of Health, 2015). Such programs have been found to be effective in retaining medical graduates in rural areas of Canada and South Africa (Mathews, Heath, Neufeld & Samarasena, 2013; Reid & Conco, 1999).

Working smarter

To work smarter means to produce more outputs per unit of time – that is, to bring about the same or better outputs with the same or less workforce. This can be achieved through more training and skills development (to improve quality, efficiency, safety and breadth of work per employee), better work organisation (such as a reduction in time spent on administrative work and more time spent on clinical work) and technological progress (such as a reduction in operating time and a move to day surgery, brought about by more effective techniques).

Working longer

More working hours mean that workers are able to produce more outputs over a certain period of time (a day, a week or a year). For example, a general practitioner may be able to see three or four more patients in every additional hour of work tacked on to the current working day, which would create a marginal cost for the business but an improvement in productivity.

Workforce plasticity

Workforce plasticity means that the workforce is encouraged to constantly review the traditional boundaries of set roles and to be flexible in the tasks they are capable of doing. For example, an assistant in nursing can take on some of the tasks of the enrolled nurse, who can take on some of the tasks of the registered nurse, who may then pick up tasks of the doctor, who if necessary may complete tasks of all those employees if they have the capacity; for example, the doctor can clean the dressing trolley while the nurse assists the patient to dress and leave the room.

Summary

- Australia has around 600 000 healthcare workers and a rapidly growing demand for more healthcare. Current workforce-planning estimates suggest that the nation could have a shortage of 2700 doctors and 109 000 nurses by 2025.
- To ensure an efficient and effective health workforce, the right people with the right skills must be in the right place at the right time and at the right cost.
- Workforce-planning is a complex process requiring strong human resource management systems, leadership, partnership, finance, education and policy.
- An effective workforce-planning framework will involve a continuous action cycle of environmental scanning, scenario-based projections, demand and supply gap analysis, strategy development and implementation, and monitoring and evaluation.
- Strategies to increase the capacity and capability of the health workforce include automation of monitoring and evaluation systems, working smarter, working longer, working more flexibly and improving recruitment, retention and satisfaction in the workplace.

Reflective questions

1 What are the greatest threats to your organisation's workforce requirements in the next five years?

2 Conduct a brief environmental scan of your organisation and identify the five key measures you would want to know to inform a workforce plan.

3 If you were able to influence your organisation to improve its readiness for the future in terms of workforce, what two specific strategies would you recommend?

4 Consider your own profession. Based on what you have studied so far, conduct a strength, weakness, opportunity and threat (SWOT) analysis of the current workforce.

5 Consider the arguments for and against a deliberate strategy to recruit part of your workforce from a developing country.

Self-analysis questions

Imagine you are the chief executive officer or professional head of your organisation and you are required to maintain your current productivity but reduce costs by 5 per cent. Where in the workforce would the most likely opportunity for reductions be found, and why? Consider the steps you would take to lead such a change.

References

Advisory Group on Reform of Australian Government Administration. (2010). *Ahead of the game: Blueprint for the reform of Australian government administration* [Plan for reform]. Retrieved from http://apo.org.au/files/Resource/APS_reform_blueprint.pdf

Australian Bureau of Statistics. (2013). *Australian social trends, April 2013: Doctors and nurses* (Cat. no. 4102.0) [Report]. Retrieved from http://www.abs.gov.au/AUSSTATS/abs@.nsf/Loo kup/4102.0Main+Features20April+2013

Australian Institute of Health and Welfare. (2013a). *Allied health workforce 2012* (National Health Workforce Series no. 5., Cat. no. HWL 51) [Report]. Retrieved from http://www.aihw.gov.au/WorkArea/DownloadAsset.aspx?id=60129544590

——. (2013b). *Nursing and midwifery workforce 2012* (National Health Workforce Series no. 6., Cat. no. HWL 52) [Report]. Retrieved from http://www.aihw.gov.au/WorkArea/DownloadAsset.aspx?id=60129545314

——. (2014a). *Dental workforce 2012* (National Health Workforce Series no. 7, Cat. no. HWL 53) [Report]. Retrieved from http://www.aihw.gov.au/WorkArea/DownloadAsset.aspx?id=60129545958

——. (2014b). *Health expenditure Australia 2011–12: Analysis by sector* (Health and Welfare Expenditure Series no. 51, Cat. no. HWE 60). [Report]. Retrieved from http://www.aihw.gov.au/WorkArea/DownloadAsset.aspx?id=60129546631

——. (2014c). *Medical workforce 2012* (National Health Workforce Series no. 8, Cat. no. HWL 54) [Report]. Retrieved from http://www.aihw.gov.au/WorkArea/DownloadAsset.aspx?id=60129546076

Australian Nursing Federation. (2013). *Submission to the Health Workforce Australia consultation paper on Nursing Workforce Retention and Productivity.* Retrieved from http://anmf.org.au/documents/submissions/ANF_submission_HWA_Retention_Productivity_May_2013.pdf

Buchan, J. M., Naccarella, L. & Brooks, P. M. (2011). Is health workforce sustainability in Australia and New Zealand a realistic policy goal? *Australian Health Review, 35*(2), 152–155. doi: 10.1071/AH10897

Buykx, P., Humphreys, J., Wakerman, J. & Pashen, D. (2010). Systematic review of effective retention incentives for health workers in rural and remote areas: Towards evidence-based policy. *Australian Journal of Rural Health, 18*(3), 102–109. doi: 10.1111/j.1440-1584.2010.01139.x

Chief Information Office. (2013). *Queensland Government Enterprise Architecture: Queensland Government ICT Workforce planning methodology; Overview* (Version 1.1.1). Retrieved from http://www.qgcio.qld.gov.au/images/documents/QGCIO/Workforce/ICTworkforceplanningmethodology/QGICTWPM_Overview_v1.1.1_2013.pdf

Crettenden, I. F., McCarty, M. V., Fenech, B. J., Heywood, T., Taitz, M. C. & Tudman, S. (2014). How evidence-based workforce planning in Australia is informing policy development in the retention and distribution of the health workforce. *Human Resources for Health, 12*(7). doi: 10.1186/1478-4491-12-7

DalPoz, M. R., Gupta, N., Quain, E., Soucat, A. L. B. (Eds). (2009). *Handbook on monitoring and evaluation of human resources for health: With special applications for low- and middle-income countries.* Retrieved from http://whqlibdoc.who.int/publications/2009/9789241547703_eng.pdf

Department of Health. (2015). *Medical Rural Bonded Scholarship Scheme information booklet for 2015.* Retrieved from http://www.health.gov.au/internet/main/publishing.nsf/Content/2AE7FFF24AB23CF4CA257BF0001ACCA6/$File/MRBS%2202015%20Student%20Information%20Booklet.pdf

Department of Human Services (2012). *Workforce planning.* Retrieved from http://www.dhs.vic.gov.au/funded-agency-channel/management-toolkit/workforce/planning

Dussault, G., Buchan, J., Sermeus, W. & Padaiga, Z. (2010). *Assessing future health workforce needs* (Policy Summary 2). Retrieved from http://www.euro.who.int/_data/assets/pdf_file/0019/124417/e94295.pdf

Health Workforce Australia. (2012a). *Health Workforce 2025: Doctors, nurses and midwives – Volume 1* [Report]. Retrieved from http://www.hwa.gov.au/sites/uploads/health-workforce-2025-volume-1.pdf

——. (2012b). *Health Workforce 2025: Medical specialties – Volume 3* [Report]. Retrieved from http://www.hwa.gov.au/sites/uploads/HW2025_V3_FinalReport20121109.pdf

Lacerda, D. P., Caul Liraux, H. M., Spiegel, T. & Neto, S. L. H. C. (2013). An approach to structuring and conducting workforce planning projects. *African Journal of Business Management, 7*(10), 789–800. doi: 10.5897/AJBM12.1429

Mak, V. S., Clark, A., March, G. & Gilbert, A. L. (2013). The Australian pharmacist workforce: Employment status, practice profile and job satisfaction. *Australian Health Review, 37*(1), 127–130. doi: 10.1071/AH12180

Mason, J. (2013). *Review of Australian government health workforce programs*. Retrieved from http://www.health.gov.au/internet/main/publishing.nsf/Content/D26858F4B68834EACA257BF0001A8DDC/$File/Review%20of%20Health%20Workforce%20programs.pdf

Mathews, M., Heath, S. L., Neufeld, S. M. & Samarasena, A. (2013). Evaluation of physician return-for-service agreements in Newfoundland and Labrador. *Healthcare Policy, 8*(3), 42–56. doi: 10.12927/hcpol.2013.23209

Productivity Commission. (2005). *Australia's health workforce* [Report]. Retrieved from http://www.rhwa.org.au/site/content.cfm?page_id=373159&current_category_code=1398

Reid, S. & Conco, D. (1999). Monitoring the implementation of community service. In N. Crisp (Ed.), *South African health review 1999* (pp. 233–248). Midrand, South Africa: Health Systems Trust.

Shacklock, K. & Brunetto, Y. (2012). The intention to continue nursing: Work variables affecting three nurse generations in Australia. *Journal of Advanced Nursing, 68*(1), 36–46. doi: 10.1111/j.1365-2648.2011.05709.x

World Health Assembly. (2010). *WHO global code of practice on the international recruitment of health personnel* (63rd World Health Assembly, Agenda item 11.5, WHA63.16). Retrieved from http://apps.who.int/gb/ebwha/pdf_files/WHA63/A63_R16-en.pdf

World Health Organization. (2008). *The WHO code of practice on the international recruitment of health personnel* (Draft for discussion). Retrieved from http://www.who.int/hrh/public_hearing/comments/en/index.html

——. (2010). *Models and tools for health workforce planning and projections* (Human Resources for Health Observer, Issue no. 3). Retrieved from http://whqlibdoc.who.int/publications/2010/9789241599016_eng.pdf?ua=1

29

Strategic planning

Sandra G. Leggat

Learning objectives

How do I:
- complete a strategic plan?
- synthesise strategic planning and management concepts to adopt strategic management in my position?
- improve the strategic planning and management processes within my organisation?
- plan the implementation of my organisation's strategic plan for my area?
- set and evaluate my achievement of meaningful goals?

Introduction

Effective strategic planning, implementation and management drive organisational performance (Rudd, Greenley, Beatson & Lings, 2008). Healthcare managers have recognised the increasing importance of strategic planning and management as the healthcare industry has become more dynamic and complex (Subramanian, Kumar & Yauger, 2011). However, development of feasible strategy can be difficult, and implementation of even well-developed strategy is often challenging. This chapter provides advice on leading and improving strategic planning and management in health service organisations.

Use of strategic planning

Strategic planning is a specific type of **planning**. Strategic planning was identified decades ago as essential for organisations competing in a variety of industries, with most of the seminal literature arising in the 1980s. More recently, strategic planning has been linked to successful operations in public sector healthcare organisations (Zuckerman, 2006) when applying previously developed concepts.

The Australian Commission on Safety and Quality in Healthcare (2011) defines 10 safety and quality standards for health services. Standard 2, which is concerned with 'partnering with consumers', requires that 'the health service organisation establishes mechanisms for engaging consumers and/or carers in the strategic and/or operational planning for the organisation' (p. 24). The standard also requires health service strategic planning as a criterion for accreditation. This is consistent with the *Australian standard: Good governance principles*, which indicates that governing bodies are responsible for ensuring the strategic direction of their organisations (Standards Australia, 2003).

> **Planning**
> Thinking about a goal and orga
> activities and resources towards
> achieving it
>
> **Strategic planning**
> 'A disciplined effort to produce
> fundamental decisions and actic
> shaping the nature and directio
> organisation's activities within le
> bounds' (Olsen & Eadie, 1982,

While there are differences in operations between public and private health services, researchers have found that for-profit and not-for-profit hospitals tend to have similar strategic capabilities (Reeves & Ford, 2004). Therefore, this chapter does not distinguish between these types of health services; the tools and techniques discussed can be used in both public and private sector strategic planning and management.

Forward-looking organisations have evolved from episodic strategic planning to **strategic management** that effectively links the identified strategies with daily operations (Zuckerman, 2006). The intent of strategic management is that the managers assist their staff to understand the strategic direction and how their positions and job responsibilities are essential to achieving the organisational strategies. This sug-

> **Strategic management**
> 'An externally-oriented philosop
> of managing an organisation tha
> links strategic thinking and anal
> organisation action' (Ginter, Sw
> Duncan, 2002, p. 13)

gests the need for communication to and involvement of staff throughout the strategic planning process, as well as during the implementation and monitoring of the strategic plan. Jasper and Crossan (2012) say that nurse managers have tremendous influence over the success or failure of a strategic plan and emphasise the need for nurse managers to translate the strategies into outcomes that will deliver high-quality care. This is true for all healthcare managers.

Framework for strategic planning

Despite the many strategic planning models available, all strategic planning follows the simple 10-step iterative process outlined in Figure 29.1 and discussed in detail in the following sections.

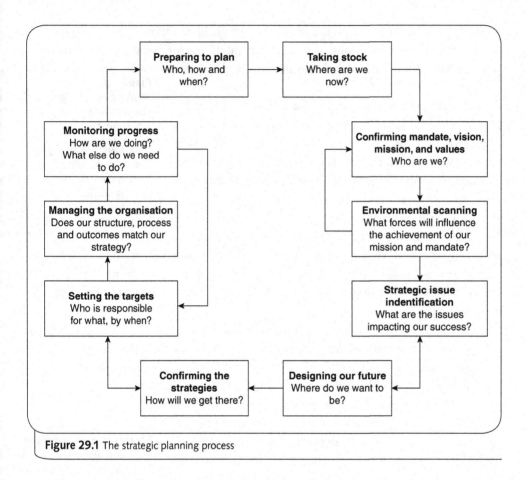

Figure 29.1 The strategic planning process

Preparing to plan

The first step requires agreement regarding the planning process. This includes identifying who will be involved, when the planning will take place, what the process will look like and the resources required. The literature suggests the need for governing board involvement in strategic planning (Nadler, 2004; Standards Australia, 2003) and for the staff responsible for the implementation to be involved (Baldwin & McConnell, 1988). In addition, as outlined above, the Australian national standards require consumer involvement (Australian Commission on Safety and Quality in Health Care, 2011). There are many recent examples of planning for new hospitals and other healthcare services in which consumers have been involved in all phases of the planning and development process.

Successful strategic planning requires a champion in a position of power in the organisation to legitimise the process; a planning team that has the time, energy and support to complete the process; willingness within the team to construct and consider a variety of arguments for the future for the benefit of the organisation; and the ability to pull information and people together at key points for important discussions and decisions (Bryson, 1988). It has been recognised that spending time at the beginning of the process outlining who should participate and how – that is, defined roles and responsibilities – leads to a strategic planning process that results in a more feasible strategic plan (Zuckerman, 2006).

Taking stock

This planning step requires an honest appraisal of the current position of the organisation in relation to similar organisations, with identification of its existing strengths and weaknesses. This appraisal contributes to the **SWOT analysis**, one of the most useful strategic planning tools identified by managers (Wright, Paroutis & Blettner, 2012). The participants consider the effects of the organisational strengths and weaknesses on the achievement of current plans. (The later environmental scanning step enables the external opportunities and threats that contribute to the SWOT to be identified.)

> **SWOT analysis**
> Strengths, Weaknesses, Oppo
> and Threats: a technique used
> identify the internal and exter
> aspects of the organisation th
> need to be addressed in the st
> plan

Confirming mandate, vision, mission and values

This step requires the confirmation of the externally imposed formal **mandate**, and the mission, vision and values. Organisational annual reports usually contain a **mission statement** and a **vision statement**. The mission and mandate need to be consistent and support each other, describing the purpose of the organisation. Many mission statements also include a **statement of values**. Organisational employees are expected to uphold the documented values in their role responsibilities.

> **Mandate**
> The formal, externally authorise
> organisational purpose that is us
> outlined in legislation, articles o
> incorporation, charters or regula
>
> **Mission statement**
> A translation of the mandate int
> the immediate purpose of the
> organisation
>
> **Vision statement**
> A description of how the organi
> will contribute to society throug
> mission
>
> **Statement of values**
> An outline of how the purpose c
> mission will be achieved: the set
> principles and beliefs that guide
> operations

The vision statement is forward-looking and is meant to answer the question of what the organisation is striving to become in the larger environment in which it functions (Bryson, 1988). Collins and Porras (1991) stress that an organisational vision needs to include both a guiding philosophy and a tangible image. The guiding philosophy should communicate the organisation's core values and beliefs, such as a religious or other foundation. The tangible image communicates the contribution the organisation will make to society if it is successful in achieving its mission.

Considering the impact of a vision statement

A review of hospital vision statements finds that many hospitals want to be known for excellence or as leaders in the field. For example, one hospital's vision is 'to lead the transformation in healthcare', while another wants 'to be the clear first choice for medical care'. But these statements do little to communicate what decisions will be made in them. They can be seen to be self-serving and do not help staff and external stakeholders understand how the hospitals will make their impacts on society.

A vision that commits to improved health for the local community is in a better position to make strategic decisions for the good of the community and not for the good of the hospital. For example, the vision statement 'Transforming lives and communities through health and wellness – one person at a time' suggests a great deal to staff about their work roles in this hospital.

Environmental scanning

The strategic plan should provide direction for the organisation over a timeframe of three to five years. Therefore, it is important that the process includes consideration of factors likely to impact on the organisation during this period. A strategic plan will be most successful if it is designed with consideration of changes in the environment; this requires collection, analysis and discussion of information gained through **environmental scanning**. Researchers have found an association between more sophisticated environmental scanning and improved organisational performance (Subramanian et al., 2011).

mental scanning
ng, evaluating and
ating information from outside
nisation to key managers within
nisation (Snyder, 1981)

The literature distinguishes between the micro-environment, or task environment, which includes direct organisational contacts such as customers and suppliers, and the macro-environment, or general environment, which includes the political, economic, ecological, societal and technological forces that surround the organisation (Subramanian et al., 2011; Vecchiato, 2012). Both must be considered in an environmental scan (see, for example, Friesen & Bell, 2007).

Organisations use a variety of environmental scanning techniques. They may be as simple as generating a list of current and future drivers of change using the framework of 'politics, economics, ecology, society and technology' to ensure all aspects are identified. The planning team reviews the list for completeness and uses it to foster discussion of the likelihood and potential impact of various changes on the organisation.

Scenario-building has been used since the 1970s in industries looking for ways to ensure that strategic planning captures future trends that may be difficult to identify. Various future scenarios are constructed that propose how the identified changes are likely to impact the organisation.

o-building
:ting future scenarios that
how the identified changes are
impact the organisation

Constructing scenarios involves defining the issues, confirming the major stakeholders, describing trends, identifying uncertainties and writing alternative scenarios (Schoemaker, 1995).

Strategic issue identification

Strategic issues are fundamental choices to be made by an organisation when there is no obvious best solution. If the solution were known, it could be operationalised and would not therefore be considered a strategic decision.

Bryson (1988) suggests that strategic issues should be identified using three elements, the first of which is a single-paragraph question used to describe the issue. For example, a strategic issue relating to the service delivery model might generate the following question: 'Economic analysis suggests that the current acute care service volumes are not sufficient to capitalise on economies of scale in resource utilisation and staff expertise. We cannot afford to expand the capacity of all of our acute services, yet all have high need. Which ones should we focus on?'

> **Strategic issues**
> Areas critical to the sustainabilit[y of]
> the organisation requiring decisi[ons]
> to be made and communicated [in the]
> strategic plan

The second element is a list of the factors that make this an important question for the future of the organisation. This might include proposed changes to casemix funding models, changing demographics of the service population, consumers' perspectives and constraints imposed by outdated facilities. The final element is an outline of the consequences of failure to address the strategic issue (such as, 'the hospital is likely to report a $15 million deficit by 2016 and be unable to attract leading medical staff').

Designing our future

While sometimes forgotten, this is an important exercise that enables the participants to be clear how the organisation will look when the strategic plan has been successfully implemented. In this stage, the participants confirm the goals and desired outcomes for the future organisation. It is difficult to envision how an organisation will look upon successful completion of the strategic plan, but creativity is required in this step. The participants should be able to predict what the organisation will be doing differently at the end of the strategic planning period – for example, 'The hospital will have increased its volume in cardiac services to 200 cases a year, have consumer representatives serving on all hospital committees and have achieved a Met with Merit rating for all 10 national standards'. This assists in the choice of strategy to achieve the desired outcomes.

Confirming the strategies

Various authors have attempted to classify strategies to assist managers in their deliberations. Three such classifications are provided here. Miles and Snow (1978) suggest that organisations adopt prospector, defender, analyser or reactor strategic stances. Prospectors search for market opportunities, tending to be the first to offer new products and services. Defenders are more conservative, competing on price and service quality; they are concerned with continually improving the efficiency of existing operations. Analysers have aspects of both prospector and defender, watching their competitors closely for new ideas and rapidly adopting the most promising. Finally, reactors lack any consistent strategy and respond to external changes only when required to do so by regulation, legislation or financial position. While there have been many studies supporting this typology, there is also concern that it does not capture all possible strategies for public and not-for-profit sector organisations (DeSarbo, Di Benedetto, Song & Sinha, 2005).

Porter (1985) identifies three generic strategies that drive competitive advantage within an industry: cost leadership, differentiation (unique products or services) and focus (or niche). More recent strategy researchers suggest that differentiation and cost leadership together can be a fourth strategy in this list (Kumar, Subramanian & Strandholm, 2001). However, competition does not operate in the same way among public sector services as it does among those in the private sector, which may limit the applicability of Porter's strategies to public sector healthcare organisations (Hodgkinson & Hughes, 2014), as these are more likely to pursue a mix of strategies, aiming to address conflicting goals (Boyne & Walker, 2004).

Hodgkinson and Hughes (2014) provide empirical support for a public sector strategy typology. Their categories comprise organisations without a coherent strategy (chaotic) and three strategy stances: value differentiation, equilibrial and socially responsible. As the name suggests, those organisations without a strategy, like reactors (Miles & Snow, 1978), are disorganised, without an overall sense of direction. Value differentiators tailor services to the needs of specific groups, focusing on delivering high customer value. In contrast, the equilibrial service providers aim to meet all population needs, trying to achieve the best service at the lowest cost. Finally, the socially responsible providers aim for the lowest costs overall.

The study results suggest that organisations with a value differentiation approach tend to demonstrate better performance than those with the other strategy stances. Overall, it seems that having a defined strategy results in better performance than having no strategy, and that a strategy that focuses on responding to customer needs, such as differentiation, is likely to be the most successful (Hodgkinson & Hughes, 2014).

Setting the targets

that are Specific, Measurable, ble, Reasonable and Time-

T
that are Specific, Measurable, ble, Realistic, Timely and

This step is linked with the preceding step of confirming strategies. Once the participants have confirmed how they wish the organisation to look at the end of the strategic plan implementation, they can reasonably assign feasible targets to each of the strategies. The **SMART** or **SMARTT** acronym is often used to ensure that effective goals and targets have been outlined (Doran, 1981). Stating 'We will provide excellent care' is not a SMARTT target, yet this is the type of target most often found in strategic plans. Reframing the statement as 'Of all discharged patients or their families, 85 per cent will rate the overall quality of the acute care that has been provided as good, very good or excellent by 2015' provides better information for understanding the focus of the strategy and enabling progress to be effectively measured.

Managing the organisation

There is substantial evidence suggesting that organisations that can align their internal processes with their chosen strategy are better performers than those that cannot (Garcia & de Val Pardo, 2004; Kumar & Subramanian, 2011). It is essential that the strategic plan is backed up with internal annual operating (or business) plans that outline priority actions and support resource allocation (Baldwin & McConnell, 1988).

Two implementation frameworks are provided in this section. The first is the **7-S Framework**, designed to assist managers to consider all of the organisational factors that may need to be modified to implement the chosen strategy (Waterman, 1982). The framework suggests that there is a need for consistency between the *strategy* of the organisation and the following six organisational factors: structure, systems, style, staff, skills, subordinate goals. For example, if the strategy focuses on improving customer service and satisfaction, the staff will need to be chosen and rewarded for their skills in customer service. The organisation's systems will need to be able to measure what customers think of the service, and the internal system will have departments for direct service and support, focused on the needs of customers. While a cost leadership strategy, aiming for the lowest costs, would not totally negate the need for customer service, the system and staff expectations would be different from those relating to the customer service strategy. While this framework has face validity and has been used by management consultants for years, it is difficult to understand the interactions between the factors and has not been empirically tested (Okumus, 2003).

> **7-S Framework**
> A system designed to assist man to consider all of the organisatio factors (Structure, Systems, Styl Staff, Skills, Subordinate goals a organisational Strategy) that ma to be modified to implement th strategy (Waterman, 1982)

Okumus (2003) has developed a detailed implementation framework that comprises strategic content, strategic context (including organisational structure and culture), operational processes (including planning, resources, communication, people and control) and intended outcomes. The suggestion is for managers to document the current and the required aspects of the context and processes to enable identification of needs to be addressed in implementation in order to achieve the desired outcomes of the chosen strategy.

Monitoring progress

While there are many ways to measure progress on the implementation of a strategic plan, in recent years the **balanced scorecard**, a strategic management system that enables organisations to monitor the processes needed to implement their strategies (Kaplan & Norton, 1996b), has been confirmed as an effective approach in healthcare (Inamdar & Kaplan, 2002; Zelman, Pink & Matthias, 2003). Generally, the scorecard tracks performance measures in relation to the targets set in the strategic plan within four or more perspectives. These perspectives include financial, customer, business and clinical processes, learning and growth, with the intent that the financial measures focused on the shorter term are balanced with the perspectives that force a longer term, more strategic focus (Kaplan & Norton, 1996a). The balanced scorecard is an effective tool for ongoing monitoring of the achievement of a strategic plan.

> **·d scorecard**
> ;ic management system that
> organisations to monitor the
> tional processes needed to
> nt the organisational strategies
> & Norton, 1996b)

Summary

- There are 10 steps that are usually completed as part of any strategic planning process. These steps comprise a generic process that includes setting the scene, gathering and analysing the data, outlining the strategies, and implementing and evaluating the plan.
- All healthcare managers need to fully understand the strategic plan of their organisation, as it is their job in strategic management to interpret the plan for their employees.
- Without SMART or SMARTT goals and effective monitoring systems, strategic plans are often not successfully implemented.

Reflective questions

1 Who should be responsible for strategic planning in your organisation?

2 How could the planning team detect strategic opportunities and strategic threats for your organisation?

3 Complete a SWOT analysis for your department.

4 What are the differences between a strategic plan and operating or business plans?

5 Using the three strategy classifications provided in this chapter, describe your organisation's current strategy.

Self-analysis question

Drawing upon your understanding of mission and vision as described in this chapter, write a two- or three-sentence personal mission statement. It should reflect your purpose, beliefs, personal values and approaches to your life and your job. Clarifying your personal mission is an ongoing process and should be regularly revisited and updated.

References

Australian Commission on Safety and Quality in Health Care. (2011). *National safety and quality health service standards*. Sydney: Author.

Baldwin, S. R. & McConnell, M. (1988). Strategic planning: Process and plan go hand in hand. *Management Solutions*, (June), 29–36.

Boyne, G. A. & Walker, R. M. (2004). Strategy content and public service organizations. *Journal of Public Administration Research and Theory*, 14(2), 231–252. doi: 10.1093/jopart/muh015

Bryson, J. M. (1988). A strategic planning process for public and non-profit organizations. *Long Range Planning*, 21(1), 73–81. doi: 10.1016/0024-6301(88)90061-1

Collins, J. C. & Porras, J. I. (1991). Organizational vision and visionary organizations. *California Management Review*, 34, 30–52.

DeSarbo, W. S., Di Benedetto, A. C., Song, M. & Sinha, I. (2005). Revisiting the Miles and Snow strategic framework: Uncovering interrelationships between strategic types, capabilities, environmental uncertainties, and firm performance. *Strategic Management Journal*, 26(1), 47–74. doi: 10.1002/smj.431

Doran, G. T. (1981). There's a SMART way to write management's goals and objectives. *Management Review*, 70(11), 35–36.

Friesen, K. & Bell, D. (2007). Regional health authorities, disaster management, and geomatics: Opportunities and barriers. *International Journal of Emergency Management*, *4*(2), 141–165. doi: 10.1504/IJEM.2007.013987

Garcia, C. M. & de Val Pardo, I. (2004). Strategies and performance in hospitals. *Health Policy*, *67*, 1–13. doi: 10.1016/S0168-8510(03)00102-7

Ginter, P. M., Swayne, L. E. & Duncan, W. J. (2002). *Strategic management of health care organizations* (4th ed.). San Francisco, CA: Jossey-Bass.

Hodgkinson, I. & Hughes, P. (2014). Strategy content and public service provider performance in the UK: An alternative approach. *Public Administration*, *92*(3): 707–726. doi: 10.1111/padm.12090

Inamdar, N. & Kaplan, R. S. (2002). Applying the balanced scorecard in healthcare provider organizations. *Journal of Healthcare Management*, *47*(3), 179–195.

Jasper, M. & Crossan, F. (2012). What is strategic management? *Journal of Nursing Management*, *20*, 838–846. doi: 10.1111/jonm.12001

Kaplan, R. S. & Norton, D. P. (1996a). *The balanced scorecard*. Boston, MA: Harvard Business.

——. (1996b). Using the balanced scorecard as a strategic management system. *Harvard Business Review*, (January–February), 75–85.

Kumar, K. & Subramanian, R. (2011). Porter's strategic types: Differences in internal processes and their impact on performance. *Journal of Applied Business Research*, *14*(1), 107–124.

Kumar, K., Subramanian, R. & Strandholm, K. (2001). Competitive strategy, environmental scanning and performance: A context specific analysis of their relationship. *International Journal of Commerce and Management*, *11*(1), 1–33. doi: 10.1108/eb047413

Miles, R. E. & Snow, C. C. (1978). *Organizational strategy, structure, and process*. New York, NY: McGraw-Hill.

Nadler, D. A. (2004). What's the board's role in strategy development? Engaging the board in corporate strategy. *Strategy & Leadership*, *32*(5), 25–33. doi: 10.1108/10878570410557633

Okumus, F. (2003). A framework to implement strategies in organizations. *Management Decision*, *41*(9), 871–882. doi: 10.1108/00251740310499555

Olsen, J. B. & Eadie, D. C. (1982). *The game plan: Governance with foresight*. Washington, DC: Council of State Planning Agencies.

Porter, M. E. (1985). *Competitive advantage: Creating and sustaining superior performance*. New York, NY: MacMillan.

Reeves, T. C. & Ford, E. W. (2004). Strategic management and performance differences: Nonprofit versus for-profit health organizations. *Health Care Management Review*, *29*(4), 298–308.

Rudd, J. M., Greenley, G. E., Beatson, A. T. & Lings, I. N. (2008). Strategic planning and performance: Extending the debate. *Journal of Business Research*, *61*(2), 99–108. doi: 10.1016/j.jbusres.2007.06.014

Schoemaker, P. J. H. (1995). Scenario planning: A tool for strategic thinking. *Sloan Management Review*, (Winter), 25–39.

Snyder, N. (1981). Environmental volatility, scanning intensity, and organizational performance. *Journal of Contemporary Business*, *10*, 5–17.

Standards Australia. (2003). *Australian standard: Good governance principles* (AS 8000–2003). Canberra: Author.

Subramanian, R., Kumar, K. & Yauger, C. (2011). The scanning of task environments in hospitals: An empirical study. *Journal of Applied Business Research*, *10*(4), 104–115.

Vecchiato, R. (2012). Environmental uncertainty, foresight and strategic decision making: An integrated study. *Technological Forecasting and Social Change*, *79*(3), 436–447. doi: 10.1016/j.techfore.2011.07.010

Waterman, R. H. J. (1982). The seven elements of strategic fit. *Journal of Business Strategy*, *2*(3), 69–73.

Wright, R. P., Paroutis, S. E. & Blettner, D. P. (2012). How useful are the strategic tools we teach in business schools? *Journal of Management Studies*, *50*(1), 92–125. doi: 10.1111/j.1467 -6486.2012.01082.x

Zelman, W. N., Pink, G. H. & Matthias, C. B. (2003). Use of the balanced scorecard in health care. *Journal of Health Care Finance*, *29*(4), 1–16.

Zuckerman, A. M. (2006). Advancing the state of the art in healthcare strategic planning. *Frontiers of Health Services Management*, *23*(2), 3–15.

30

Health service planning

Chaojie Liu and John Adamm Ferrier

Learning objectives

How do I:
- understand when and why health service planning is required and initiated?
- identify important stakeholders and consider how they may be engaged in health service planning?
- develop critical thinking regarding the implications of various approaches and instruments used in health service planning?
- improve my skills in effective health service planning?

Introduction

Matching available health resources to consumer needs is challenging. Governments and health bureaucracies with finite resources face increasing demands from their client populations, which often have complex health issues. No country has sufficient resources to meet every single health need of every citizen. Consequently, health service planning is important to maximise population health outcomes and ensure value for the available money.

Due to the inherent contradictions existing between the high demand for and the limited responsive supply capacity by health services, health service planning is often characterised by negotiation, lobbying and compromise among various interest groups. A consensus can best be achieved if stakeholders agree upon a set of core values and all involved in the process endorse principles and the procedures of planning.

Definitions

Health service planning may stem from the perspective of consumers (population-based) or from the perspective of providers (institutional-based) (Eagar, Garrett & Lin, 2001). The ultimate choice between these two options often depends on who is responsible for performing the planning and the rationale.

> **Health service planning**
> The planned process of aligning and future health services and r to the changing health patterns demographics of a given area o

Population-based planning

Population-based planning claims to adopt a bottom-up approach and usually involves multiple organisations. Such an approach requires authority and ability from planners to achieve cross-boundary cooperation. Resources ought to be allocated to health facilities in a way that can best meet consumer need. Planners – usually government agencies or joint councils – must develop a good understanding of the competency, capacity and willingness of various providers and consumers to execute the plan (Coakes & Kelly, 1997). Population-based planning tends to regard health promotion and disease prevention as priorities rather than focusing on treatment of diseases (Issel, 2009).

> **Population-based planning**
> A bottom-up planning approach considers the current and future resource utilisation of a given po

Institutional-based planning

By contrast, **institutional-based planning** adopts a top-down approach and is often anchored on a single organisation or group of organisations aiming to maximise gains (in terms of finance or health outcomes or both) from the invested resources. Such planning usually focuses on the extent to which a difference is made to those who receive or would receive the services (Issel, 2009) and tends to ignore those who are not covered by the services. Therefore, the benefit to overall population health may be limited and dependent on the scope of services that may be able to be delivered by the organisation. Many health organisations perform institutional-based planning for reasons of efficiency and/or cost-effectiveness (Eagar et al., 2001).

> **Institutional-based plannin**
> A top-down planning approach often anchored on a single orga or group of organisations, aimin maximise gains (in terms of fina or health outcomes or both) fro invested resources

Public health planning of Victorian local governments

Municipal public health planning was made compulsory by the Victorian government in 1988. Local councils have since been required to identify the risk factors affecting the health of their populations and to develop strategies to prevent and minimise the identified risks. The planning process is repeated every three years.

The intention of local public health planning is to encourage councils to respond to and manage local population health. Because health service provision is largely the responsibility of state governments, emphases have been placed on establishing partnerships between the state, the market and civil society, on building social capital and on enhancing health promotion (Edwards, 2012).

Reasons for planning

There are many reasons why health managers perform health service planning. Firstly, the health market is easily manipulated and distorted, and population health is simply too important to be left unplanned (Gage, 1979). The human population is characterised by rapidly changing morbidity and health needs due to prolonged life expectancy and scientific advancements. Despite this, many health technologies and products brought to the market lack scientific evidence support in terms of their efficacy (Vayda, 1977). Health provision is an example of a free market approach being problematic, because there is a distinct power and knowledge imbalance between consumers (patients) and suppliers (health professionals). Consumers often feel disempowered in health consumption decisions, as they often do not have a complete understanding of the issues. Suppliers have significant power, not only because of their inherent specialist knowledge, but also because they act as gatekeepers to treatments and drugs.

Secondly, a society can only offer services it can afford, and governments often have to meet competing demands from other services, such as defence and social welfare (Semple, 1977). Escalating health expenditure has become a public concern in Western countries, regardless of whether the method of financing is socialised or privatised, or a mixture of the two. Health service planning enables people within the system to collect anecdotal evidence of program effectiveness (Issel, 2009) and rationalise health expenditure.

Thirdly, there are several control measures growing out of planning, 'from a centralized and directed kind to a decentralized, negotiating and bargaining type' (Anderson, 1969, p. 345) for the purpose of achieving better quality care and reducing waste. And finally, in countries where public spending on health accounts for a large proportion of total health expenditure, health service planning becomes a political signal for accountability: by the end of 1970s, most developed nations had produced and commenced implementation of national health plans (Anderson, 1969; Gage, 1979).

Health service planning can be triggered when a particular health problem emerges as a public concern, when periodic strategic planning is performed in an organisation or when new funds have become available – or a new willingness to release them has emerged (Issel, 2009). It can also be triggered on the emergence of new evidence in relation to a particular service program.

In recent years, breast cancer screening services have attracted a great deal of debate among researchers, politicians and consumers. One would expect a screening program to reduce the overall mortality associated with this cancer; otherwise, it might produce the unnecessary burden of overdiagnosis and potentially unnecessary treatment to consumers (Gotzsche & Jorgensen, 2013). Although the World Health Organization acknowledges the effectiveness of mammography-screening for a 25 per cent reduction of mortality of breast cancer (Weedon-Fekjær, Romundstad & Vatten, 2014), this was challenged by some researchers in a Cochrane Review (Gotzsche & Jorgensen, 2013). Two research articles on the subject of mammography for reducing mortality of breast cancer were recently published in the *British Medical Journal*, with one claiming no effect (Miller et al., 2014) and the other claiming a significant effect (Weedon-Fekjær et al., 2014). Meanwhile, consumer demand for breast-screening services remains high, especially with the recent advent of high-profile celebrity disclosures increasing demand (Evans et al., 2014) and with breast-screening being one of the most successful of all cancer-screening programs (Sullivan et al., 2003). This has led to a potentially awkward situation for managers in deciding whether resources allocated to breast cancer screening should continue unchanged or perhaps be diverted to other services. The debate is expected to continue and is unlikely to be settled in the short term.

Management and health service planning

Health service planners

Health service plans ought to reflect the needs of target populations, which means that planners have to consider and balance the interests of various stakeholders (Gagliardi, Lemieux-Charles, Brown, Sullivan & Goel, 2008). The constantly changing models of service delivery add to the complexity. (Gauld, 2002). Issel (2009) argues that at least three areas of expertise are critical to health service planning: expert knowledge and experience of the health problems; research skills in epidemiology, social and behavioural science; and skills in fostering agreement across diverse constituents, capabilities and interests.

Consumer participation is essential in health service planning (Eagar et al., 2001; Issel, 2009; Thornicroft & Tansella, 2005), because it is an opportunity to foster effective provider–recipient interaction, with ideas and energies flowing towards the services, and results and respect from the services. Such two-way interaction facilitates implementation and, it might be hoped, contributes to ultimate consumer acceptance and satisfaction.

Participation of frontline health workers in planning processes is increasingly valued (Dyck, Tiessen & Lee, 2013; Thornicroft & Tansella, 2005). Medical practice in the Western setting has a long tradition of individual-based decision-making (Liu, Bartram, Casimir & Leggat, 2014). Since the very inception of health service planning, the failure of 'government authorities' to include frontline health providers has attracted criticism, because ultimately these personnel provide the services. Richards (1981) argues that general practitioners are best placed for participating in local health planning. There are many barriers to engaging consumers and frontline health workers in a meaningful way. A lack of trust, skill, time and effective mechanisms for provider participation is common in many health systems (Gagliardi et al., 2008; Liu, Liu, Wang, Zhang & Wang, 2013).

Decision-making

Health service planning often requires difficult decisions: priorities have to be established, and limited resources need to be directed towards identified priorities or needs. These decisions should reflect core values and principles that guide the overall planning processes. Those core values usually include accessibility, equity, efficiency, quality and effectiveness. Some (for example, efficiency versus accessibility) may come into conflict in planning (Eagar et al., 2001).

The pattern of stakeholder participation in planning processes dictates the values and principles adopted by planners. Issel (2009) summarises six approaches to stakeholder participation (see Table 30.1). Although these are not mutually exclusive, it is not uncommon for a responsible authority to favour one more than others, leading to a particular approach in the manner in which planning exercises are conducted. It would be more useful to see those 'approaches' as skills that are required under different circumstances to reach consensus.

Various stakeholders are given different opportunities to voice their concerns within these six approaches. A comprehensive rational approach pays particular attention to the balance and equality of stakeholder participation in planning. Both the communication action and advocacy approaches place significant weight on the concerns of those who experience the problems targeted by the planning, although the latter often depends on planning experts, who may misunderstand their constituents. Health professionals generally shape the incremental and apolitical approaches, whereas collective interests of health professionals are addressed in the strategic planning approach.

There is a consensus that governments should not intervene in the internal management decisions of service providers (Liu et al., 2014); however, it is hard, if not impossible, to avoid political influence, especially if the government is the primary funder of the service. Governments often want service providers to align their planning with a set of unified goals (Department of Health, 2011). Political agenda may also shape priority settings. For example, in the late 1990s, the Clinton administration in the United States put racial and ethnic disparities on the public agenda, leading to increasing service programs aiming at eliminating ethnic disparities (Issel, 2009).

Cultural values shared by the general public have a significant influence on decision-making in health service planning. For example, medical care services are more likely to be seen as an individual responsibility by people residing in the United States,

Table 30.1 Comparison of various approaches to decision-making in health service planning

Approach	Description	Advantages	Disadvantages
Comprehensive rational	A textbook-written idealistic planning approach, with a systematic and logical sequence of thought processes and actions	Obtaining information from all stakeholders; taking into account all contingencies and peripheral influences; addressing issues facing the entire service delivery system	Failure to consider individual values; separation of planners from political reality; heavy reliance on planner's understanding of means and ends that may not be substantiated or endorsed by others
Incremental	Isolated and disjointed efforts addressing small and immediate concerns, with a hope that accumulated effect will eventuate	Strong tolerance of uncertainties and knowledge gaps; rapid response to concerns	Lack of coordination and integration that is likely to lead to conflicting or mismatched programs
Apolitical	An evidence-based practice that is built on best available scientific knowledge	Strong focus on technical aspects for high efficacy; dependence on objective information	Ignoring of political aspects and subjective experience of those with the health problem; difficulties in dealing with evidence bias and knowledge gaps
Advocacy	A planning approach that is pushed by experts who speak for or on behalf of those with certain health problems	Raising awareness and acting on behalf of those disadvantaged who are not empowered to convey their concerns	Likelihood of misinterpretation of the problem of those concerned and of conflicts and confrontations with other interested parties
Communication action	An approach of working in partnership with those with the concerned health problem through communication and empowerment	Interactions between those who are affected and those who are managing and delivering services, with a hope of achieving consensus through mutual adaptation of attention, beliefs and trust	Time-consuming; high requirement of communication and negotiating skills in those involved in the planning
Strategic planning	A service-planning process that is guided by and aligned with a strategic plan of the organisation	Consideration of organisational contexts, both internal and external; services aligned with the vision and future direction of the organisation	Lack of flexibility to respond to new environmental opportunities or threats

whereas in Australia, Canada and many European nations, people would regard the provision of health services as a universal and therefore public good. In the Global Burden of Disease Study, people of workforce age used to be valued higher than the others (Sabik & Lie, 2008). This has recently been abandoned (Australian Institute of Health and Welfare, 2014), because of oppositions from some countries who argue that human dignity and social solidarity should not be displaced by economic productivity (Rosen, De Fine Licht & Ohlsson, 2014).

Frameworks for health service planning

Before detailed planning commences, a working group, often in the form of a consortium, needs to be established which ideally comprises from five to seven people (Issel, 2009). The group is responsible for devising a set of principles and core values to guide the planning process. This is perhaps the most important and most often neglected step. Failure to adequately define the scope of the planning will ultimately lead to a quagmire of well-intentioned but ultimately useless plans.

The ultimate goal of health service planning is to assure that the resources available to various health programs achieve the best possible outcomes with the greatest efficiency (Eagar et al., 2001; Gaston, 2005); however, defining outcomes in isolation is often difficult. Internationally, there is a trend to incorporate ideas generated from the public and communities into health planning goals (Issel, 2009).

Once desired outcomes are defined, they will be measured with indicators. Each indicator offers a certain perspective by measuring the effectiveness of the interaction

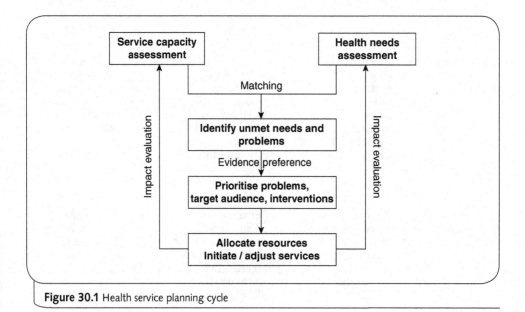

Figure 30.1 Health service planning cycle

aimed at the health problem. Common indicators used in health service planning measure frequency (prevalence and incidence) of problems, severity and duration of problems, and cost and frequency of use of services (Fazekas, Ettelt, Newbould & Nolte, 2010; Department of Health, 2011).

Health service planning is usually conducted in a cyclical manner, involving assessment of problems, prioritisation and implementation decisions (Fazekas et al., 2010; Gaston, 2005). Evaluation also forms an integral part of planning. It not only demonstrates the effectiveness of planned actions but also feeds into a new cycle of service-planning (see Figure 30.1).

Assess health needs and health service capacity

The health service planning process must commence with the clear identification of existing resources, programs and known problems or gaps in service provision. Occasionally, targeted problems have been determined, usually by funders, prior to the planning. Three types of assessment may be involved, though not necessarily all at once, in health service planning: needs assessment, organisational assessment and marketing assessment.

Needs assessment

A needs assessment defines the gaps, lacks and wants relative to a predetermined health problem or a certain population (Issel, 2009). Perhaps the most commonly used definition of needs (Asadi-Lari, Packham & Gray, 2003) is Bradshaw's (1972), according to which there are four types of needs: normative, felt, expressed and comparative. Service data and administrative records usually capture normative, expressed and comparative needs, but they have often failed to reveal the felt or perceived need, which may be obtained from sources such as qualitative population surveys. Benchmarking and spatial analysis (for example, geographic information systems) are two commonly used tools that identify comparative need (Brijnath, Ansariadi & de Souza, 2012; Eagar et al., 2001).

Normative need is defined by professionals using scientific concepts and notions.

Felt need examines what consumers want, wish and desire.

Expressed need describes vocalised needs or how people use services.

Comparative need indicates gaps between groups of people.

Organisational assessment

An organisational assessment determines the willingness and capacity of the organisation to provide the defined health services. A SWOT analysis offers a useful framework to guide organisational assessment (but is by no means the only tool available). Internal strengths and weaknesses, as well as external opportunities and threats, are assessed in comparison with other providers through staff consultation and use of existing organisational records (Eagar et al., 2001; Issel, 2009).

Marketing assessment

A marketing assessment intends to understand to what extent the target audience is interested in the service program and how it can be drawn into the program. Pricing and packaging design may be involved in a marketing assessment.

Set priorities

Priority-setting is an exercise involving both rational and political processes. The initial concern of the planners should be to satisfy themselves that they fully understand firstly what health needs should be considered and how they should be ranked, according to the size and seriousness of the problem, and secondly the likelihood of the problems being solved using effective interventions open to the providers. To assist with prioritisation of these issues, a scoring system can be developed to rank health problems. Problems with a larger size and higher levels of seriousness and those that are more likely to be solved are given higher scores. For example, a formula (Issel, 2009) has been adopted by the United States Centers for Disease Control and Prevention for its planning process:

> priority score = [(score of problem size) + 2 (score of problem seriousness)] × (score of effectiveness of intervention)

Many indicators have been developed to assist with decision-making in health service planning. The magnitude of a health problem is usually assessed using incidence (magnitude of newly occurring cases) and prevalence (quantity of cases in the community). The seriousness of a problem can be assessed from physical perspectives (morbidity and mortality) and functional impacts (activities of daily living), or using a combination such as burden of disease (quality-adjusted life years and disability-adjusted life years) and health-related quality of life (Price, 1999; Snow, Walker, Ahern, O'Brien & Saltman, 1999).

Effective interventions in relation to a defined health problem are usually determined on scientific research evidence that has tested the outcomes (Greenhalgh, Howick & Maskrey, 2014). Cost benefit and cost-effectiveness analyses are often used to compare and contrast alternative options. In resource-poor settings, additional indicators beyond the normal measures might be needed to rank priority populations according to need (Gherunpong, Sheiham & Tsakos, 2006). The evidence-based medicine movement has developed an increasing influence over the past two decades, because this provides planners with an independent and impartial defence against charges of favouritism or discrimination (Greenhalgh et al., 2014).

The next step moves from a focus on the problem to a focus on people and clients. A priority score does not provide an answer to the question of who should be looked after by society. Certain population groups often bear disproportional burdens of ill-health. Responsible planners will ensure they understand and quantify the distribution of health problems among peoples of differing age, sex, racial identity, socioeconomic status and any other differentiation relevant to the target population. From a political, cultural and economic perspective, it is important that resources and services are allocated to the right people by the right providers at the right time in the right amount in the right frequency at the right geographic location for the right outcome in a culturally acceptable manner and at the lowest possible delivered cost. Unfortunately, considerations from these differing perspectives do not always result in consensus; for example, it is difficult to argue for extra resources to treat prisoners, who commonly exhibit the lowest levels of health in any society, if this might mean the diversion of resources from other, more 'politically worthy' interests.

Issel (2009) argues that five dimensions are likely to be considered by politicians, planners, managers and consumers:

Propriety refers to the role of planners: whether the planners are obligated to address those problems and look after those affected.

Economic feasibility considers costs associated with actions.

Acceptability describes the willingness and frequency of use of potential services from the cultural and financial perspectives of consumers.

Resources refers to the capacity and availability of resources that are needed for delivering services.

Legality examines obligations imposed by laws, or regulatory conditions.

Implement decisions

Management arrangements have been proven to be associated with quality of healthcare and patient outcomes (Aiken et al., 2014). It is naive to consider technology as a silver bullet that can bring an automatic end to a problem. Resource commitment and adequate incentive mechanisms are equally important for realising the desired goals of any service plan. A recent study conducted in nine European countries revealed that an increase in nursing workload by one extra patient is associated with a 7 per cent increase in patient mortality within 30 days of hospital admission (Aiken et al., 2014). Over the past decade, high-performance work systems – a series of participative measures of human resource management – have attracted increasing attention from healthcare managers as a result of evidence that supports the link between these systems and improved patient care (Leggat, Bartram & Stanton, 2011; Liu et al., 2014). Health service planning standards (for example, doctors, nurses and beds per 1000 of the population) and role delineation of services (for example, levels of qualification) may assist managers in ensuring that services are provided safely (Eagar et al., 2001).

Evaluate impact

The outcome of health service planning through the delivery of services ought to be demonstrated by impact evaluation. The term 'impact' means, in this case, the desired outcomes of a health service plan, such as the changed health status of the target audience, the changed service capacity of the provider, or both (Eagar et al., 2001), but it could, conceivably, also include unintended or negative outcomes. The potential impact of a service on non-users should not be ignored.

Since the target audience is deliberately selected and biased to those who most need the service through health service planning, the health impact on those actually exposed to the service is often greater than on an average population (Lance, Guilkey, Hattori & Angeles, 2014). For example, restricting varieties of medicines in the provision of primary care may reduce the pharmaceutical expenditure of individuals who seek medical attention from primary care providers at that instance; however, it may encourage some patients to bypass primary care in favour of tertiary providers such as hospitals, resulting in more expensive care (Yang, Liu, Ferrier, Zhou & Zhang, 2013).

Appropriate evaluation design is critical for demonstrating the effectiveness of a service program. Theoretically, the impact of a planned service program can be confirmed only through a comparison of changes between those who are randomly assigned to a group of intervention (exposed to the service) and a group of control (not exposed to the service). Unfortunately, such randomisation is not intrinsically possible in health service planning, because service recipients often self-select or are selected into a service program. Furthermore, the effects of service may not be straightforward: it may in some respects interact with many other health determinants, such as education and income. As a result, complicated statistical analyses (such as multiple regression, matching and propensity score estimation) may be required to estimate the impact and allow for the adjusting due to the possibility of confounding influences of factors other than the designed service on the outcome indicators (Lance et al., 2014).

People responsible for evaluation may also influence the way evaluation is conducted and impact on the results. Evaluators may be internal or external. It is important to note that internal evaluators are more likely to be biased in favour of a particular process; but they cost less and can facilitate the implementation of the plan (Issel, 2009).

Summary

- Health service planning has become an important instrument for improving quality and efficiency of healthcare. It is also seen as a core component of health system governance (Fazekas et al., 2010).
- Plans need to be well executed. The increased use of planning has attracted concerns about coordination and coherence among the plans (Hall, 1981; Wright & Sheldon, 1985).
- Things do not always happen as planned. Contingency plans are needed in case emergencies or disastrous events occur, whether natural or manmade (Lees, 1981).

Reflective questions

1 What are the differences between population-based planning and institutional-based planning?

2 What is the goal of health service planning?

3 Who should be involved in health service planning, and what roles can they play?

4 What would you do if consensus were hard to reach among key stakeholders?

5 What dimensions are usually considered in determining priorities, and how are they measured?

Self-analysis questions

What are the key values (in terms of funding, availability and accessibility) associated with the provision of healthcare that Australians have endorsed? As a manager, how do you ensure that those values guide the practice of health service planning?

References

Aiken, L. H., Sloane, D. M., Bruyneel, L., Van den Heede, K., Griffiths, P., Busse, R. ... Sermeus, W. (2014). Nurse staffing and education and hospital mortality in nine European countries: A retrospective observational study. *Lancet, 383*(9931), 1824–1830. doi: 10.1016/s0140-6736(13)62631-8

Anderson, O. W. (1969). Planning health services, American style. *Medical Care, 7*(5), 345–347. doi: 10.1097/00005650-196909000-00001

Asadi-Lari, M., Packham, C. & Gray, D. (2003). Need for redefining needs. *Health and Quality of Life Outcomes, 1*(34). doi: 10.1186/1477-7525-1-34

Australian Institute of Health and Welfare. (2014). *Assessment of global burden of disease 2010: Methods for the Australian context.* Canberra: Author.

Bradshaw, J. (1972). A taxonomy of social need. In G. Mclachlan (Ed.), *Problems and progress in medical care: Essays on current research* (7th series, pp. 69–82). Oxford, United Kingdom: Nuffield Provincial Hospital Trust.

Brijnath, B. P., Ansariadi, M. & de Souza, D. K. P. (2012). Four ways geographic information systems can help to enhance health service planning and delivery for infectious diseases in low-income countries. *Journal of Health Care for the Poor and Underserved, 23*(4), 1410–1420. doi: 10.1353/hpu.2012.0146

Coakes, S. J. & Kelly, G. J. (1997). Community competence and empowerment: Strategies for rural change in women's health service planning and delivery. *Australian Journal of Rural Health, 5*(1), 26–30. doi: 10.1111/j.1440-1584.1997.tb00231.x

Department of Health. (2011). *Victorian Health Priorities Framework 2012–2022: Metropolitan health plan*. Retrieved from http://docs.health.vic.gov.au/docs/doc/7BD7DBD50AAEFF8FCA 25794B0019A388/$FILE/1104014%20VHPF_2012-22_FA7%201%20June.pdf

Dyck, K. G., Tiessen, M. & Lee, A. M. (2013). Integrating health care providers' opinions into mental health service planning for underserved populations. *University of Toronto Medical Journal, 90*(4), 143–149.

Eagar, K., Garrett, P. & Lin, V. (2001). *Health planning: Australian perspectives*. St Leonards: Allen & Unwin.

Edwards, D. (2012). *Local public health planning as a form of social action to achieve better health outcomes: What can be learned from the Victorian experience?* (Doctoral dissertation, La Trobe University). Retrieved from http://arrow.latrobe.edu.au:8080/vital/access/services/ Download/latrobe:34966/SOURCE01

Evans, D., Barwell, J., Eccles, D., Collins, A., Izatt, L., Jacobs, C. ... Murray, A. (2014). The Angelina Jolie effect: How high celebrity profile can have a major impact on provision of cancer related services. *Breast Cancer Research, 16*(442). doi 10.1186/s13058-014 -0442-6

Fazekas, M., Ettelt, S., Newbould, J. & Nolte, E. (2010). *Framework for assessing, improving and enhancing health service planning*. Santa Monica, CA: RAND.

Gage, R. W. (1979). Planning for health services. *Journal of the American College Health Association, 27*(6), 279–280. doi: 10.1080/01644300.1979.10392870

Gagliardi, A. R., Lemieux-Charles, L., Brown, A. D., Sullivan, T. & Goel, V. (2008). Barriers to patient involvement in health service planning and evaluation: An exploratory study. *Patient Education & Counseling, 70*(2), 234–241. doi: 10.1080/01644300.1979. 10392870

Gaston, C. (2005). *Health service planning and policy-making: A toolkit for nurses and midwives*. Manila, Philippines: World Health Organization.

Gauld, R. (2002). From home, to market, to headquarters, to home: Relocating health services planning and purchasing in New Zealand. *Journal of Management in Medicine, 16*(6), 436– 450. doi: 10.1108/02689230210450990

Gherunpong, S., Sheiham, A. & Tsakos, G. (2006). A sociodental approach to assessing children's oral health needs: Integrating an oral health-related quality of life (OHRQoL) measure into oral health service planning. *Bulletin of the World Health Organization, 84*(1), 36–42. doi: 10.1590/S0042-96862006000100012

Gotzsche, P. C. & Jorgensen, K. J. (2013). Screening for breast cancer with mammography (review) [Intervention review]. *Cochrane Database of Systematic Reviews, 6*(Cd001877). doi: 10.1002/14651858.CD001877.pub5

Greenhalgh, T., Howick, J. & Maskrey, N. (2014). Evidence based medicine: A movement in crisis? *British Medical Journal, 348*. doi: 10.1136/bmj.g3725

Hall, T. L. (1981). The Planning of Health Services: Studies in Eight European Countries [Book review]. *Health Services Research, 16*(1), 103–105.

Issel, L. M. (2009). *Health program planning and evaluation: A practical and systematic approach for community health* (2nd ed.). Sudbury, MA: Jones & Bartlett.

Lance, P., Guilkey, D., Hattori, A. & Angeles, G. (2014). *How do we know if a program made a difference? A guide to statistical methods for program impact evaluation.* Chapel Hill, NC: MEASURE Evaluation.

Lees, W. (1981). Health service planning for war. *British Medical Journal (Clinical Research Edition), 282*(6273), 1401–1402.

Leggat, S. G., Bartram, T. & Stanton, P. (2011). High performance work systems: The gap between policy and practice in health care reform. *Journal of Health Organization & Management, 25*(3), 281–297. doi: 10.1108/14777261111143536

Liu, C., Bartram, T., Casimir, G. & Leggat, S. G. (2014). The link between participation in management decision making and quality of patient care as perceived by Chinese doctors. *Public Management Review* (September). doi: 10.1080/14719037.2014.930507

Liu, C., Liu, W., Wang, Y., Zhang, Z. & Wang, P. (2013). Patient safety culture in China: A case study in an outpatient setting in Beijing. *BMJ Quality and Safety, 23*, 556–564. doi: 10.1136/bmjqs-2013-002172

Miller, A. B., Wall, C., Baines, C. J., Sun, P., To, T. & Narod, S. A. (2014). Twenty five year follow-up for breast cancer incidence and mortality of the Canadian National Breast Screening Study: Randomised screening trial. *British Medical Journal, 348*. doi: 10.1136/bmj.g366

Price, E. (1999). Functional status and health service planning. *Journal of Quality in Clinical Practice, 19*(4), 224–225.

Richards, B. W. (1981). Health service planning [Letter]. *Journal of the Royal College of General Practitioners, 31*(232), 694.

Rosen, P., De Fine Licht, J. & Ohlsson, H. (2014). Priority setting in Swedish health care: Are the politicians ready? *Scandinavian Journal of Public Health, 42*(3), 227–234. doi: 10.1177/1403494813520355

Sabik, L. M. & Lie, R. K. (2008). Priority setting in health care: Lessons from the experiences of eight countries. *International Journal for Equity in Health, 7*(4). doi: 10.1186/1475-9276-7-4

Semple, A. B. (1977). Health Service Planning [Book review]. *British Medical Journal, 1*, 1342. doi: 10.1136/bmj.1.6072.1339

Snow, L., Walker, M., Ahern, M., O'Brien, E. & Saltman, D. C. (1999). Functional status and health service planning. *Journal of Quality in Clinical Practice, 19*(2), 99–102. doi: 10.1046/j.1440-1762.1999.00309.x

Sullivan, S. G., Glasson, E. J., Hussain, R., Petterson, B. A., Slack-Smith, L. M., Montgomery, P. D. & Bittles, A. H. (2003). Breast cancer and the uptake of mammography screening services by women with intellectual disabilities. *Preventive Medicine, 37*(5), 507–512. doi: 10.1016/S0091-7435(03)00177-4

Thornicroft, G. & Tansella, M. (2005). Growing recognition of the importance of service user involvement in mental health service planning and evaluation. *Epidemiologia e Psichiatria Sociale, 14*(1), 1–3. doi: 10.1017/S1121189X00001858

Vayda, E. (1977). Health Services Planning [Book review]. *Canadian Medical Association Journal, 116*, 847.

Weedon-Fekjær, H., Romundstad, P. R. & Vatten, L. J. (2014). Modern mammography screening and breast cancer mortality: Population study. *British Medical Journal, 348*. doi: 10.1136/bmj.g3701

Wright, J. & Sheldon, F. (1985). Health and social services planning. *Social Policy and Administration*, *19*(3), 258–272. doi: 10.1111/j.1467-9515.1985.tb00238.x

Yang, L. P., Liu, C. J., Ferrier, J. A., Zhou, W. & Zhang, X. P. (2013). The impact of the National Essential Medicines Policy on prescribing behaviours in primary care facilities in Hubei province of China. *Health Policy and Planning, 28*(7), 750–760. doi: 10.1093/heapol/czs116

Index

the United States
Taylor Publisher Services